BLINDNESS RESEARCH: THE EXPANDING FRONTIERS

Proceedings of the National Consultation Concerning Needed Research in the Behavioral Sciences and the Humanities with Reference to Problems Related to Blindness. Held April 9–12, 1967, at University Park, Pennsylvania.

Co-sponsored by:

The American Association of Workers for the Blind

The Center for Continuing Liberal Education of the Pennsylvania State University College of the Liberal Arts

The Committee for Research in Problems Related to Blindness

The State Office for the Blind, Department of Public Welfare, Commonwealth of Pennsylvania

The Vocational Rehabilitation Administration, The United States Department of Health, Education and Welfare

BLINDNESS RESEARCH:
THE EXPANDING FRONTIERS

A LIBERAL STUDIES PERSPECTIVE

edited by
MAXWELL H. GOLDBERG
with
John R. Swinton

THE PENNSYLVANIA STATE UNIVERSITY PRESS
University Park & London 1969

Standard Book Number 271–00073–2
Library of Congress Catalog Card Number 68–8179
Printed in the United States of America
by The Colonial Press Inc., Clinton, Mass.

Designed by Marilyn Shobaken

FOREWORD

It is altogether fitting that the Pennsylvania State Office for the Blind should be a co-sponsor with The Pennsylvania State University's Center for Continuing Liberal Education of a conference which addressed itself to the needs of blind people and workers with the blind for the next decade and beyond and, in so doing, produced this significant volume.

Scientific research into the difficult problems of today's life is often taken for granted; so it is important to stress the contributions of a conference such as this, which demonstrates both that research in a special field can advance all knowledge and that timely application of the findings of research to today's problems is imperative.

I am most gratified to endorse heartily this study of the research needs in the area of problems related to blindness on so broad, so scientific and, above all, so human a basis.

MARY E. SWITZER
Administrator, Social and Rehabilitation Service
Department of Health, Education and Welfare

CONTENTS

INTRODUCTION

At the 1959 annual meeting of the American Council on Education, Dr. John W. Gardner, then President of the Carnegie Corporation of New York, made what has since become an historic observation. In his keynoting address, on "The University in our Civilization," he declared: "The role of the universities is undergoing a remarkable change. They are thrust into a position of great responsibility in our society—a position more central, more prominent, more crucial to the life of the society than academic people ever dreamed possible . . ." *

The papers that follow provide ample documentation of the accuracy of Dr. Gardner's 1959 statement, and of the advances, since 1959, made by the process he then described as vigorously under way. At that time, Dr. Gardner further remarked: "With increasing frequency the rest of the nation is turning to the universities for guidance and giving them unprecedented opportunities to play a formative role in our society." In the present instance, several outside groups turned to The Pennsylvania State University—more specifically to its College of the Liberal Arts and its Center for Continuing Liberal Education—for basic collaboration; and the University responded in a way, if not altogether unprecedented, at least so distinctive as already to have become the model for at least one similar venture elsewhere.

Speaking for the non-academic co-sponsors—the Vocational Rehabilitation Administration (U.S. Department of Health, Education and Welfare); The American Association of Workers for the Blind; the Committee for Research in Problems Related to Blindness; and the Department of Public Welfare of the Commonwealth of Pennsylvania—Dr. Norman M. Yoder, Pennsylvania Commissioner for the Blind, stated: "Somehow we must relate the university-based research with the agency needs, and we must relate agency research to the knowledge of the total university." The University Park Research

* *Educational Record,* Vol. 41, Jan. 1960, p. 5.

Consultation which has produced this collection of papers suggests the gains that can be made for certain groups within our society, and hence for the common good, through the interrelationships Dr. Yoder has specified.

For this collaboration and these gains, one despairs of an adequate inventory of appreciation. It has to be at once so deep and inclusive of so many. Dr. Yoder himself and his staff, (Miss) Mary E. Switzer, Administrator, Social and Rehabilitation Services, U.S. Department of Health, Education and Welfare; Dr. William M. Usdane, Chief, Research Grants and Demonstration; Dr. Douglas C. MacFarland, Chief, Division of Services to the Blind, and their staff in the Vocational Rehabilitation Administration, HEW; Louis H. Rives, Jr., President of the American Association of Workers for the Blind, and Sidney Cohen, Executive Secretary of that organization; Mary K. Bauman and the other members of the Committee for Research in Problems Related to Blindness—particularly, Francis M. Andrews (Chairman of the Committee), Joseph Kohn (past Chairman), and Robert S. Bray, Chief, Division for the Blind, Library of Congress; the other participants in setting up the program and in the Consultation itself (Stewart E. Armstrong, President, American Association of Instructors of the Blind, being illustrative); the writers of the basic and analyst papers and the session leaders; and, finally, the other University people involved.

Concerning the writers of the basic and the analyst papers, a special note is in order. The format for the Consultation called for these papers on relatively short notice and to meet relatively close deadlines. From the beginning, this was regarded as a real risk; and, even though calculated, a risk judged by some as quite dubious. It meant eliciting, from busy scholars and other professionals, a total quantity of manuscript which would be the makings of a large volume. However, the risk was overcome, and the cooperative spirit of the contributors went far to insure the success of this crucial phase of the venture.

More than a hundred years ago, Alexis de Tocqueville marveled at the speed and vigor with which we Americans set up voluntary organizations; and at the practical success of such groups once formed. In the Committee for Research in Problems Related to Blindness, de Tocqueville would see this impulse still successfully asserting itself; and he would find in it telling instances of how much, within such voluntary cooperative enterprise, the "significant individual" counts—a noteworthy example being Mary K. Bauman. As with the other collaborators, so with those from the University: members of the staff of our Continuing Education Services, in particular Robert E. Beam,

Conference Coordinator; the staff of the Center for Continuing Liberal Education, in particular John Swinton, Research and Editorial Assistant; the session reporters; the session leaders—all of them taking time from busy schedules; some of them, as Dr. Robert G. Bernreuter (Vice President for Student Affairs, Professor of Psychology, Emeritus), responding beyond the call of professional incentive or duty.

There are at least three more names, all connected with the College of the Liberal Arts, to be mentioned: Dean Kenneth G. Roose, who brought to his chairing of the opening general session both an official word and his personal concern; Dr. Cyril F. Hager, Associate Dean for Continuing Education, and Director of the Center for Continuing Liberal Education; and Dr. Roy C. Buck, Associate Director for Social Sciences at the Center, and Professor of Social Science. Dean Hager gave his Godspeed to the decision to have a Humanist serve as chairman and program developer for a project in which the behavioral-social sciences, as it turned out, were so largely involved. From the initial exploratory talk to the beginning of his sabbatical leave, Dr. Buck set his mark upon the shape taken by the planning.

Finally, a word is in order with regard to the opening paper in canvas for the deliberations of the conference. Arnold Barach was asked to provide a projective screen which would, in turn, serve—not as backdrop—but, as a "foredrop" for the future-oriented research papers to follow. His "Technological and Social Changes Ahead" proved a worthy addition to his past contributions and provided a suitable foredrop for the exploration of the Consultation theme: *Stress—catastrophic and continuing—as related to research problems associated with blindness*. Specifically, the Barach paper furnished both background and projective context for setting up the conceptual framework and presenting the research syntheses of the Consultation: I. Dependency (1. Childhood and Adolescence; 2. Old Age); II. Transition (3. Motivation; 4. Education; 5. Counseling); III. Public Life and Responsibility (6. Social Participation and Citizenship; 7. Occupation or Vocation); IV. Integration (8. Reaction to Loss; 9. The Multiple-Handicapped Blind; 10. Social Resolution—Bureaucracy: The Agency and the Person).

The opening presentation, then, sought to depict the sort of world—the sort of society—that both the blind and the sighted will be in, so as to provide for the other participants a picture to which to address such questions as: what are the implications of this (1) for those working with the blind; (2) for research in problems connected with blindness; (3) for particular agencies and organizations working with the blind?

The attempts, in turn, to answer such key questions as these would substantially contribute, it was hoped, toward gaining the major objective of this Consultation concerning needed research in the Behavioral Sciences and the Humanities with reference to problems related to blindness. The goal was to bring together the scholarly resources of the liberal arts and sciences and those of agency research and the understanding and expertise of those dealing, specifically, with problems related to blindness; and, thereby, to gain the following specific outcomes:

1. Produce a practical publication describing new ways of attacking research in problems associated with blindness and new concepts and new directions for such research.
2. Encourage and stimulate research proposals.
3. Provide guidelines for a ten-year national plan of relevant research.

MAXWELL H. GOLDBERG
Associate Director for the Humanities
Center for Continuing Liberal Education
Program Chairman

University Park, Pennsylvania

WELCOME ON BEHALF OF THE COMMITTEE FOR RESEARCH IN PROBLEMS RELATED TO BLINDNESS

I want to offer a welcome on behalf of the Committee for Research in Problems Related to Blindness and to devote a short amount of space to a discussion of the background of the Committee.

As many of you know, work with the blind experienced a spurt of growth during the World War II years when a number of younger people, earnestly interested in work with the blind but without experience, came into the field. They demanded information and answers to questions; and so, quite informally, in the late forties, they began to design and implement some research of their own. During this period there was not quite so much federal support for research. They started out hoping that by their own efforts, time and a very little money, they might be able to accumulate the information that was needed.

One of these initial efforts culminated in a meeting and a report which seemed fruitful and enlightening and replete with efficient, cheerful, constructive cooperation. To disband at this point seemed destructive, so a lasting organization was formed. This was really the beginning of what is, today, a grass roots committee of people on the firing line as far as work with the blind is concerned.

On the whole, this is not a very theoretical group. Instead, it is a group which, in the schools and in the agencies—day in and day out —gets the job done. Yet someone was still needed to find the facts and supply the answers. And so we, the members of the Committee for Research in Problems Related to Blindness, have chosen to act as a catalyst between the workers and the researchers rather than as another research group, so that we can encourage one group to solve specific problems and the other to apply the results.

The Committee is not a fund raising organization; it is rather an advisory organization—provided it can find someone who wants its advice. It is an organization that points to areas where research is needed.

We members have, for some time, wanted the opportunity to pool many greater minds than our own and so we have dreamed about and planned a national conference on problems related to blindness. The planning has been extensive; but at last, under our auspices as well as with the cooperation and support of the American Association of Workers for the Blind, the United States Vocational Rehabilitation Administration, the Pennsylvania Department of Public Welfare, and The Pennsylvania State University Center for Continuing Liberal Education, we have reached the point where we are gratefully able to welcome all of you to this National Research Consultation Concerning Needed Research in the Behavioral Sciences and the Humanities with Reference to Problems Related to Blindness.

MARY K. BAUMAN
Director of the Personnel
Research Center
Philadelphia, Pennsylvania

THE INDIVIDUAL, STRESS, AND THE NEW WORLD OF SOCIAL AND TECHNOLOGICAL CHANGE

TECHNOLOGICAL AND SOCIAL CHANGES AHEAD

Arnold B. Barach

My purpose in this paper will be twofold: first, to sketch, in fairly loose form, the outlines and the nature of technological and social changes ahead; and, second, by implication, to demonstrate how the shifts and turns of these two mainstreams of current life may affect the individual and his place in society.

Perhaps my function should be regarded more as that of a catalyst than of a generator of new concepts and ideas. What I mean to contribute is a judgment or an appraisal of the many diverse and varied predictions that one reads with increasing frequency, and which originate with a multitude of authorities or, if you will, pseudo-authorities.

The profession of prediction, if one may call it that, is a wide open field, limited neither to the academic nor the business world, exclusive to no single group or occupational category. These days, in particular, there is an outpouring of publications, statements, books, and so on, all dealing with a profusion of projections for the future, and every one of them pretending to have the final or almost-final word on where we are heading.

Recently I received a scholarly new tome titled *The American Economy to 1975,* read a stimulating discussion of trends of tomorrow in *Fortune* magazine, heard the Columbia Broadcasting System bravely talk about life in the twenty-first century, perused a series of scholarly papers on coming challenges for the city emanating from a distinguished seminar sponsored by the Smithsonian Institute, examined a weighty government document from the Joint Economic Committee of Congress on the 1970's, found myself the recipient of a handsomely published magazine from the Kaiser Aluminum Company exploring "probable changes in the world we live in in the next two decades," and received in the mails speeches by the acting Secretary of Commerce, the Secretary of Labor, and the Secretary of Transportation, all much concerned with the world of tomorrow. I am concerned that so many people are getting involved in the future and may neglect the very-important present.

The point that must be made is that we are no longer a people content to let the future take care of itself. There are too many individuals in all categories of activity who are concerned about where we are headed, what problems are likely to emerge, and how we can cope with them. It is the concern of educators, city planners, demographers, poverty workers, those in transportation and communication, and literally hundreds of other specialists and professionals. The approach is as practical as making our air and water free of pollutants and as idealistic as dissolving the barriers that divide nations as effectively as they divide neighborhood from neighborhood.

WHERE WE HAVE COME

Of the many reasons that explain this maturing responsibility of planning for the future, two seem to stand out in terms of their impact on our political and social structure: (1) the swift pace of change of the past quarter century; (2) the swifter pace of progress that confronts the nation as it heads into the 1970's.

The reaction to these trends is exactly in tune with our culture and traditions. Gerhard Colm and Theodore Geiger expressed it well when they wrote:

> American society since its beginning has been characterized in greater or lesser degree by such attitudes as an orientation toward the present and future and not toward the past; a predisposition to base thought and action on the facts of the existing situation rather than upon inherited custom or abstract doctrine; a deep confidence in the power of rational thought and human action to solve personal and social problems; and a willingness to compromise or accommodate competing group and individual interests. By and large, American society has been optimistic, pragmatic, rationalistic, open-minded, and cooperative. It has tended to value conscientious work, material well-being, technical skill, individual flexibility, and social and geographical mobility. These values have contributed to American economic success and in turn have been strengthened by it.[1]

The economic performance of the past few years has been remarkable indeed.

In 1960, there were just under 67 million people at work. Today, we approach a total employment of 75 million.

Personal incomes have risen from about 401 billion dollars to over 580 billions in the last six years.

The nation's gross national product went from $503.7 billion to $739.5 billion in the same period.

Behind this remarkable economic growth is a long and upward period of national expansion that is unprecedented either in the annals of this country or any other. Today's worker produces, on average, three and a half times as much in an hour's labor as his grandfather did. The significant fact is that the true acceleration of this growth in productivity came after World War II, when the average annual rate of increase was 3.4 per cent, as against 2.6 per cent in the period since the crisis year of 1929. The net result has been a tripling of production, and the country now stands in the posture of the world's greatest economic power—comprising only six per cent of the world's population while accounting for about one-third of its production.

The obvious fruit of such a rich cultivation of economic resources has been a standard of living the level and dimensions of which are unprecedented in history. Let us look first at the spread of this economic wealth and the extent to which it is shared by everyone.

THE ROAD TO RICHES

There was a time when the concentration of wealth in this country was not so far removed from the days when the lords of the manor raked in the cash while the serfs merely raked. As recently as 1929, five per cent of American families received 30 per cent of the nation's income. In this decade, the top five per cent still get a disproportionate share of income, but the share is almost down to half of what it was less than 40 years ago; it is now about 18 per cent.

This redistribution of income at a time when total income was rising at a rapid rate has elevated bank accounts for millions and produced a scale of living that now embraces for the ordinary man everything from his own sailboat and color TV set to air conditioning and a second car in the garage. While there is much to be done, the fact is that whereas about 30 per cent of all families had incomes of less than $2,000 in 1929, fewer than 11 per cent are in that bracket today, measured by 1964 dollars. That, I submit, is progress and indicative of our potential.

We are a nation which indulges itself to the hilt, both in material things and, I am glad to report, in the non-material. Travel abroad is becoming almost as commonplace as a Sunday afternoon drive. Purchase of goods is fantastic; we buy more than any other people in the world, and few of these things that we spend so freely on are indispensable to a happy and full life.

We also indulge ourselves in medical care, recreation, cultural pleasures, and education, all of them further manifestation of the quality of life made possible by our economic renaissance of the past 20 years. At the turn of the century, four out of every 100 young people between 18 and 21 were enrolled in college; this year it is almost 11 times that ratio—44 out of 100. We can boast that nowhere in the world is higher education available to so many young people as here.

Along with our material enrichment has come a new awareness of a devotion to the public welfare. The billions spent on rebuilding our cities, even though they seem like a very small drop in a very big bucket, are a recognition that the urban society cannot exist as a healthy and sound organism unless it is carefully protected and enhanced both in its architectural appearance and in its social structure. One may argue with the results, but it is apparent in dozens of cities that a rebirth has taken place in areas which previously would have been considered slums and forgotten. The redevelopment program stands as a prime example of how aroused citizens, distressed by the neglect and degradation of their environment, can do something about it if the hand is willing and the purse able. And yet, none of it could have been done without the great resources of technological and economic riches which we have collected in the past generation or two.

For another example of this dedication to the social welfare, we can cite the Poverty Program which, with all its faults, has nevertheless established itself as a milestone in our society.

Our involvement in health programs, calling for the expenditure of huge sums for research, public health services, better hospitals, mental health centers, is a third evidence of how this country's great wealth is being invested in undertakings far removed from the accepted government activities of a few decades ago. It is significant enough that the work is being done, but more significant is the fact that a new group of priorities have appeared on our national scene involving not only the welfare of the individual family but that of society as a whole. It is a recognition of how the great expectations of this society can be realized.

"THE PAST IS PROLOGUE"

I have digressed here a bit simply to make the point that as we look at the world of tomorrow, we must keep in mind the directions of today, for here are found our goals and purposes. Franklin Roosevelt may have been anathema to the political outs when he used the power of his office to give the country such things as social security, rural conservation, jobs for its unemployed, protection for its investors, help for its handicapped and aged and stabilization of its agriculture; but when the political outs became the political ins, they retained all of these new functions of government, and even added to them. They discovered not only that there was political popularity in them, but also that they held some of the answers to the problems that rose out of our new and complex society.

It is reasonable, therefore, to propose that what we are doing now in urban renewal, eradication of poverty, and medical care—to mention but three government concerns of the 1960's—represent continuing programs, surely to grow in the years ahead once we return to a period of peace.

Our concerns of tomorrow will be increasingly ecological—the pollution of our cities and landscapes, the spoiling of our soil through the irresponsible use of pesticides and insecticides, the scarring of our countryside by six- and eight- and now ten-lane highways, the strains on our water supplies and agriculture and other resources by a population explosion which, although it has slowed in the past couple of years, will likely be felt again by the 1970's.

Whether the available means that are used to wrestle with these challenges will be equal to the dimensions of tomorrow's problems is a highly disputable point. Speaking at the Columbia Seminar on Technology and Social Change, Donald Michael may have exaggerated a bit; but nevertheless he posed the old issue in fluent terms when he said:

> The problems, whether they be urban renewal, air pollution, education for the new age, Medicare, international development programs, the exploitation of the oceans, assigning technology development priorities, etc., will be too complicated to be dealt with effectively by the techniques that have characterized our society to date. And the issues will be too critical, the potentials for and scale of disaster too great to stake our social survival upon conventional approaches—even when they are undertaken (as they rarely are) with the best of disinterested goodwill. All we have to do is to look at the looming disaster our cities represent, to recognize that we are going to have to do much better.
>
> The tasks we face, then, will require the full use of whatever rationalized techniques we have, and these techniques will proliferate in the years ahead with advances in the social sciences, with increasing use of computers, data banks, simulation, system analyses, operations research, and so on.

In consequence, planners and decision makers will be confronted with a set of circumstances that will also suggest important changes in the democratic process. The competing demands for human and physical resources, necessarily expended over long periods of time, will require the development of ways to assign priorities and to revise costly efforts, even if it's politically uncomfortable and institutionally disruptive. At present we have neither the priority scheme nor the means for efficiently and reliably transcending convention and institutional restraints. Yet, obviously, we will have to be able to choose between major technological developments, and we will have to be able to maintain or alter these decisions more in the light of their real accomplishments, rather than in the light of political commitments.[2]

TOMORROW: THREAT OR PROMISE?

Our times are prosperous ones, challenging, exciting, disruptive of many old values (including, certainly, the Puritan Ethic), and overlaid with concerns of social responsibilities and how to deal with them within the dimensions of the world we will live in. The shape of that world comes to life in statistics (how many people we will be, how much money we will have, how many cars we will own, how many students we will enroll, how many babies we will rear) and in sometimes real, sometimes fanciful predictions of the kind of technology ahead. What follows is a judgment which, hopefully, is balanced enough to make sense within the realities at hand. It is not enough just to extrapolate for, as experience has shown, extrapolation is but one step removed from oversimplification. Ignored completely may be the value judgments that must be made as to whether this trend or that curve is likely to be maintained in the face of shifting influences and environments.

At the 1939 World's Fair, one of the biggest auto manufacturers asserted that auto output would reach "impossible" levels over the next quarter century. We would, he said, have an unheard-of 32 million cars on the road by 1964! There were gasps of disbelief and plenty of skepticism. In fact, the skeptics should have been skeptical in the opposite direction, for by 1964, this nation simultaneously boasted and complained about its 70 million car population—a figure which now, incidentally, has risen to over 80 million, better than one car for every three people.

And who can ignore the colossal blooper of one of our leading social prophets of the 1930's, Henry Wallace? Wallace was sneered at, called a Socialist and worse, and considered a dangerous man in some circles because he had the audacity to predict 60 million jobs for Americans in another generation. Mr. Wallace was indeed a conservative seer, as events have proven. For here we are, a generation later, with 75 million people at work and more being added every week.

This habit of understatement about what is to come seems to be deeply ingrained in the nation's fabric. Is it likely that Americans, even the most sophisticated among us, are fearful of being too optimistic about tomorrow because they don't want to cling to expectations that may not be fulfilled? Could the reason be that we don't want to be let down by disappointment? Or are there other reasons for this tempered optimism?

In this nation, human enterprise and daring have built great monuments to technical achievement and skills, yet there is a guilt that goes along with these monuments, a fear that we are desecrating the human soul with material obsessions, upsetting nature with the spread of our cities, putting a priority on ugliness in our architecture and design. Thus, to look ahead to a world even more embellished with buildings and machinery and highways may compound the guilt that already exists.

The historian Herbert Muller observes that there is in man's nature an "ancient habit of overrating the past." Men are romantics about the past—they think of childhood as a blissful period of happiness devoid of problems or frustrations. But they cannot bring the same romanticism to their dreams about the future, unless all is good and all is beautiful. Remember the wonderful creature of Langston Hughes which he named "Simple," and which he made a repository of all the common sense in humankind.

"Do you believe in fortune telling?" asked Mr. Hughes.

"Sure," said Simple, "when the fortunes are good."

The fortunes have not always been good, nor will they be consistently good in the future. Troubles and agonies are part of human experience. Thus, to the fear that the future may not turn out to be all that is hoped for, and to the sense of guilt involved in the making of a world that gets constantly more overwhelming in its technological complexity, there must be added a third element that makes men reluctant to face up to the future. This is the underlying sense of the unknown that has always beset mankind's dreams and hopes.

All nations and races have significant groupings of people who are content with life as it is or, in the extreme instances, with life as it was. They are not interested in change, they often resist it, and their reasons for this attitude are not necessarily without logic. Better to live in a present that is understood and manageable than to anticipate a future that can upset all the basic patterns of life. Tradition has much in its favor, and continuity of tradition most of all. By not anticipating change and, in fact, by sidetracking it before it is too late to stop it, the status quo is undisturbed. Given this kind of approach, it is indeed a simple matter to underrate the trends towards tomorrow and to underestimate with profound error the kind of world that lies just over the horizon.

WORLD OF THE FUTURE

We talk about a political consensus, Johnson-style, in the hope of achieving some sort of unanimity on our goals and attainments ahead. Can we not also obtain some sort of consensus as to where we go in the years ahead?

The Rand Corporation sought to achieve a consensus of prophets not long ago when it compiled the views of 82 experts on their timetable for specific attainments in various areas of human endeavor including scientific breakthroughs, population control, automation, space progress, war prevention, and weapons systems.

The credentials of these authorities are above challenge—their ideas represent the most advanced thinking and knowledge in their various areas of competence. I would like to mention just a few of their predictions.

In the immediate future—that is to say, within the next four or five years—they predict we will have achieved useful desalination of sea water for drinking, irrigation and industry.

Also in this period will come development of new synthetic materials for ultralight construction. Who is to say what effect this will have on our traditional methods of architecture and engineering?

Effective fertility control, so desperately needed in certain countries, is only a few years distant.

Automated language translators are close to perfection, say these experts.

We are very close to the time when transplants or substitutes for many of the vital organs of the human body will be routine.

And finally, in this interval of the next few years, reliable weather reports will be possible, according to this scientific consensus. Today, the odds are about two out of three that the prediction will be right.

As we move on into the decade of the 1980's, this scientific consensus foresees even more startling developments. The use of non-narcotic drugs will be socially acceptable and widespread for the purpose—and I quote—"of producing specific changes in personality characteristics."

There will be implanted artificial organs made of plastic and electronic components in common use. Controlled thermonuclear power will be a reality, and mining of the ocean depths will become an established industry. But the most startling development of all in the decade of the 1980's will be the initial development of a primitive form of artificial life. The moral implications of this are overwhelming.

Looking ahead to the final decade of the century, we are told that regional weather control will be a very real possibility. We will have the economic feasibility of producing synthetic proteins for food, and the use of biochemicals to immunize against bacterial and viral diseases will be commonplace.

In other medical areas, psychotic diseases will be cured by physical or chemical therapy. It will be possible to exercise control over genetic defects by modification of genes through chemical engineering. The injection of biochemicals to stimulate regeneration of damaged organs and limbs may be possible by then—man will not necessarily be able to recreate a mangled arm or leg, but he will have greater possibilities of restoring to use a limb that has been crippled by accident or disease.

What happens after the year 2000? Again quoting the results of the survey, we or our children will be living in a world where, through use of biochemicals, we will actually be able to grow new limbs and organs. Drugs will be available to upgrade levels of intelligence. (Tentative experiments in recent months have already demonstrated that such drugs are possible.) Life expectancy will possibly be stretched another 50 years. It is probable that communication on an extra-terrestrial basis will be accomplished. There is an odds-on chance that control of gravitation will have been achieved through modification of the gravitational field.

In the 1980's will come automatic medical diagnosis through computers, use of robots for such things as trash collection or sewer inspection, a universal language for automated communication, tax collections and tax withholding through computers. And in the 1990's or a bit later we will develop automated highways for controlling traffic, automated voting (you vote from your home), newspapers and magazines printed right in the home. Inevitably in this interval will come international agreements guaranteeing minimal economic needs to the world's population as a result of high production from automation.

Looking at everyday life and work over the next 20 or 30 years, the survey found strong expectations that banks and stores will be linked by computers for handling credit charges. Automation in office and service centers will displace about 25 per cent of our workers. There will be a widespread use of teaching machines, automatic libraries, automated rapid transit, and widespread involvement in education as a leisure time activity.

Technologically, the world will be turned topsy-turvy. There will be little that is recognizable in terms of what we are now familiar with.

The science of today will be displaced by new and daring innovations which will change not only the appearance of the world men live in, but the intellectual and the emotional climate in which he functions. He will have to discard many of his old values and find new ones. He will have to make peace with the conflict of the two cultures and discover ways of blending them into one culture. Otherwise, he may be drowned in a world of cold technological wonders.

POPULATION EXPLOSION

Fundamental challenges will be posed to all that we have accepted up to now as the established nature of society and social organization. Look at what will happen to population between now and the end of the century: three and a half billion people now, at least double that by the year 2000. Reflect a moment on what that means in terms of the design, the size, and the basic comforts of our cities. What does this imply for metropolitan development, transportation, housing, food supply, recreation space, use of the world's goods? What does it mean as a measure of the total political structuring of the world, a world in which the have-nots are multiplying at a rate far in excess of that of the haves?

Our cities and our political institutions will change under this pressure and there will be new appraisals of resources of energy and raw materials. For about 6,000 years man's most exclusive source of energy was in his muscle power; in about two-thirds of the world, that is still the case. But the industrialized nations long ago discarded muscle power in favor of steam, electricity, and other forms of electro-mechanical energy. We have at our disposal tens of trillions of mechanical-electrical horsepower to aid us. In this nation, containing 6 per cent of the world's population and consuming 35 per cent of the world's energy output, the rate of increase for energy requirements has been 3½ per cent a year.

A reasonable question is: how long can we indulge ourselves in so rich a feast of fossil fuels? In the next 35 years we will consume about 500 billion tons of coal, and it is estimated that there is more than enough to meet the need. Our oil consumption is even more extravagant, and while there is no visible shortage now, this cannot last forever. Furthermore, as the newer nations of the world attain the technological heights, they will demand their share of the available energy resources. Obviously, new energy sources will have to be found and developed. Atomic power will play a far more dominant part in the creation of energy than it does today. Uranium and thorium, the vital nuclear fuels, will increasingly replace diminishing fossil fuels.

Likewise, we cannot depend forever on our present resources of metals, minerals, and other raw materials. The skills of the inorganic chemists have paid off tremendously in the synthesis of new materials which even nature cannot duplicate. But the day is approaching when we will have to recycle our wastes so that they can be reused over and over to supplement what we can still extract from the earth.

Water is a prime example. More than 97 per cent of our water is in the oceans, unusable for most human purposes. Two per cent is frozen in glaciers and ice caps. The one per cent left is so poorly distributed that the margin between aquatic affluence and aquatic poverty is thin indeed.

In the next 20 years the world's demand for fresh water will double. Residents of the west know well what happens when demand outruns supply, but in much of the nation, the experience of a water shortage is so rare as to be virtually unknown.

Our needs for water are overwhelming. Almost 50 per cent of what we use goes for irrigation. Another 40 per cent is needed by industry. The water that we drink, bathe in, wash our car with, or use for watering the grass makes up the remaining 10 per cent. One wonders where the shortage hits worse—in the bath tub or, for example, in a steel mill, where 65,000 gallons of water are needed to produce a ton of steel.

So the world that we now move into will be unlike anything that we have ever known before. It will be a compound of riches and problems. It will have the promise of technological achievement and the threat of profound scarcities of the essentials of life.

ONWARD TO A YOUTHFUL COUNTRY

The technological revolution will manifest itself in many ways. Life expectancy may be extended because of it. The quality and diversity of life will be enhanced as its dividends begin to be enjoyed. Systems of communication and transportation will be created in different form, and people may travel in 2,000-mile-an-hour airplanes or electronically controlled automobiles as casually as they watch television in three dimensions or read newspapers delivered over the air waves. There will be new intrusions into space, with results which can be anticipated only in terms of what the science fiction writer foresees.

In a more practical sense, the technological revolution will have to do with people, with industry and work, and with education. For it is in these three areas that its changes will make themselves most dramatically felt and create their most lasting effects.

If we project the population mix ahead 10 or 15 years (and it is not hard to do since the people involved are already here except for those who will be very young), then we get a picture of a shifting pattern between the old and the young. We are a nation in which the number of young—those under 25—just about exceeds everyone else, a trend which is true in many parts of the world. This tipping of the population seesaw is already of priority importance to the marketing experts and the demographers on Madison Avenue. And while one may be somewhat amused by the cry "Don't trust anyone over 30," this surge of youth into the ranks of the political effectives is not amusing, particularly to gray-beard politicians who are not so sure what the youthful chatter is all about, but who nevertheless feel bound to turn an aged ear in its direction.

A quick reading of the Census Bureau's projections makes the point. In the mid-sixties, it is the people in the 35 to 44 age group who are the most numerous of all those from 25 to 65, divided into ten-year groupings. There are almost 25 million of those, about two million more than the number in both the 25 to 34 age group. And the numbers decrease, proportionately, as the groupings advance up the population scale. It is at the lower end of the scale, the early 20's and under, where one can find evidence of changes to come.

By 1980, the picture will be drastically different. Instead of a mere 23 million between 25 and 34 there will be 40 million—roughly one-sixth of the total population of 1980 concentrated in this youthful age bracket. To their numbers must be added another 21 million or so between 20 and 24. In other words, 61 million Americans just about old enough to vote and young enough to be on the bright side of 35. The over-35's will be a declining proportion of the nation's populace—with one exception. Instead of about 18 million who have now passed 65, there will be about 25 million, most of them retired, most of them a liability for the nation's health and retirement facilities.

Only the middle-aged will be in decline—those from 35 to 55 or 60. There will be fewer of them in 1980 than there are today. While they will carry the full brunt of the job of managing the country and its economy, they will be forced to do it while occupying a minority position in terms of numbers.

There is one further observation to be made, and that concerns the shift in family formation, with all of its implications for housing, birth rate, community needs, and so on. In recent years, new marriages have been occurring at the rate of about 500,000 annually, and while the figure has risen slightly, the big jump will occur in the next few years when 700,000 new families will set up housekeeping each year. By the middle or late 1970's, the country can expect about 850,000 weddings a year. If households formed by the unmarried are included in this count, the number of new households that are established in the early 1970's is estimated to rise to 1,200,000 annually. The population explosion is about to make itself felt.

Where will these millions work? What will they do? Just as the population mix is shifting, so is the economic mix, with some of the changes already visible.

The total mix and the composition of the mix are two different but nevertheless related consequences of the technological revolution. By total mix is meant the gross national product—the total value of goods and services produced in the country. Colm projects three different possibilities in 1964 dollars, all reachable—given certain assumptions.

His first, what he calls the "target project," visualizes a gross national product of one trillion, 400 billion dollars in 1980 (compared to about 760 billion in 1966). He argues that such a potential is "feasible under our economic and social institutions," assuming unemployment is maintained at about a 3½ per cent rate.

His second projection, which he calls the "judgment projection," assumes a government policy in support of economic growth and counteracting recessions. "This projection realistically assumes some human failure in economic diagnosis and prescription and some slippage in political implementation." Given these failings Colm nevertheless anticipates a GNP of one trillion, 200 billion dollars is possible for 1980.

His third, and lowest projection foresees a GNP of slightly over a trillion dollars, assuming continuance of present fiscal and monetary policies. He sees in these policies the implication of an unemployment rate of 8.5 per cent and higher because of failure to provide for the millions of young workers who enter the labor force in the next decade.

Whichever of the three Colm projections one leans towards, the fact is that, measured by constant dollars, our gross national product stands to increase from something over 25 per cent to as much as 100 per cent in the next 12 or 13 years. Twenty years from now, based on the projections above, the factor of progress will be twice or three times what it is today. We are in a historic phase comparable to the lifting of a rocket from its pad: lift-off has been achieved, the rocket is in flight, but the full blast of the engines has not yet taken effect.

CONSEQUENCES OF THE ECONOMIC EXPLOSION

One immediate consequence of this growth will be a higher living standard for millions. Average family income, measured in 1963 dollars, is now close to $8,000 a year. It should exceed $10,500 by 1980. The number of families with incomes below $2,000 will still be significant enough to cause concern, but can be expected to drop below 8 per cent.

The upgrading of the American style of life will be accompanied by a reduction in working hours, which in the past 75 years dropped from more than 60 hours per week to something under 40 hours. Again citing Colm, we can expect an average work week of 35.9 hours in 1980. Even assuming this modest drop in the work week, it can be anticipated that vacations will be lengthened, holidays multiplied, and even sabbatical leaves provided millions of workers in the fashion of academia and the steel industry.

Industrial growth will not be shared equally by all businesses, and some will certainly shrink. A Department of Labor analysis suggests that these industries are likely to expand most rapidly as the nation moves through the seventies: atomic energy, banking, aviation, electric power, electronics manufacturing, foundries, hotels, industrial chemicals, iron and steel, automotive, petroleum and natural gas. Government—the growingest industry of them all—will show big expansion in education, health services, hospitals, sanitation, and police services, mainly concentrated at the local level.

As is not surprising, the fastest-growing businesses will not necessarily be the sources of the major job opportunities. Automation and use of computers will displace hundreds of thousands of workers in such industries as electric power, metal foundries, iron and steel, petroleum and natural gas. Agriculture, where employment has dropped about 42 per cent in the last 20 years as a result of mechanization and advanced agricultural engineering, will reflect another reduction of about 20 per cent in job openings between now and 1975.

Which skills, then, will be in greatest demand? The Labor Department foresees these: accountants, advertising and market research, personnel experts, purchasing agents, clergy, vocational and rehabilitation counselors, engineers in some areas of the profession, health service specialists, mathematicians, physical scientists, biological scientists, social scientists, social workers, lawyers, doctors, teachers, librarians, technicians. Service occupations will expand almost as fast as professional ones and there will be continued high demand for restaurant help, building service workers, domestic employees, clerks, business machine operators, real estate, insurance, sales, and such protective service workers as firemen, policemen, and guards. Mechanics and repairmen have excellent prospects. So do such building trades workers as glaziers, structural metal workers, operators of earth moving machines, sheet metal workers, cement masons, electricians, plumbers, and pipefitters. But the unskilled worker—no matter in what industry he is employed—will find a decreasing demand for his services as further automation takes over the manual tasks.

EDUCATION A TOP PRIORITY

It is almost a redundancy to observe that the capable individual of the 1970's and 1980's will require, above all, the educational indoctrination suitable for functioning in and adapting to his environment. Without this intellectual reinforcement, a person may find himself buffeted about by the rapid changes and frustrated by a world that is only half understood. It will be challenge enough grasping the simple essentials of the new technology. The real challenge will be in a new orientation of personal value systems and goals so as to live successfully in our world of the future.

The acquisition of knowledge will truly test our educational resources and techniques. Paul Ylvisaker of the Ford Foundation quotes Richard Meier's contention "that the major problems of 1980's megalopolis will not be such graspable nettles as food and water shortages, but an overloading of the human communications system—its capacity to absorb infinitely proliferating signals and still to respond rationally." The knowledge explosion has within it a fantastic potential for upsetting all of our previous criteria of the educational process, for never before has the sum of human wisdom accumulated and compounded itself at such a breakneck pace.

One expert witness at a colloquium on the Challenge of Curricular Change estimated that half of what a graduating engineer studies today will be obsolete in ten years. It was at that same colloquium that Joseph Jackson Schwab, of the University of Chicago, observed: "If a biologist today were to go into outer space and stay there for four years, he would have a desperate time catching up with his fellow biologists when he returned. After eight years of absence, he would hardly be able to communicate with them."

More than 300,000 articles are published each year in about 6,000 scientific and technical journals in the United States alone—and this is a fraction of the 2,000,000 articles written by some 750,000 scientists in about 50 languages around the world every year. Dr. Glenn Seaborg, chairman of the Atomic Energy Commission, estimates that in another 50 years the total of scientific articles published each year in the world will be 20,000,000, written by some 8,000,000 scientists!

The fact of the matter is that educators are well aware of what is to come and, for that matter, what is happening right now. The Office of Education just recently announced the establishment of a Policy Research Center Program, whose purpose will be, in cooperation with educational institutions around the country, to "analyze future educational needs and resources and, in light of these analyses, provide policy makers with relevant information and techniques for decision making." Through a series of centers to be established in selected universities, the Office of Education will probe such problems as curricular objectives for the future, the implications of new technologies for education, the economic and political resources available for education and the place of the schools in the social structure of the country. Within this framework, projects will be launched on such diverse problems as the changing role of teacher and professor, the need to educate for leisure time roles, the future roles of the military and industry as educational forces, the shape of the urban complex of tomorrow, advances in biophysical knowledge of factors related to intelligence and learning, and so on. It is a development that may be fundamental to the future course of education in this country.

THE CALL FOR LEADERSHIP

Education cannot do the job by itself. An indispensable need will be a leadership endowed with great wisdom, a sensitivity to the needs and wants of fellow men, and, above all, the courage to choose, and choose correctly, among the various alternatives that will be available in the brave new world ahead. There will be a mandate to avoid the imposition of a Big Brother mentality on a newly structured political organism reflecting the technological and social revolutions that are less than a generation ahead. I have not spoken here of such new concepts as a world much more tightly bound together than now, of the new modes of living, leisure, and recreation—and our ability to share them equally, of the urban chaos that exists now and that will worsen without desperate measures in the next few years. Nor has the continuing encroachment of urban sprawl on our unspoiled countryside been examined.

All are peripheral to the main issue, and that is—how the individual can live happily and successfully in a world that may produce inordinate stresses and tensions. This conference will, hopefully, generate some of the answers to the dilemma, particularly as they apply to the handicapped blind.

NOTES

1. Gerhard Colm and Theodore Geiger, *The Economy of the American People* (Washington: National Planning Association, 1967).
2. D. Morse and A. W. Warner, eds., *Technological Innovation and Society* (New York: Columbia University Press, 1966).
3. R. L. Hill, ed., *America 1980: The William A. Jump—Thomas McKillop Memorial Lectures in Public Administration* (Washington: U.S. Department of Agriculture, 1965).
4. Von Neumann Sarnoff, *et al., The Fabulous Future—America in 1980* (New York: E. P. Dutton and Co., 1956).
5. U.S. Department of Labor, "Technological Trends in Major American Industries," *Labor Bulletin No. 1474* (Washington: Government Printing Office, 1966).
6. ———, *Occupational Outlook Handbook* (Washington: Government Printing Office, 1966).
7. 88th Congress Joint Economic Committee, *State and Local Public Facility Needs and Financing* (Washington: Government Printing Office, 1966).
8. ———, *U.S. Economic Growth to 1975: Potentials and Problems* (Washington: Government Printing Office, 1966).

DIMENSIONS OF BLINDNESS

Mary K. Bauman

Just what is blindness? The answer is far from simple.

It is quite impossible to develop reliable statistics with regard to blindness on an international basis because of the great variations in the definition of blindness from one country to another. In countries with less economic and industrial development, the word tends to apply only to total lack of vision, but in this country and in some others such as Canada and Great Britain, the term "blindness" is by no means synonymous with "total blindness."

Even in the United States, the confusion is great, and the best we can do is say that it was far greater before 1935. The Social Security Act of that year defined blindness as visual acuity for distant vision of 20/200 or less in the better eye, with best correction; or visual acuity of more than 20/200 if the widest diameter of field of vision subtends an angle no greater than 20 degrees. In simpler terms, we describe as "blind" an individual who cannot see at 20 feet what a person with normal vision can see at 200 feet, or an individual whose field is so restricted that he can see only a very limited area at one time. This is often referred to as "legal blindness." Every new law, both state and federal, can of course redefine blindness for its own purposes and some of this has occurred. Also, if agencies serving blind people function strictly along the lines of the 1935 definition, they must refuse some services to people who could use them while they offer some to people who may not need them. This results in much criticism of the legal definition and, in recent years, much discussion of change. However, at this time, most grants and therefore the guidelines for most research—our area of concern—are based on the 1935 definition.

The legal definition of blindness causes a great deal of difficulty for research workers because it embraces people so heterogeneous with regard to vision that they form nothing like one group. From my own experience I would say they more nearly form three groups:

1. Those for whom vision is of no practical use in a testing or working situation. This obviously includes the totally blind, but it also includes those who can distinguish objects only when held between their eyes and the source of light. Few jobs and, to my knowledge, no tests are done this way.

2. Those for whom vision is helpful in a testing or working situation but who cannot read even moderately enlarged ink print really effectively. These people often supplement their vision with touch in a very effective way—so effectively and so habitually that they may say they scarcely distinguish the information they get tactually from that which they get visually when using these two senses together. They have no difficulty orienting themselves in a work space, seeing where an object lies on a table, distinguishing the shapes of blocks, or using vision to guide their hands in gross movements required by a job. They may distinguish very large print, such as newspaper headlines, and perhaps with great difficulty and for short periods of time they may read what we ordinarily refer to as "large type," but this size of ink print is not really useful to them as a major part of a job, day after day.

3. Those who use ink print effectively although it may have to be large type, or held very close to their eyes, or used with a special and perhaps cumbersome visual aid and under special lighting conditions.

In most research related to blindness, these differences in vision play a very significant part. If the research involves any use of materials, printed or concrete, people in groups (2) and (3) as defined above function very differently from those in group (1). Even those in (3) function somewhat differently from those in (2)—enough to affect test results materially. People in (2) and (3) might be thrown together as a research population but (1) can never be included without separate statistical treatment.

What about research which does not involve printed or concrete materials—research on attitudes or personality? The way in which the subjects respond to the research stimulus may be unaffected by differences in vision, but the life experiences about which they are reporting have been. Many people regard partially seeing people as less well-adjusted to "blindness" than the totally blind, and the partially seeing themselves feel that they have more difficulty being understood and accepted. In addition they are rootless people, having no sense of belonging either with the seeing or the blind. Even the term, "partially seeing," may not clearly be the property of those whose acuity lies between object vision and 20/200. There has been some suggestion that these people be called "economically blind" with the term "partially seeing" applying to persons with acuity between 20/200 and 20/70.

Another factor in vision which importantly affects research is the age at which vision was lost. The person who retained vision until the teens or later shares the description "blind" with people whose condition is congenital, but the latter cannot share with him many of the concepts he developed during the years when he could see.

DEMOGRAPHIC DIMENSION

Not only because of differences in definition of blindness, but also because a real census is impossible, all statements about the number of blind people are estimates. In recent years such estimates have been made available by at least three rather responsible sources. I am choosing to use, for this paper, the figures produced by the National Society for the Prevention of Blindness,[5] in part because they are very recent, in part because they give more kinds of information than do the other estimates.

These estimates indicate that in 1940 there were, in the U.S., roughly 230,000 blind people; this represented a rate of 1.75 per thousand in the population. By 1950 the estimate rose close to 300,000, by 1960 to 385,000, and by 1965 to 416,000. By this latter date, the rate had risen to 2.14 per thousand, partly because of the greater percentage of older persons in the population. If we assume no change in rate, the increasing population represented by projected estimate of the Bureau of Census will result in 446,500 blind persons in 1970 and 519,200 in 1980. Thus, in four decades the number of blind persons in the U.S. will have more than doubled.

Blindness is not distributed equally throughout the states. Instead, it appears most frequently in the southern states and Hawaii, least frequently in North Dakota, Minnesota, Connecticut, Wyoming, Idaho, and Utah. Nor is it distributed equally in all age groups; less than 10 per cent of blind persons are under 20 years of age while nearly 50 per cent are 65 or over. Indeed, 38 per cent are 70 or over. It is estimated that: slightly more than 30,000 new cases of blindness occur each year, there are more blind men than women, and blindness appears more frequently in the non-white population.

HISTORICAL DIMENSION

With some variations, society as a whole has passed through three stages in its attitudes toward blind people: (1) the stage of mendicancy, when blind people were regarded as liabilities; (2) the stage of the asylum, when blind people were regarded as the wards of society; and (3) the stage of integration, when blind people were accepted as members of society. Some evidences of all these stages are still to be found in our handling of blind people today.

Ancient writings suggest that mendicancy was regarded as the natural and proper condition of the blind. The blind beggar was frequently met on the streets of Athens, Rome, Carthage, and Jerusalem, and in some cultures he was not allowed to work even if he demonstrated that he could. Indeed, he might be an untouchable whose blindness was regarded as a curse, a visitation of the gods, and it was feared that blindness could be transmitted by touch. It was believed that the blind person was suffering punishment for his sins, or perhaps for the sins of his parents, and any effort to alleviate his condition would be to pit oneself against the gods. This concept of blindness as punishment for sin is still with us to some extent. In 1949 Simmons[8] carried out a study of attitudes of seeing people toward blindness and found that 7 per cent held this view. In the study of Adjustment to Blindness, done about the same time through interviews with blind people, we found that 22 per cent felt, or had at some time felt, that their blindness was a punishment. In recent meetings with staff members of an agency for the blind, I found that several of them had experienced situations in which sighted people had been unwilling to touch a blind person because they feared the mere touch would communicate some disease to them.

The asylum seems to have originated in the Middle Ages, when some of the blind beggars banded together in "brotherhoods." It is not clear whether the asylums, supported by society, represented a practical way to meet their real need for housing, or whether a society, proud of its attainments, was trying to hide what seemed to be an area of failure. At any rate, such custodial institutions did arise as early as the fourth century. A very famous one was the Quinze-Vingts in Paris which, according to tradition, was founded by St. Louis.

The asylums of the Middle Ages did not encourage the blind to work; today many of our "homes" do encourage employment within the institution and are set up to offer both a place of employment and a place to live.

Even when not segregated in "homes," blind people enjoy certain privileges. In many states there is a "blind pension," a special aid program which is administered according to the plans of the individual states but subject to the approval of the Social Security Administration and with a substantial amount of the monthly grant coming from the federal government. The American Foundation for the Blind [1] reports that about one-half of all blind persons in the U.S. receive such financial aid with an average monthly payment in 1963 of $81.50. Also, since 1948, blind persons have been allowed an additional exemption of $600 on their income tax. In 1953, Barker, Wright, Meyerson, and Gonick[2] wrote:

> No group among the physically handicapped in the United States has been so favored by special legislation as the "legally blind." Examination of a recent survey of federal and state laws relating to the handicapped shows that of 15 pages of text devoted to summarizing Acts of Congress in this area, 6 pages are concerned specifically with legislation for the blind. By contrast, legislation concerning crippled children, the only other disabled group given a major heading, is summarized in one-half page.

We like to think that our culture has reached the stage of integration where blind people are completely accepted; their value being determined on the basis of ability and personality. Blind children are no longer forced to attend residential schools but may, and in many cases do, attend local schools. Blind people find more employment opportunities open to them, and also assume roles of leadership in both political and non-political organizations. But many doors are still closed.

THE DIMENSION OF ATTITUDES

Without meaning to minimize the real difficulties which blindness creates, many blind people say that what most troubles them, what most holds them back from goals they seek, is not blindness itself but attitudes of sighted people toward it. But many are quick to admit that the attitudes of blind people are part of the problem. Recently the agency serving the blind in Pennsylvania felt that this matter of attitudes was important enough to devote a complete workshop to the subject. Some of the dimensions of attitude discussed there are given below.

If we carefully consider their behavior, we cannot doubt that many of the lay public have misconceptions regarding blindness. One of the most irritating is the notion that sight is the equivalent of intellect, therefore that loss of sight equals loss of mind. This appears to be the reason waitresses, elevator operators, and so on, ask the companion of a blind person what the blind person wants when he is right there to answer for himself. Others seem to think that loss of sight means loss of all the senses, including hearing, for they talk loudly to a blind person, as if he were deaf; at other times they stand right beside him and talk to others about him, as if he could not hear what was being said. The reverse of this is the belief by some that when a person loses his vision, his other senses become super-acute. At one time this was a belief held even by scientists, but a number of experiments by psychologists such as Seashore and Hayes disproved this many years ago. One kind of sensory compensation in which many people believed until recent years was called "facial vision." This referred to the fact that many blind people can tell when they are coming to an obstacle or when they have passed some object as they walk along. Careful studies by Dallenbach, Worchel [10] and their supporting group proved that if hearing was completely blocked, "facial vision" was lost. This was, then, just a special method of using auditory information, a method sharpened by many blind people who had no other way to get evidence concerning their environment. This could be accomplished by sighted people, also.

Another misconception of the public is that all blind people are totally blind; consequently there is a marked lack of understanding of those who can see a little, but not enough to read a street sign or the number on a bus.

Frequently the public looks upon blindness as darkness, a concept which is encouraged by some publicity of agencies serving the blind. Others think that blindness necessarily equals unhappiness. This was another of the questions Simmons asked in his research on attitudes of the seeing public, and 24 per cent of his respondents said that they believed blind people could never be happy. As a result of this mistaken concept, some members of the public are surprised and even resentful when they find blind people cheerful and obviously enjoying themselves. Certain people appear to *want* to pity the blind and they feel very frustrated when they find no reason to do so.

Blindness is also curiously entangled in people's minds with concepts of both superiority and inferiority. Some think that blind people can do only very easy things. We find a reflection of this in a familiar phrase: "It is so easy I could do it with my eyes shut." On the other hand, many think a blind person is "simply wonderful" no matter what he does—even simple, ordinary things. The public has little knowledge of what the blind are able to do. A small excursion in this direction was made by Barbara Bateman[3] who found that sighted children thought that blind children could *not* swim, enjoy television, or tell time, but thought that they *could* readily write their names. Just the reverse is true, of course.

Tied in with these misconceptions are the open reactions of the public. Many look upon blind people as objects of curiosity, sometimes just to be stared at, but often to be addressed and questioned. If braille is written or read in public, many people seem to feel that this gives them the privilege persistently to question a total stranger. The public also regards all blind people as objects of charity.

The public is closer to being right when they regard blind people as objects of protection. Many times blind people do need assistance in travel, especially in the crossing of busy and unfamiliar streets and the offer of a seeing person to act as a guide is welcome—if he knows how to be a good guide! It is less desirable when teachers feel that they should protect blind children by giving them marks they have not earned, defending their action by saying the work was "good for a blind child." It is equally troubling to know that some employers set lower standards in the case of blind workers but, at the first sign of a drop in business, let the blind worker go because he produces less than other workers. Workers with the blind feel that a double standard never really benefits the blind person.

Above all, I think that blind people are a source of anxiety to many. People tend to feel responsible for a blind person, even for a stranger on the street, but they do not know how to carry this responsibility. They feel guilt about not being helpful but do not know how to be helpful. Many project their guilt by blaming the blind person, by trying to avoid him or by letting him know that they wish he were not there.

It is difficult to impress upon the public and employers that blind people can make an equal contribution with the seeing, while agencies put on campaigns for contributions to help the blind, playing up the tragedy and helplessness of blindness. It makes little sense to most employers to hire with one hand and donate with the other. Some blind people are suspicious and regard all seeing people as enemies and objects of prey. Their attitude is that they will get as much as they can out of all seeing people, that the world owes them a living just because they are blind. If they work, they do not expect to produce as much as their neighbors and, if they can manage it, they will not work at all.

THE PERSONAL DIMENSION

Blindness is something which happens to an individual and, indirectly, to his family; it is deeply personal and is never quite the same for any two people. Blindness is a factor in a total life system, more or less affecting all other factors in that system. Some will be greatly and obviously affected; others are affected in a more subtle way and the individual may think for years that he has avoided that particular effect, only to have it catch him when he is least prepared for it. Sometimes we like to protest that the blind person is just like every other person except that he cannot see, but that oversimplifies the problem.

In the brief space of this paper I can mention only a very few of the possible details in the personal dimension of blindness. No one blind person will have experienced all of even the few that I list—nor will any blind person have been free of all of them.

Blindness is certainly something different to the person who has no visual memories from what it is to the individual who loses his vision in his teens or later.* The congenitally blind child, or one who lost his vision in infancy, does not, in the beginning, realize that he is different from other people. He does not know what blindness is because he does not know what seeing is. He does not know what darkness is because he does not know what light is. If he grows up in a loving family but one which does not overprotect him, he experiences his environment through sound and touch and for some time he does not know that others experience it in some other way. To the young child who is not forcefully told otherwise, "normal" is what *he* is. It does not occur to him that other people are different. He does learn that there are certain ways in which he must conform to the society in which he lives. He learns that he must go from place to place by walking although it may seem more natural and less dangerous to crawl; he learns that he must eat with a spoon or fork although he finds food more readily with his fingers. These are the rules to which he must conform and he learns to do so, not realizing that others can do these things more easily than he.

* I am greatly indebted to Louis Rives for this account of the feelings of the young blind child.

Then, as he gets a bit older, he begins to notice that other boys can do things he cannot do and he wonders why. Why can they catch a ball when he cannot? Why do they say there is a bird in the tree when he cannot hear it sing? Why do they speak of clouds when he knows only that he does not feel the warmth of the sun? Sooner or later someone tells him it is because he is blind, but the word still means little.

Only very gradually, through one experience after another, does blindness take on meaning, and much of the meaning it takes depends upon the people around him. If his family is ashamed of his blindness, hides him and rejects him, he will be ashamed of his blindness and try to deny it, or to overcompensate for it, or to withdraw from society. Other relatives, childhood companions, teachers, indeed, many people contribute to his view of blindness and of himself as a blind person. All of these people will not treat him in the same way, of course. If those who are close to him handle the matter well, he in turn will find the strength to handle most of the others; but whether he pities himself, whether he overprotects himself, whether he expects special privileges—these, and many other attitudes grow out of his experiences as he matures.

His own success in solving the problems presented by blindness also contributes greatly to what blindness means to him. Three major areas of living which are inevitably affected by blindness are mobility, communication, and skills of daily, or shall we say, social living. The experience of blindness will be very different for the person who early learns some method of independent travel, some skill in reading, in making records for himself, and in writing to others. While at times dependence may be unavoidable, mastery of these skills, and of the graces which make one an acceptable social companion, go a long way towards enabling the blind person to meet the seeing world as an equal. These skills save him from going only where someone chooses to take him, free him from feelings of insecurity and inferiority in groups of seeing people, enable him to express himself and his own personality.

For someone who loses his sight after he has formed a concept of himself, the reactions of his family and perhaps of others in his immediate environment will still have their effect, but he must first of all deal with his own feelings. If the most satisfying elements of his self-concept as a seeing person centered on something which is absolutely impossible for him as a blind person, such as being an excellent shot, blindness will be much harder to bear. If what he valued most in himself was the ability to write, he will realize that he can still write. Also, if as a seeing person he had formed very unfavorable views of blindness, he will now suffer a great emotional struggle as he tries to change either his view of blindness or his view of himself. Many people report that they consciously experienced an inability to accept themselves as being blind until they met a blind person whom they liked and could admire.

The personal dimension of blindness includes many other practical elements. To the person still in school, it may mean being taken from regular school classes, from school friends, perhaps even from the family, to be placed in a residential school. It means being unable to read one's most personal mail unless friends and family are willing to learn braille. It means never again seeing beloved people and things. It may mean giving up career goals or losing a job. It certainly means never driving one's car again, and it is interesting to note that this is one of the things blind people frequently regret. But there are sometimes far greater losses. Unfortunately, not all wives react to visual loss with understanding; so for a certain number of men who lose their vision, there is the loss of the wife and perhaps children as well—a whole new and very lonely life.

And for some, whose visual loss occurred because of some foolish behavior on their own part, blindness is the lasting reminder of that foolishness until they die.

Much as this personal dimension of blindness varies from one individual to another, one element is common although its intensity varies: the element of stress. In a world of increasing stresses, the blind person shares those with the rest of us—the rushing, impersonal, too automated world with its highly competitive quality. In addition, blindness itself is a source of stress. If the individual wishes to take an equal place in society he usually has to work twice as hard. To get through college he must put in many more hours of study because braille reading is much slower than ink print reading and few college-level books are available in braille. With the student acquiring most of his information by listening, "reading" as it were, he spends more than double the time he would spend reading ink print. Nor is it easy to skim. There are problems in finding good readers and matching one's time with theirs, although tape recorders have eased this considerably.

To be nearly self-sufficient in a job, the blind person must constantly be on the alert for auditory cues for things other workers can see. He must often spend time with cumbersome record keeping that would have been a note or two for a sighted person; and the blind person may have to live with the frustration of knowing he will never be moved ahead. Blindness is an endless series of frustrations, little frustrations that one can laugh off, at least on one's good days, big frustrations which look tragic and sometimes change the whole pattern of a life. Even walking down the street independently is an obstacle course of bruised shins from the unexpected trash can or baby carriage in the path to the real threat to life itself on a busy street corner.

The inner tensions of living with blindness vary from minute to minute but they are always there, fluctuating with the environment and the moods of the individual.

GOALS OF THIS CONFERENCE

Recently I had dinner with friends from several of the universities in Philadelphia and they were comparing oral examination procedures in their several graduate schools. One said that, in her university, candidates for the Ph.D. in sciences took an oral examination in which they were asked to suggest solutions to problems which were unsolvable. The candidates knew before they entered the examination that the problems to be presented were regarded as not capable of solution and that they would be evaluated on their originality, their creativeness, the quality of their logic, and the excellence and complexity of knowledge with which they attacked the problems. Let us, in our meetings, not fall short in originality and creativeness, in clarity of logic, and in applying the best of our present knowledge, and surely some of the problems of blindness will find solutions.

NOTES

1. American Foundation for the Blind, *Blindness—Some Facts and Figures* (New York, 1963).
2. R. Barker, Beatrice Wright, L. Meyerson, and M. Gonick, *Adjustment to Physical Handicap in Illness: A Survey of the Social Psychology of Physique and Disability,* Bulletin No. 55 (New York: Social Science Research Council, 1952).
3. Barbara Bateman, *Sighted Children's Perception of Blind Children's Abilities,* Research Bulletin No. 8 (New York: American Foundation for the Blind, 1965).
4. Milton D. Graham, *Toward a Functional Definition of Blindness,* Research Bulletin No. 3 (New York: American Foundation for the Blind, 1963).
5. National Society for the Prevention of Blindness, *Estimated Statistics on Blindness and Vision Problems* (New York, 1966).
6. U.S. Public Health Service, *Statistical Report: Annual Tabulations of the Model Reporting Area for Blindness Statistics* (Washington: Government Printing Office, 1964).

7. Irvin P. Schloss, *Implications of Altering the Definition of Blindness,* Research Bulletin No. 3 (New York: American Foundation for the Blind, 1963).
8. Harry E. Simmons, "The Attitudes of the Sighted Toward the Blind," *Proceedings of the American Association of Workers for the Blind* (Washington, 1949).
9. P. Worchel, "Space Perception and Orientation in the Blind," *Psychological Monographs: General and Applied,* Vol. 65, No. 15 (1951).
10. ——— and K. Dallenbach, "Facial Vision: Perception of Obstacles by the Deaf-Blind," *American Journal of Psychology,* Vol. 60, No. 4 (October, 1947), 502–553.

SESSION REPORT

John R. Swinton

Following the presentation by Mrs. Mary K. Bauman of her analyst paper, Arnold Barach drew some relationships between the future of the blind population and the future of the general population.

He noted that the anticipated increase in the number of blind people in the nation is probably in approximate proportion to the expected increase in the population overall. Blindness, he pointed out, is therefore a problem which we will live with even more in the coming decade.

Mr. Barach noted that the changes in technology, art, society, youth, vocational opportunities, and human values are all nicely woven into the format of the Conference. These changes will have to be faced equally by the blind and by the sighted population. He continued:

> Particular stresses are already apparent: Youth lives under tremendous pressure right now—witness the proliferation of drugs and delinquency which are symptoms of stress and reflections of the environment in which we are raising our children. Kiplinger studies reveal that our youth is a product of the affluent society, but doesn't like it. When they grow up they have no sense of personal recognition, and their responsibilities are not clearly defined. They grow long hair, wear weird clothing, and drop out of college.
>
> Many of them join the Peace Corps and VISTA to discover what, in this very comfortable, posh way of life, there is that can give them identity. They can't find it here so they journey to Africa and Asia and seem to find it there. There they are worthwhile, they can perform jobs responsibly, they can win recognition, and they can get out of the parental nest.
>
> What are the results of this forsaking of the structured life of parents? About half of these young people change their career plans. They come back wanting to serve their fellow man. They come home relatively uninterested in making a buck, acquiring a color television, and collecting two or more cars. They have found some solutions to the problems of the world in which they are going to have to live.
>
> Their answers lie, interestingly enough, either in service or in education. (Education, they discover, is better than they thought it

was and many of them return to college and seek graduate degrees.)

These young people are growing in number. In fact, their segment of the population will soon outnumber the rest of us. They will be a powerful political force. They will be the innovators, rejecting many of the material values of our generation and involving themselves with the rest of the world and with the people at the other end of the economic spectrum. They are very likely to have more sympathy and compassion.

Tensions are also developing in the area of jobs and careers. What will happen to people when the new computerized technology gains its full impetus? We all know the computer can successfully replace workers.

Cybernation produces problems of training people to live in an environment where they will have more leisure. Do you stress continuing education? How do you help the man who wakes up one morning, goes to the office, and discovers that the machine has replaced him? This is not an isolated problem. As a reaction to it some companies are sending their employees back to school for up to a year, either up-grading them or teaching them a new skill. A doctor today would not consider himself competent ten years from now unless he were systematically exposed to the new techniques. Lawyers have already begun to use computerized law libraries.

These trends indicate a world which will be more advanced than our present world, with increasing tensions. Knowledge of these trends and, specifically, of the new technology, is important because we must learn to cope with larger numbers of blind people who will require services. The challenge will be severe; it will involve the need for better education and the need for more facts.

Data banks may soon carry quick answers to such questions as these: Who are the blind? Where are they? What are their needs? What are their potentials? Is it right to apply the types of education we are now using as against other options? Does the new technology offer some substitute for the means of communication which are now used?

These are proper and important questions but they have to be examined in terms of the techniques available and the expertise with which they can be applied.

I hope that some insights will flow from this Conference reflecting the fact that we cannot hope to live in the same environment in the next ten years that we live in now. Communications, transportation, and everything around us is developing so quickly that inevitably values will have to be revised and approaches will have to be changed. Probably the era of the innovator will take hold in every area. Perhaps here some new approaches will be forthcoming to prepare the profession for what the future is likely to bring.

During the ensuing discussion period, Commissioner Elias Cohen, noting that his field is geriatrics and that 50 per cent of the blind are in the old age group, asked whether this fact is attributable to blindness' late arrival or to the increasing survival rate.

"Is there," he asked, "within our grasp the prevention of blindness in this large population? Are there techniques that can be applied? This is the kind of question which is ripe for the epidemiological studies that are traditional in the field of public health."

Dr. Geraldine Scholl raised other problems: "While increasingly we have business and industry willing to establish educational installations," she said, "these same people continually vote down additional taxes and bond issues meant to implement more farsighted programs within the schools. Then, of course, there is the additional problem of parents who are convinced that education should proceed exactly the way it has since they were in school: one classroom, one teacher. Perhaps what we really need is the help of sociologists ready to work with attitude change."

Speaking from the viewpoint of a "hard core" research scientist, Dean George G. Mallinson expressed the opinion that too much emphasis was already being placed upon social science research. The real promise, he asserted, lay with the contributions his field could make.

Both the Consultation Chairman, Dr. Maxwell H. Goldberg, and Mrs. Bauman explained that the Conference, by plan and agreement, was to be devoted to behavioral science research and that no slight was intended to the acknowledged contributions of the hard sciences. Dean Mallinson nevertheless cautioned that some of the answers to the problems that would be discussed in a social science framework could be solved more readily by recourse to the hard sciences.

Miss Yvonne Agazarian praised the idea of a data bank, discussed briefly by Mr. Barach, but she noted that "data transfer" remained a generally unsolved problem. "How do you," she asked, "get the information out of the books and repositories and into the people?"

Charles Gallozzi mentioned that the United States Office of Education's Council on Exceptional Children has made some tentative progress in the field of information retrieval and dissemination.

Dr. Elena Gall remarked that she considered discussions of "large numbers and percentages" of blind people to be less important than a concentration on individual cases of blindness. "In planning for the future," said Dr. Gall, "we haven't really used effectively the tools we have. There stands before us a long list of failures. Do we have parent education? intensive follow-ups? individual treatment? No. While of course we must deal with the next generation, the need to predict is less pressing than the need to perfect the art of teaching the blind. Let us not concentrate so much upon the new ways but upon where we have failed in using the ways already available to us."

PARENT-CHILD RELATIONSHIPS

FAMILY STRUCTURE, PARENT-CHILD RELATIONSHIPS, AND DISABILITY

Marvin B. Sussman

INTRODUCTION

In this analysis, the specific problems of disability in the family—particularly the problems of the blind child and the relationships among members of his family—are approached from a sociological perspective. Two themes—one a description of the structure of the family system in American society and the factors which make it a viable and primary system, and the other an explanation of intra-family processes—encompass both the macro and micro levels of the problems. Included are such topics as the concept of reciprocity, unequal exchanges, and the processes of bargaining, power, and influence. These topics provide a theoretical backdrop for consideration of disability in the family, of related questions, and of suggested treatment and solutions.

The first focus is upon the frequently neglected fact that the majority of American nuclear families are active with other units within a kin-related network. This familial system is capable of providing for its members economic, emotional, educational, welfare, and other supports complementary to or competitive with those furnished by other societal institutions. This is a condition affecting intra-family relationships and an individual's or his family's relationships with other kin-related nuclear families and societal institutions. The kin network is a voluntary social organization and as such competes for the interest and participation of its members.[1]

THE STRUCTURAL UNITS OF THE EXTENDED NUCLEAR KIN FAMILY SYSTEM

The basic unit of the kin system is the nuclear unit (subsystem) composed of husband and wife and their issue—found usually in an independent household apart from kin. The kin system is composed of an x number of subsystems. For this discussion I will limit the analysis of structure of four basic subsystem types. Murdock has delineated three basic types of units: the nuclear family of *procreation,* the nuclear family of *orientation,* and the *affinal* family.[2] Hill has suggested a fourth type, the family of *gerontation.*[3]

The nuclear family of procreation is created by marriage and is composed of husband, wife, and offspring. The family of orientation is the one in which the individual is reared; it is composed of the individual's parents and siblings. Each spouse of the family of procreation belongs to a family of orientation. The gerontation nuclear family consists of these generationally linked nuclear units of parents, children, and grandparents. The affinal family consists of parents and siblings of the individual's spouse. During his lifetime an individual may be a member of all four of these subsystems. Upon marriage the individual creates the nuclear family of procreation. If his parents are living, he is a member of the family of orientation. He marries into the affinal family, and he is linked to the gerontation family as a grandson in kin obligations with his living grandparents.

The four nuclear units are independent of each other, but are also linked on the basis of affection, choice, and reciprocity. With the expectation that each family unit can maintain its independence and unity, relationships between these subsystems are entered into voluntarily.

The boundary of each nuclear unit encompasses the internal affairs of the subsystem. These include role relationships and the associate processes concerned with the maintenance of the system. The inter-nuclear-unit-linked boundary may envelop two or more nuclear subunits. Within this boundary, role relationships and expectations and joint activities are governed by norms relative to the situation. All four nuclear units may form a kin system boundary within which the roles played vary according to situations, objectives, maintenance of the larger structure, and internal and external stresses produced by subsystems other than the family.

THE CONCEPT OF RECIPROCITY

One of the key concepts for explaining the bases of the network and intrafamily relationships is reciprocity,[4] an exchange whereby the individuals in the dyadic relationship do things for one another, and which is a commonly shared expectation. Individuals engage in reciprocal acts because they expect to be rewarded. Yet there pervades in the family field a certain alarm and fear about this type of analysis, because the idea that marital partners engage in activities resulting in rewards for themselves is contrary to the romantic myth about such relationships—namely, the predominant belief that individuals in a marriage relationship act according to some moral code which requires each partner to be completely "other" oriented.

Reciprocity is based upon activity for which one is rewarded; and, as George Homans[5] has suggested, the more the individual is rewarded as a consequence of his action in any situation, the more likely he is to engage in the same or similar related activities later on. In contrast, as the individual engages in activities for which he is unrewarded, he disengages himself from these activities or reduces their infrequency.

UNEQUAL EXCHANGES

One common misunderstanding about reciprocity is the implied assumption that exchanges between two individuals must be equal or approach equality; that eventually there is a reckoning; and that if the exchanges are unbalanced, there results a severing of the relationship. Undoubtedly, in any relationship with another person or a group, each individual makes such an evaluation; but in all probability it is not a closely calculated one. In evaluating the bases for reciprocity, however, most of the reciprocal relationships which exist among individuals are based upon exchanges which are unequal, and which often involve unspecified, perceived obligations for which the individual giver can never be certain of the appropriate returns.

The bases for this unequal exchange are two: the powers of attraction which relate individuals to one another; and the existence of social and cultural structures based upon differentiation of influence, power, status, and prestige. Attraction implies that one individual desires to be associated with another, and that from this association the individual will be rewarded. In some instances, because this is his best available alternative, a person may stay in a relationship where he must give more than he receives. Rewards may come not only from the other person in the reciprocal relationship but from others outside who confer status based on the association. The attractive person has some qualities or resources which can be released if there develops a mutually attractive relationship.

A corollary principle is the voluntary behavior of the individual who is attracted to another person. He enters into this relationship on his own volition; and consequently, in subsequent exchanges, he has a legitimate right to expect an exchange of equal quantity. Even within the family, where norms obligate the individuals to each other, a voluntary character to a relationship exists; for members can "reject" transactions even though they are physically or mentally forced to participate in them. In a reciprocal relationship a participant's desires and expectations may not be in consonance with reality. He may be in a subordinate position, and he may be giving a great deal more to the attractive person than he is receiving; yet he is satisfied and motivated to continue this exchange.

Another characteristic of the reciprocity process is that exchanges need not be made in the same medium. In an exchange, an individual receiving financial reward may give, in return, deference, honor, prestige, and respect.

THE PROCESS OF BARGAINING

Related to reciprocity is the process of bargaining, which has as its objective obtaining some advantage in a transaction with another individual. It is difficult to delineate the specific motivations for the bargaining process. By the same token, it is obvious that each interaction involves some degree of bargaining. Each party to the interaction consciously—or more often subconsciously—directs his behavior in relation to his perception and expectations of what the other individual will accept in order to reach an agreement. The intriguing feature of the bargaining process is that the individual has perceptions and expectations of what the other person will accept but never is completely certain of what is an acceptable arrangement. Consequently, the bargaining which ensues is actually an effort to determine what are acceptable expectations and to give to the other person a minimum concession in order to obtain a greater advantage. Mechanisms of bargaining involve not revealing one's real intentions. Often the verbal communication is expressed to indicate falsely that the individual is thinking primarily of the other person rather than of himself.

Bargaining which occurs in relationships between individuals or between families is less formal and visual, but it does take place in a very real and significant way. In taking an adamant position on an issue, the husband evaluates his wife's initial response in order to determine what mileage he can get by standing firm or making concessions. His wife, in turn, is trying to find the bases for his demand, to evaluate his expectations, and to give minimal but sufficient compliance so that she can bargain more effectively on another issue or in another situation. As Shelling[6] points out, it is obvious that the continuous process of bargaining, guided as it is by expectations, results in the compounding of expectations, and becomes the source of conflict and tension among individuals.

In discussing both reciprocity and its correlate of bargaining, our use of expectation needs clarification. Expectation is very closely linked with reciprocity and bargaining. However, in those instances when we talk about reciprocal relationships, the expectation of reciprocity is not expressed; whereas in our common usage of bargaining—as between formal structures—the expectation is expressed.

PROCESSES OF POWER AND INFLUENCE

A discussion of reciprocity cannot be concluded without some reference to the processes of power and influence. It has already been demonstrated that reciprocal relationships may be asymmetrical, in that individuals in subordinate or superordinate positions are in a reciprocal relationship, engaging in exchanges of unequal quantities and of different items. As Simmel[7] suggests, the location of individuals in a structure where they can command a larger share of the exchanges indicates an active reciprocity, with orientation and influence even in the apparently one-sided superordinate-subordinate relationship. Especially in discussing reciprocity between family members or between families, it is helpful to differentiate the terms "power" and "influence." Influence as exercised by an individual is his ability to persuade others to do things in such a way that benefit is accrued to him. Power, on the other hand, implies a legitimate use of force to compel a one-sided reciprocity. Influence has little effect upon anyone except a receptive person, and in this sense is a voluntary reciprocity rather than a compulsory one. It is apparent that, among family members and among families, reciprocal relationships are based more upon the subtle expression of influence than upon the outright effects of power.

RECIPROCITY AND THE KIN NETWORK

The existence of social exchange or reciprocity in human relationships cannot be disputed, and there is no question that this fundamental and pervasive process is a basic element in integrating member nuclear family units within the urban kin family system and intra-family relationships. In the relationships between member units on intergenerational or bilateral kin lines, reciprocal relationships emerge partly out of tradition and feelings of familial responsibility and partly out of opportunity and the rewards that ensue from effective bargaining. Exchanges between member family units are not equal; nor do they occur, nor are they expected to occur, about the same time. In looking at intergenerational exchanges, one can make a case for serial reciprocity. Parents will do a variety of things for their married children and grandchildren with the expectation that at a later time, when they are in their declining years, these young married children —now middle-aged and established—will take care of their needs as they become less and less independent. In turn, having taken care of aged parents, the middle-aged couple engage in various activities to launch their young children into marriage and careers, expecting that, when they themselves reach their threescore and ten, they will be looked after by their children.

It is suggested that one cannot continue indefinitely in a reciprocity relationship without receiving some reward in return. The service perspective can be followed only so far, after which it loses its ability to sustain the individual in the relationship. In a study currently being completed concerned with the distribution of property after the death of a family member,[8] it is found that kinship relations are undisturbed when dispositions of property go according to traditional patterns. In our society, upon the death of the male head of the household, property is usually distributed to the surviving spouse and the couple's progeny. Perhaps 90 per cent of the property settlements are of this kind. However, in those cases which do not follow this typical model, it appears that kinship patterns are severely disturbed and dismembered. Potential heirs and legatees have specific views on who should be rewarded according to the reciprocities based upon services rendered to the deceased. The child who has labored long and hard to care for the aged parent discovers that another favored child or nephew or some distant relative is given the legacy. The consequence is dismemberment of kinship relations because of the failure to fulfill expectations. The point of this illustration is that the service orientation must in time become integrated with the self-orientation in order to sustain a reciprocal relationship. Obviously both the service and self-interest motives exist. Just how important they are and how they work are still unknown.

In any network the individual or family unit can choose to be involved in kinship relations and theoretically can withdraw from the network. Members within a family have no such choice. They cannot easily withdraw physically, but they can do so in a psychological sense. Moreover, there are societal expectations that family members will be involved with one another; and the culture prescribes responsibilities of parents, children, and so on. Among member nuclear families in a kin network, however, involvement on a voluntary basis quite rapidly takes on the trappings of tradition and commitment. The more involved one becomes, the more one builds credits and debits and becomes cemented to the viable kinship network. As this problem is studied more carefully, one will detect parallels to the commitment process of novices entering a profession or religious order. It becomes easier to extricate oneself from reciprocal relationships of the kin network earlier in development of the network than later on. With each transaction the individual becomes more committed to the structure, while the relationships take on increasing meaning for him.

Parent-child interaction occurs within a matrix of inter-family and inter-institutional relationships described above. These external relationships place restraints upon the form and shape of internal transactions of family members. The prescriptions of the world outside of the family have real meaning to those inside it. Family members bring into their relationships with one another attitudes, perceptions, values, and beliefs gained from varied institutional and organizational sources and promulgated by numerous influential agents of socialization.

Socialization is one of the most important activities of the nuclear family; and while all family members engage in socialization activities, some do so more than others. Socialization is the learning of roles the mastery of which enables the individual to associate with others in groups. Roles involve behaviors according to group norms or rules; and with each role there is described model behavior. The major agents of socialization in the nuclear family are parents. Most research has focused upon the mother's role, and only recently have we begun to look upon the father, the siblings, and other adults in the household as possible significant agents of socialization.

A concern for the growing importance of the father and the sibling (oldest child) roles in role learning is based on the patent observation, and seemingly irreversible trend, that in increasing numbers, married women are being gainfully employed outside the home. Also, the focus on "momism" has neglected the father's role in the socialization process. There is no denying that the mother has the major responsibility for performing expressive roles—those involving the emotional, social, and physical needs of their children and her spouse. In many instances she must perform instrumental roles as well—those involving achievement of specific objectives and the making of important decisions. A review of research in this area indicates that husband and wife share both types of roles, and that the particular shared arrangement of roles depends upon a large number of situational, personality, and sociological variables.

Intra-family behavior or studies tend to ignore the consequences of parent-child relationships upon the marital relationship. Current ideology stresses primary concern for the child, with all other matters subordinate. The implied assumption is that, for all practical purposes, the needs and satisfactions of marital partners dissolve, or at best become unimportant, after the birth of a child. Furthermore, attention to them suggests a selfishness unbecoming in view of the needs of the child. It is important to recognize these vagaries of perception and values; for efforts to understand the meaning and significance of parent-child relationships are futile without consideration of the needs, interaction patterns, and expectations of marital partners, and the effect of the parent-child relationship on these other relationships.

ROLE EQUILIBRIUM—CRISIS RELATIONSHIPS

In studying the nuclear family, it is appropriate to conceive of it as a system in a state of dynamic equilibrium. At first blush, this seems to be a self-contradictory statement; but when examined closely, it appears to be consistent with the notion that any system is organized around a core of common activities, and that within it there are constant pushes and pulls which unsettle the stability of existing relationships. Role definitions, allocations, and expectations provide the structural elements of stability. Modifications in roles are a consequence of interaction within the family and of those transactions the family has with other systems in the society. When the family is faced with some type of crisis or emergency—such as that caused by the illness of a family member—the family's role structure is modified, and the members' capability to perform their usual roles is temporarily reduced. The family is in a state of disequilibrium and goes through the experience of readjusting power and role relationships as well as resocialization of its members into new roles. In time there is re-established a dynamic equilibrium with the rearrangement of subordinate-supraordinate relationships within the family. The length of time needed to re-establish equilibrium is often dependent upon the type of crisis, the members' definition of crisis and the family's resources to meet the crisis. Studies show that crises which occur from the outside, and which are sudden, unanticipated and short in duration—such as those as a consequence of a tornado or flood—effect a very rapid readjustment to a new equilibrium. Crises occurring within the family as a result of alcoholism of a member, birth of a mentally retarded child, or disability of a member—such as blindness or deafness—may have serious effects upon the family's equilibrium, effects which require a long time before a new equilibrium is established. In this situation the stress is upon the individual who often perceives the cause of the crisis to be his or some other family member's failure. Recrimination, attributions of guilt, expressions of abandonment and helplessness are characteristic behaviors in such situations, and are severe psychological barriers to the resocialization now required. On the other hand, crises precipitated outside tend to enhance reintegration of the role structure rather quickly as the family moves along spontaneously to meet the tasks of maintenance and continuity.

From a theoretical perspective, one can demonstrate the importance of crisis in affecting interpersonal relationships wherever they exist, especially those within the family. In spite of much "clinical evidence" and interest in this area, the evidence is not altogether clear regarding the effects of crisis within the family and upon the equilibrium of the system. One major reason for this difficulty is in determining whether the crisis is extra- or intra-familial in origin. This is almost impossible to determine by objective standards, since one must rely upon the family's definition of the situation. One family, for example, may feel that a member's failure to obtain a promotion is completely beyond their control and is related to the politics and other behaviors of the work system. Another may attribute this failure to the personality and other characteristics of the individual family member. In their perception of the situation they determine whether it is a crisis; and, if viewed as a crisis, it precipitates other events. How they rationalize and explain the situation determines whether it is a crisis and whether its origin is regarded as extra- or intra-familial. Especially in reviewing the impact of a disability, such as blindness, upon intra- or extra-family relationships, this distinction should be kept in mind.

In most of the studies associating crisis with reorganization of family structure and behavior, the major conclusion is that crises have a very specific effect upon the capabilities of the role system to function and upon the utilization of the talent of the nondisabled, as well as of the disabled, members of the family. In studying the problems of the alcoholic family members, Jackson[9] found that families had extreme difficulties in re-establishing a functioning role system on as high a level as existed prior to the onset of alcoholism.

The physical handicaps of children often produce conflict and disagreement between parents, especially in areas concerning appropriate child-rearing practices and family attitudes. It appears as if the physical handicap draws attention to these divergencies because the handicapped child presumably must be given special attention and offers the opportunity for greater disagreement. One can not overestimate the potential source of marital conflict stemming from having a physically disabled member in the family. The work done by Farber[10] on the severely mentally retarded child and Korkes'[11] work with parents of the mentally ill child indicate that, because of self-blame or attribution of blame to one's partner, parents of such children have difficulties in effecting appropriate marital relationships. Work with families of diabetic children indicates that the presence of diabetes in a child is related to lower marital integration, less agreement on how to handle the child, and greater marital conflict. The diabetes of a child produces an intrafamilial crisis; but it has not yet been proved conclusively that the resulting marital integration is due to the chronicity and the lack of a ready-made solution to the crisis.[12]

DISABILITY IN CHILDREN: SOME THEORETICAL CONSIDERATIONS

One striking finding on the impact of disability upon children is their lowered self-concept when they are compared with nondisabled children. In a recent study 54 blind children and sighted children matched for mental age were administered the Bialer-Cromwell Children's Locus Control Scale. The results indicated that blind children scored lower for internal control than sighted children. Age was correlated with one's position on the control scale. On this characteristic, younger children scored lower than older children. As it is in many others, control was used in this study as an indicator of the individual's ability to perceive himself in control of the events around him.[13] Work concerned with difference in perception between diabetic and nondiabetic children produced similar results.[14] There is a striking resemblance to these findings in those obtained from studies of minority group children. Lowered self-concepts are characteristic of ethnic and racial minorities who have not been given the opportunity to participate in the race towards the goal of occupational and social mobility. In addition, these same minorities have had a long tradition of being subordinate, and over the centuries have taken on the value of hopelessness. They often believe that events cannot be changed, and that one's actions will do little to achieve desired objectives or goals. Things come about because they are "in God's hands." [15]

The parallels between the expressed hopelessness of the child who has a physical disability and the child who has a self-induced psychological or "cultural" disability differ more in the potentialities for changing the conditions which produce a lowered self-concept than in their effects. Society is almost incapable of doing away with the stigma it attaches to the physical disability, which is given the label of "deviancy." On the other hand, changes in the structure of society can be brought about—namely, to remove some of the blocks in the way of minority children in obtaining equal opportunities. Such changes are already under way. The significant point is that the child with the lowered self-concept caused by any set of circumstances or reasons is likely to be an underperformer who requires the therapeutic efforts of members of his family and those of other organizational systems.

The disabled child with a lowered self-concept is in obvious need of help; but, in providing him with too much help, there are dangers for the family unit and often for the child himself. A number of researches and exhortations by students in the field of disability indicate that a disabling condition of a family member has a tremendous emotional impact on the whole family. It is likely that, in varying degrees, members of the family will experience feelings of disappointment, anger, and guilt. Such feelings become real and meaningful when the family comes face to face with society's expressions of ambivalence about their problem.[16] In addition to society's expression of unconcern, and its labeling and stigmatizing, parents themselves view the birth of a child as an extension of themselves; and when the production is less than perfect, they suffer from deflated egos and find it difficult to understand why their child is physically imperfect.

PROBLEMS AND TREATMENT

The raw fact is that the present world is predicated on "normalcy." This reality has serious consequences for effective therapeutic dealing with the handicapped child. The emphasis on normality often leads to the exertion of pressures upon the handicapped child that exceed those placed on the nonhandicapped. Such pressures for achievement frequently produce emotional instability. This response is the result of extreme feelings of guilt and shame by parents and normal siblings. Sometimes these responses are the result of an overwhelming pity for the child. Even in instances when, on an intellectual level, parents can accept the disability and its handicapping aspects, the strong feelings often prove to be uncontrollable and provide the bases for the formation of negative attitudes towards the disability and the child. This often is the cause of the lowered self-concept of the blind child and of instability in family relationships.

Concentrated attention on meeting the needs of the blind child often becomes a burden and leads to a state of dependency accompanied by feelings of hostility. If the blindness of a child is not the cause of such a situation, it at least aggravates the burdens of family relationships which are already in a precarious condition of excessive dependency or alienation. The dilemma is that the blind child needs emotional support, encouragement, supervision, and education, which suggest a dependent relationship upon other members of the family; and at the same time, like nonblind children, he needs the development of capabilities to become independent and to establish his own identity. This problem of the relationship between dependence and independence is a universal one; it is the outcome of socialization. Disability aggravates the struggle between independence and dependent strivings and often magnifies the incapability of family members to use the appropriate socialization mechanisms in order to meet both the dependent and independent needs of the blind child.[17]

The nature and the type of family interaction patterns are related to the etiology of childhood blindness. In conditions of congenital blindness—as a result of congenital cataracts, optic atrophy, cerebral deficiencies, congenital glaucoma, and albinism—parental response is usually traumatic and is related to feelings of shame, guilt, self-blame, and self-recrimination. The suggested therapeutic approach is intensive case work and psychiatric care, in which the therapist provides support for the socialization agents in order to meet the needs of this child for mothering, fathering, and sistering.[18]

If blindness occurs as a consequence of an accident, the family members' response will vary drastically according to the experience it has had with crises, the level of affectual relationships within the family, and the intellectual capacities and psychological capabilities of its members. The family, including the individual who suffers the accidental loss of sight, has practically no preparation for this loss. Consequently, for resocialization into new roles, it is necessary to begin in the emergency room or during the first few days in the hospital, and especially during the period of outpatient department treatment.[19] In work with diabetic children,[20] it was discovered that after the diagnosis of diabetes in the child, there was the usual disbelief and grief period, so that any effort at resocialization was practically useless. The only result was the beginning of rapport between the parents and the physician and others of the treatment team. Actual education into the meaning, significance, and treatment for the diabetic child did not occur, however, until a week after diagnosis.

Immediately after the onset of a disability, there is a heightened emotional response coupled with a temporary allocation of roles in order to meet the emergency now confronting the family. In most cases these role allocations and expectations are temporary; and once the "heat" of the emergency is off, a more permanent reallocation occurs. This is based upon the family member's perception of what is reality and what has to be done in this situation. It should be stressed that when a child has been visually impaired role allocations are functionally related to the degree of impairment suffered by the child. The response to the accidental loss would vary widely if the loss were in one eye as compared with the loss of vision in both eyes. Partial loss of sight may precipitate a temporary reallocation of roles; but, after the correction is made, there will be an effort to reconstitute role allocations as they once existed, while acknowledging the fact that role distributions change by themselves over time.

In some accidents involving loss of function and—in some instances—disfigurement, there is the need to prepare the afflicted individual for the period of immobility and for the potentially stigmatizing response of the nondisabled. Preparation is also required of the other family members. They now have to divert many of their activities and energies to patterns of physical care and social action which will not imperil the recovery of the disabled family member, and which, after recovery, will maintain him on a level of functioning achieved through rehabilitation. From observing the impact of the loss of a part or function of an individual, it is obvious that his family is likely to be incapable of handling their own or the disabled person's psychological care. The current pattern in medical practice is to make the diagnosis and to prescribe therapy and then to expect the family members—and, in the case of the child, the parents in particular—to devote practically their whole lives to this therapy. This is a philosophy which is not in consonance with reality, and it undoubtedly precipitates failures in rehabilitation of the disabled individual. A more realistic and probably more successful approach to handling the problem of the severely handicapped is to develop a more complete sharing of responsibility for care of the individual between the family and other organizational systems. In making such an arrangement, one would consider the needs of the nondisabled as well as of the disabled individual.

Diseases in which the prediction is fatal present additional problems in reference to the allocation of roles, the formation of appropriate attitudes, acceptance of this eventuality, and appropriate behavior. Our knowledge on how to handle the end of life is limited. It is obvious that role allocations are temporary, and that it is necessary—let us say in the instance of a child with leukemia or other diseases which may lead to blindness or hearing loss before death occurs—that we provide this child the best possible experience during his lifetime. At the same time, we must limit the psychological disturbance in other family members, so as to prepare them for their normal functioning after the death of the child. Suggested here is a program of education which will enable the individuals to move quickly to new roles after the sad event occurs.

QUESTIONS AND SOLUTIONS

From a review of the social case work literature, one arrives at the general conclusion that the social worker requires that, when involved in the socialization of the visually impaired child, the parents depart from the usual child-rearing methods that have evolved out of generations of experience. The obvious conclusion is that parents need to learn and accept new teaching methods and new patterns of interaction geared to the child's handicap. Case work practice involves providing this viewpoint along with the nourishment of parental capabilities and capacities in undertaking this very special task of socialization.

Social workers are quick to admit that the visually impaired child may drain parents of their inner resources, leaving them with many unmet needs and with difficulties in fulfilling parental roles to their nonblind children. The solution proposed is family-centered case work.[21] The basic approach is to handle the tensions that can result from parental reactions to the visually impaired child, as well as the almost impossible demands upon their time and abilities. A more logical approach would be to develop institutional arrangements and mechanisms whereby other organizational systems can share with members of the family these difficult tasks of socializing the blind child to a level of competence that is satisfactory to the child, the members of his family, and the reference group.

In a recent study Robert Scott concludes that in the city of New York, most of the agencies concerned with helping those with visual impairments concentrate their efforts on a relatively small number of cases which are in need of help; and that the group they service are largely "good" cases which have optimum expectations of making a successful adjustment.[22] Even when service agencies share this responsibility of socializing the child, little consideration is given to the problems of socializing the normal children, which also involves the time and energies of parents.

Conclusions from work on the structure and functions of the kinship network in urban society[23] suggest that, in the treatment of the visually impaired child and his family, one should consider how members of this network may participate effectively in the therapeutic process. A social diagnosis involving the social relationships between members of nuclear families in a kinship network, as well as study of the reciprocity and exchanges of these individuals, may result in the discovery of other socialization agents who can share with parents the difficult problems involved in the education and socialization of the handicapped child. Some of these kin members may become effective agents, capable and willing in the therapeutic process to assume responsibility unencumbered by feelings of guilt, shame, pity, and hostility.

Regarding the needs of the non-impaired child or adult members of the family on a level of equal importance to those of the impaired child enables the establishment of realistic socialization outcomes in which are considered the talents of all family members, the availability of economic and social resources, the interests of other organizational systems, the motivations of family members, and the like. If these factors are considered in determining a rehabilitation program for a blind child, one avoids the more than usual phenomenon of the blind child's failure to meet levels of achievement expected by parents and other family members; and, in families where there is disability, the condition of underachievement of normal children as a consequence of parental concern and time spent with the impaired child. Moreover, the disabled child no longer needs to sense himself an entity isolated by his unique capacity to obstruct the goals of all around him.

In much of our thinking and planning about the rehabilitation of a handicapped child, we seem to ignore a commonly observed phenomenon. This is that, when individuals are successful or moderately successful in achieving objectives established for themselves and by society, and when they feel that they are accomplishing something, it is only then that they "can afford" to behave constructively in regard to the problems of other individuals. By being successful they feel assured, secure; they approach dilemmas more objectively, and are willing to give time, energy, and their resources to the degree that their own success and security are not threatened. In this connection, the established individual's output might be considered as "risk capital." If in helping and working to solve the problems of others, he loses, he has suffered a minimum loss, one which he can absorb because he still has his success, security, and integrity. If he wins, he receives enriched payoffs which enhance his ego, status and prestige.

On an operational level this notion means, in effect, that the blind child will "make it" at the highest level permitted by his handicap, if those around him are successful in achieving their own objectives and, in relation to the blind child, do not perceive what they are doing as deleterious to the achievement of these personal and family goals. If this analysis is correct, then therapies must be directed towards delimiting the number of obstacles placed in the way of individual family members, especially parents, in their achievement of desired goals. This type of analysis is devoid of the emotionalism which surrounds much thinking concerning disability and family relationships. Implied is a need for families who have a visually impaired child to establish for themselves realistic goals of rehabilitation which are in consonance with their own values, capabilities and ambitions.

SUMMARY AND CONCLUSIONS

In this analysis, the urban kinship network, its structure and behavior, have been explored with particular emphasis upon intrafamily interaction. The family kinship system, which is based upon the concept of reciprocity and within which exchanges occur via bargaining, is a voluntary organization. As such, it competes with other societal institutions for members—a process which affects intra-, inter-, and extrafamily relationships.

Socialization, the learning of roles; the effects of parent-child interaction on other relationships, such as the marital one; and the retention or establishment of role equilibrium during critical stress periods are sociological aspects relevant to the problem of disability in the family. A disabled child has specific difficulties in functioning socially in a world predicated upon "normalcy." Encountering increased pressures to achieve, together with society's pity and stigmatizations, he must often combat emotional insecurity and a lowered self-image. Furthermore, his parents not only must assist with the child's socialization into new roles, but also must deal with his siblings' needs, as well as their own adjustment, including perhaps feelings of guilt or hostility.

Within a theoretical framework of the structure and activities of the family kinship system, suggestions have been made concerning the therapeutic process. Essentially, a realistic socialization and re-socialization should proceed from the standpoint that the needs of the non-impaired children and adults are as crucial as those of the disabled child. Such an approach would more effectively mobilize the entire family's helping resources as well as decrease the handicapped child's pressures to achieve and his feelings of isolation from the "normal" functioning world.

NOTES

1*a*. Marvin B. Sussman, "The Help Pattern in the Middle Class Family," *American Sociological Review* (February, 1953), 22–28.

1*b*. ———, "Family Continuity: Selective Factors Which Affect Relationships Between Families at Generational Levels," *Marriage and Family Living* (November, 1955), 338–341.

1*c*. ———, "The Isolated Nuclear Family: Fact or Fiction," *Social Problems* (Spring, 1959), 333–340.

1*d*. ———, "Intergenerational Family Relationships and Social Role Change in Middle Age," *Journal of Gerontology* (January, 1960), 71–75.

1*e*. ———, and Lee G. Burchinal, "Parental Aid to Married Children: Implications for Family Functioning," *Marriage and Family Living* (November, 1962), 320–332.

1*f*. ———, "Relationships of Adult Children with Their Parents in the United States," *Family, Intergenerational Relationships and Social Structure,* ed. by Ethel Shanas and Gordon Streib (Englewood Cliffs: Prentice-Hall, 1965), 62–92.

1*g*. ———, "The Urban Kin Network in the Formulation of Family Theory," *Yearbook of International Sociological Association,* ed. by Rene Konig. Forthcoming.

2. George P. Murdock, *Social Structure* (New York: Macmillan Co., 1960).

3. Reuben Hill uses this family form in studying three generational families.

4*a*. Marvin B. Sussman, "Theoretical Bases for an Urban Kinship Work System," Paper given at the annual meeting of the National Council on Family Relations (Minneapolis, October 29, 1966).

4*b*. Marcel Mauss, *The Gift, Forms and Functions of Exchange in Archaic Societies,* trans. by Ian Cunnison (London: Cohen and West, Ltd., 1954).

4*c*. Claude Levi-Strauss, "The Principle of Reciprocity," *Sociological Theory,* ed. by Lewis A. Coser and Bernard Rosenberg (New York: Macmillan Co., 1957), 204–294.

5. George Homans, *Social Behavior: Its Elementary Forms* (New York: Harcourt, Brace and World, 1961), 53–59.

6. Thomas C. Shelling, "An Essay on Bargaining," *The American Economic Review* (June, 1956), 281–306.
7. Georg Simmel, *The Sociology of Georg Simmel,* ed. by Kurt H. Wolf (New York: The Free Press of Glencoe, 1950).
8. Marvin B. Sussman, Judith Cates, and Dave Smith, *The Family Inheritance,* The Russell Sage Foundation. Forthcoming.
9. J. K. Jackson, "The Adjustment of the Family to Alcoholism," *Marriage and Family Living,* 18 (1956), 361–369.
10. B. Farber, "Effects of a Severely Mentally Retarded Child on Family Integration," *Monographs of Society for Research in Child Development,* Vol. 24, No. 2 (1959).
11. L. Korkes, "A Study of the Impact of Mentally Ill Children Upon Their Families," Trenton: New Jersey Department of Institutions and Agencies, 1955 (mimeographed).
12*a*. Alan J. Crain, Marvin B. Sussman, and William B. Weil, Jr., "Effects of a Diabetic Child on Marital Integration and Related Measures of Family Functioning," *Journal of Health and Human Behavior* (Summer, 1966), 122–127.
12*b*. ———, "Family Interaction, Diabetes, and Sibling Relationships," *The International Journal of Social Psychiatry,* Vol. 12, No. 1 (1966), 35–43.
13. Shirley L. Land, and Shalom E. Vineberg, "Locus of Control in Blind Children," *Exceptional Children* (September, 1964), 257–260.
14. Marvin B. Sussman and William B. Weil, Jr., "Social Environment of the Diabetic Child," working paper 44.
15. Fred L. Strodtbeck, "Family Interaction, Values, and Achievements," *Talent and Society* (Princeton, New Jersey: Van Nostrand, 1958), 259–266.
16. G. H. Zuk, "The Cultural Dilemma and Spiritual Crisis of the Family with a Handicapped Child," *Exceptional Children,* 28 (September, 1962), 405–408.
17. S. Finestone, Fern Lowry, Martin Whiteman, and Irving Lukoff, *Social Casework and Blindness* (New York: American Foundation for the Blind, 1960), 127–140.
18. Ada Kozier, "Casework with Parents of Blind Children," *Social Casework,* 43 (1962), 15–22.
19. These notions were suggested by remarks made by H. Robert Blank, M.D., at a meeting of the Subcommittee on Behavioral Sciences, National Institute of Neurological Diseases and Blindness, Washington, D.C., February, 1967.
20. Marvin B. Sussman and Lillian B. Weil, "Processes of Acceptance of Disability," working paper 45.
21. Ada Kozier, "Casework with Parents of Blind Children," *Social Casework,* 43 (1962), 15–22.
22. Robert A. Scott, "Selecting Clients for Welfare Agencies," *Social Problems,* 14 (Winter, 1967), 248–257.
23. Marvin B. Sussman and Lillian B. Weil, "Processes of Acceptance of Disability," working paper 45.

PARENT-CHILD RELATIONSHIPS AND VISUAL LOSS

R. Paul Thompson

Among the trauma-laden complexities facing the parent and educator of the present day is the visually impaired child, a living crossword puzzle of challenges and needs. This youngster, entering as it were into a kiln of knowledge and opportunities for experience as he approaches life, comes complete with physical variations and psychosomatic perplexities all encapsulated into one enigmatic organism. This organism appears to wait almost instinctively for further direction or activation from an outside source. As such a source, a parent or teacher, holding a guidebook in one hand and destiny in the other, is in position to make the next move. How this move will be made is our present concern.

Too frequently the "teaching" proceeds through comfortably selected patterns—the regimentation of "course of study" outlines which "must be followed," pragmatic postulates and antiquated axiomatics which rest for footing upon the "tradition of the fathers," and upon conformities, stereotypes, and delimiting objectives. More hopefully, directions for this child may be determined with consideration of him as an independent, distinctive personality, who awaits extrication, sometimes even from himself, by the perceptive parent, case worker, and educator. It is to the end of looking more deeply into the uniqueness of each visually handicapped child and to explore at least peripherally the peculiarities and potentialities of which he is constituted, that this paper is directed.

RESEARCH COMPLETED

The sociological perspective presented by Dr. Sussman[26] concerning family structure, parent-child relationship, and disability has been thought-provoking and stimulating. In his global view of the impact which disability of an offspring brings upon a parent, we must recognize that mere cursory concern cannot be tolerated. The extent of the influence caused by blindness on the interfunctioning of the family subsystems of procreation, orientation, gerontation, and affinity needs insight and informed action.

The scarcity of research related to visually handicapped children is appalling. Scott notes that "certain areas have been more thoroughly studied than others. A great deal more is known about the mechanical problems of education and training than is known about the psychosocial development of blind children." [22] The likelihood that we can find only 320 instances of blindness in a sample of one million persons under the age of 18 years seriously limits research possibilities, but does not lessen our need for information. Particularly needed is behavioral research, even though such research "always deals with a partial measure of a small segment of the behavior of a very small percentage of all blind people." [2] Although understanding of outcomes is valuable, insight into causes can be even more significant in that action is suggested which may greatly improve the quality of the end product.

Lowenfeld [15] points out frustrations and suddenly shattered objectives of the parents into whose household has come the visually handicapped child. He depicts these parents as "confused because they have no idea how to bring up a blind child and not [seeing] any way to lighten the 'darkness' in his life, anxious because they fear what they do not know and not [trusting] their own abilities in coping with the unknown, and guilty because they believe they have failed their child since they are the ones who produced him being blind or were unable to do anything to prevent his becoming blind, and because in a vague way we carry the Biblical idea that the sins of the parents are manifested in the children."

The emotional adjustments which parents must make when they have a child who is handicapped either physically or mentally are often extreme and of long duration. Cohen[5] identifies four stages through which such a parent generally passes in accepting the child's handicap: "(1) experiencing a period of grief, (2) acknowledging and learning to handle their anger, (3) dealing with the anxieties aroused by the impact of the child's handicap on their usual adaptive patterns, and (4) making certain adjustments in their way of life that will affect not only the handicapped child but the total family unit."

Needs, aspirations and frustrations of parents are noted by Telson[27] as the principal problems presented before the counselors in relation to a blind youngster. In testing 68 boys and 75 girls with no useful vision, ages 14 to 21, who had lost their vision before six years of age, Sommers found that, in respect to personal and social adjustment, as a group they fell below the norms of the seeing. In connection with this testing, interviews with parents disclosed that "the majority of mothers studied experienced frustrations or feelings of conflict because of having given birth to a blind child." [23] Langley says that the most important aspect influencing the adjustment of children who are blind is parental attitude[13] Cerulli and Sugarman[3] agree with this observation.

One difficulty commonly observed in the parent of a blind child is that of overprotection. "As the child grows up, it may become evident that the mother is not encouraging normal development of self-care, independence in feeding, freedom to explore, freedom to develop peer contacts, and to compete in the ways appropriate to the child's age. This can be what is called 'reaction formation,' where the mother's true feelings are guilt and rejection, feelings which she hides even from herself by constant overt devotion, a dedication of herself to the child." [12] Elonen and Zwarensteyn emphasize that "only too often the children have been confined to a bed, to a playpen, to the backroom, to the boundaries of the trailer, or at most to the house. . . . For those who are permitted out of the crib, very often the next step is into a space cleared of all objects. Having removed all obstacles and articles with which the child might injure himself, the parents have thus also effectively removed all sources of stimulation." [7]

Maternal rejection, expressed in hostile handling of the child, is cited by Newell [30] as resulting in aggression. This finding is supported by Wittenborn[30] in his study of adopted children, and reflected in a 1958 study of adjustment in adolescents by Verrillo.[28]

In a review of research on maternal deprivation, Ainsworth[1] concluded that maternal deprivation without physical separation can be as devastating as maternal deprivation with separation. She found evidence indicating that maternal deprivation could greatly influence the development of the intellectual processes such as language, abstraction, and certain aspects of personality. Yarrow came to a similar conclusion in his review of the literature, noting that maternal deprivation in early life tends to be associated with later disturbances in intellectual and personal social function.[31]

Ourth and Brown[19] compared a group of newborn infants who received impersonal hospital attention with a group whose mothers were instructed to hold and rock their babies for 30 to 60 minutes at each feeding period during the first four days of hospitalization following birth. The results indicated that the non-mothered group cried much more than the mothered group, with the greatest difference in crying taking place between the feeding periods when there seemed to be no observable reason for the crying, except that the infant appeared to be unhappy or felt insecure and unsatisfied by his impersonal treatment.

An interesting study was conducted by Harlow[9] in which "mother surrogates" were used with monkeys. One "mother" consisted of a roll of wire mesh, adequate to support the monkey infant, warmed by radiant heat, topped with a block for a head, and with a bottle built in for feeding. The other, the cloth mother, was made from wood covered with sponge rubber and sheathed in tan cotton terry cloth; a light bulb behind her radiated heat, a ball with a painted face served as her head, and again a bottle was built in for feeding. "The result was a mother, soft, warm, and tender, a mother with infinite patience, a mother available twenty-four hours a day, a mother that never scolded her infant and never struck or bit her baby in anger." The findings indicated "that contact comfort was an important basic affectional or love variable [overshadowing], the variable of nursing; indeed the disparity [was] so great as to suggest that the primary function of nursing as an affectional variable is that of insuring frequent and intimate body contact of the infant with the mother." When the infant monkeys were in test situations designed to arouse fear, they always clung to the cloth mother, never to the wire mother, even when she was their source of food. When placed in a new environment, the infants would use the cloth mother as a source of security, exploring the strange area, trying some of the toys, and then returning to cling to the mother for a while before going forth again.

Parents of visually handicapped children are encouraged by Lowenfeld [14] to show their affection in tangible ways. "If your child cannot see you smiling, he needs to become more aware of your love and interest in him by your talking to him and by other ways in which you can let him feel your affection. . . . Your baby senses your feelings about him by something in your voice—not so much by what you say, but by the feeling tones in your words."

Studies by Dennis[6] relate to maternal deprivation in pointing out that institutional children were extremely immature in motor development. Provence and Lipton found general agreement with this but observed that a more prominent lack appeared in general impairment of their relationships to people and weakness in their emotional attachment. "These observations [supported] the supposition that many aspects of learning and modes of adaptation observable in the normally developing infant are intimately linked to and dependent upon maternal care." [21] Intellectual retardation was found by Goldfarb in infants who merely lie in cribs in the dormitories of institutions. Such infants evidenced impairment in their ability to develop concepts and were much less able to adapt to new situations, follow rules, perceive relationships, and speak.[8]

In a study by Kent, three groups matched for age included 60 pupils from residential schools for the blind, 43 blind pupils from New York City Schools, and 60 seeing children from the same schools. A control group included 30 blind children from residential schools. Regardless of personality type, for all groups praise was found to be more effective as a motivator than blame. Degree of achievement, in response to either motivational variable, proved to be the same for the seeing and the residential blind group. There were "no indications that the dynamics of personality development in the blind differ from those of other groups. Social factors within the home and school environment appear important in the personality development of blind children." [10]

A number of studies pertaining to the development of self concepts of the visually handicapped child indicate the influence which parents and others have in such development. Steinzor[25] interviewed two groups of visually handicapped boys and girls, one in an elementary school and one in junior high school in New York City to learn if visually handicapped youngsters think of the sighted and the blind as two opposite and irreconcilable groups with different and exclusive characteristics and functions. The interviews showed feelings of being different or inferior in respect to the sighted and at least an avoidance of unpleasant experiences with them. One boy stated, "The only thing is that my parents say, 'Just think, if you were only born two months later you would be able to see.' " Commenting further on this problem, Cohen notes, "Blindness from birth may have less consequence from the child's own psychological self-concept, once formed, but children born blind tend to be more affected by other people's attitudes toward them." [4]

Land and Vineberg conducted an investigation designed to gather construct validation data for a much used test of promising new personality construct. The Bialer-Cromwell Children's Locus of Control Scale was administered to 54 blind children and sighted children matched for mental age. The results indicated that blind children scored lower than older children on the same trait. The scale demonstrated itself to be a valid measure of a trait seemingly related to an individual's ability to perceive himself in control of events around him.[12]

A study by Steinzor[24] of 16 siblings of visually handicapped children who had been admitted or were seeking admission to a psychiatric clinic connected with an agency for the blind, included an interview during which respondents were asked to complete two sets of stories. One set had a sighted child as a protagonist; the other, a blind child. Answers to stories about sighted children were compared with those about blind children.

> Some trends were very clear. Blind children were presented as needing more help than sighted children. . . . The handicapped child was usually considered a special part of the family and was accepted as such. This acceptance took the form, especially among older siblings, of recognizing that the blind child needed particular care and could only partly participate in the usual activities of the family. . . . The feeling was expressed that blind children could share in activities, but not in an atmosphere of equality . . . Rarely was the handicapped child seen as belonging to "the blind."

Maxfield and Fjeld, in a study using the Vineland Social Maturity Scale, found that blind children as a group were retarded on specific items, appeared to be more docile, less active, and have less initiative than seeing children of corresponding ages.[17]

A number of researchers and authors have submitted suggestions for parents in working with visually handicapped children. Parmelee observed that "Mothers of blind children not realizing that their blind infants could feed themselves with their fingers continue to spoon feed these children. . . . If the parents can take the step of allowing the blind infant to feed himself, the child seems to proceed rather readily to further hand exploration and begins to differentiate between food and non-food." [20] Westlund and Palumbo[29] suggested that every service for handicapped children should be concerned with, and provide opportunity for, psychiatric help to parents. Kozier[11] recommended casework that would help parents plan for the education of their children who are blind and the integration of this casework with counseling in such areas as overprotection and sibling relationships. "Parent institutes of short duration are no substitute for the continuing services rendered by visiting preschool workers who can assist the parents individually and on the basis of their own observations about the home, the family, and the blind child's place in it," states Lowenfeld. "Attitudes can be influenced best while they are in the making. Therefore, guidance to parents while their blind child is still very young is the most effective way of promoting wholesome parent-child relations." [15]

Maloney[16] suggests sending a child-care aide into the home to assume full care of the child for three to four hours a day, five days a week for several months. She contends that while in the last analysis the parents have the most influence in their child's life, in order to effect change in a troubled family, external stimulation must be provided for a considerable portion of the time.

RESEARCH NEEDED

An inventory of the above citations and other research in parent-child relationships and visual loss indicates considerable deficiency. The research, while being scarce, is emaciated by the evident lack of correlation between existing studies, their frequent irrelevance to a total picture of needed research, and the seeming avoidance of the practitioner in making application of information already laboriously garnered. Scott accentuates this latter paradox in noting that "In work for the blind a peculiar schism exists between research and practice. Few practitioners see the relevance of research findings for their work. Conversely, the research is often resistant to, and unsympathetic towards, the practitioner's concerns. These attitudes are reflected in the customary impatience of the former with the latter." [22]

Child-Oriented Research

With unified action between theory and practice the following child-oriented research might be successfully pursued:

1. A longitudinal study of the sensory stimuli needs of the visually handicapped child (*a*) at birth, (*b*) first six months, (*c*) from six months to one year, (*d*) from one to three years, and (*e*) from three to six years of age. Such research might explore the effects of deprivation and augmentation of auditory, tactual, olfactory, and taste stimuli upon the developing child, by simulated studies on monkeys.

2. A determination of the degrees of freedom of organization and reorganization in the brain that can minimize the behavioral significance of blindness. With a more lucid understanding of the effect upon behavior exerted by blindness, and the compensatory potential

of the brain to organize or reorganize in a void of visual stimuli, procedural steps to assist such persons might be developed.

3. Techniques for teaching eating skills and finger and hand manipulation of the visually handicapped child. Guidance is needed not only by parents of these children, but also by case workers, aides, and all other agency personnel.

4. A longitudinal study of alterations and modifications in the locus of control of the visually handicapped child through the years from one to twelve. Knowledge of factors which affect development of inner control and influences which tend to decrease dependence upon outside control, could be appropriately used in parental and tutorial practices.

5. Techniques of strengthening the self concept of the visually handicapped child, viewed from the (*a*) preschool, (*b*) nursery, and (*c*) primary grade levels of experience. This study might be related to the previous one mentioned, showing relationships between locus of control and self concept structuring.

6. Construction of realistic social maturity tests and scales for more authentic assessment of the congenitally blind. With the establishment of "norms" of social competency, constructive techniques might be developed for the achievement of "goals of behavior" by congenitally blind youngsters.

7. Relationship between achievement objectives and behavioral patterns in the congenitally blind. In a given environment, the knowledge of factors that attend the development of behavior designed to achieve objectives of the congenitally blind child would be most enlightening.

8. Relationship between achievement objectives and behavioral patterns in the adventitiously blinded child, with correlations between time of accidental blindness and onset of altered objectives. Identification of influences which bear relationship with the pursuit of goals in the adventitiously blinded child, as related to time of onset of blindness, the relative speed with which such blindness developed, and the degree of change in visual acuity and usefulness, could contribute basic information to guide corrective measures.

9. How the deprivation of sight directly affects the child through changes in the brain's information handling capabilities—whether it is through the biological effects of a low number of impulses coming

into the cortex, or through the effects of experimental limitations, or as a deleterious overlay of emotional deprivation. This research, suggested by Cohen[4] could provide directions for the use of other sensory stimulation as a substitute for vision.

10. A study to gain a better understanding of the development of the blind child with particular reference to factors which promote or retard optimal growth emotionally and socially. The extension of studies such as that conducted by Norris, Spaulding, and Brodie[18] could provide additional information for the guiding of parents and others who work with the visually handicapped child.

11. What processes of development are retarded by blindness? Which processes of development are unaffected by it? Which processes are actually facilitated by it? To these questions, suggested by Scott,[22] should be added the problems of identifying those detrimental effects of blindness that are curable, those incurable effects that are improvable, and those effects that are unimprovable.

12. Relationship of early training in orientation and mobility skills to the development of social maturity, emotional stability, and scholastic success of the visually handicapped child.

13. Relative importance of visual information in the cognitive development as well as in the personality development of infants.

14. Development of the use of hands as a replacement of vision.

15. The extent and nature of development lag in children caused by blindness.

Parent-Child Research

A family unit is viewed as primal in the American society. It is upon this unit that societal advancement appears to be largely based. The birth of a blind child into this unit frequently causes much disruption to the unit and, by its extension to an interaction with other units, a discernible disruption to society in a larger dimension. Knowledge of the factors involved in this disequilibrium and directions for corrective and counteractive measures can result in greater family stability. Accordingly, improvement in society as a whole will result. The following studies therefore seem indicated:

1. The impact of the visually handicapped child on the development of relationships in the subsystems of (*a*) orientation, (*b*)

affinity, and (*c*) gerontation. The advent of the visually handicapped child causes a varied reaction in the family subsystems. The identification of these reactions and the relationship of such reactions to the development of the visually handicapped child is needed for the design of corrective action.

2. Relationship between parental acceptance of blindness in children and (*a*) place in the family occupied by the blind child, (*b*) financial standing of the family, and (*c*) emotional stability of the parental unit.

3. Relationship between religious concepts of parents and their reaction to and acceptance of visual loss in their children.

4. Effects of delayed and/or inadequate paternal acceptance of handicapping conditions in children.

5. Developmental deficiencies in preschool blind children identifiable with paternal deprivation.

6. Development and techniques of acceptance patterns of the family subsystem of orientation which includes a visually handicapped child.

7. Longitudinal study of alterations in parental expectancies of the visually handicapped child as compared (*a*) at conception, (*b*) at birth, (*c*) at one year of age, (*d*) at three years of age, and (*e*) at six years of age.

8. Identification and effects of reciprocity in parent-child relationships in instances of visual handicapping conditions in the child.

9. Effects on the nuclear family of decreased parental attentiveness and concern for siblings at the advent of a visually handicapped child.

10. Emotional problems caused by parents of organically impaired children which obstruct the child's ability to compensate for his handicap.

11. Emotional and sociological modifications affected in marital relationships upon the advent of a visually handicapped child.

12. Disequilibrium caused in the kinship subsystems at the birth of the visually handicapped child.

13. Relationship of degree of visual disability and acceptance by (*a*) parents, (*b*) siblings, and (*c*) grandparents.

14. Resocializing behavior in the kinship subsystems in accident-caused blindness in children.

Parent-Agency Research

In the complexity of adjustment patterns imposed upon parents by the birth of a visually handicapped child, parents are often found in desperate need of help. Even in the absence of marital tensions and in optimal kinship relations, the entry of a blind child into the family structure causes traumatic reactions. When society looks from the distance at a family unit in a state of disequilibrium caused by blindness and demands conformity and stability while at the same time offering no assistance, it may well be expecting the impossible. The burden as well as the enjoyment of development of potential in each "normal" child has been and is being borne by society as a whole. In the case of blindness, this is the kind of supportive strength which is needed from agencies and individuals outside the family circle. Such research as now indicated is concerned with providing a basis for and directions to such extra-familial assistance:

1. Relationships between behavior patterns in the visually handicapped child cared for without special assistance in a family unit and a child in a home where periodic assistance is rendered by a child-care specialist.

2. Identification of effective techniques to be desired in the child-care specialist working with pre-school children.

3. Personality characteristics of the child-care worker contributive to positive development of the visually handicapped child.

4. Relationship of the roles of parents and agencies in sharing the responsibility of giving socialization development to the visually handicapped child.

5. The behavioral adjustment of orphaned visually handicapped children who are placed in child-care institutions as compared with such children in foster home placement.

6. The effect on the parental acceptance and adjustments of assistance from child-care workers in the early teaching of their

visually handicapped children in such areas as: (*a*) infant mothering, (*b*) crib orientation, (*c*) crawling, (*d*) room orientation, (*e*) individual play, (*f*) toy manipulation, (*g*) eating habits, (*h*) toilet habits, (*i*) sibling relationships, (*j*) speech development, and (*k*) exploration of inside and outside environments.

NOTES

1. Mary D. Ainsworth, "The Effects of Material Deprivation: A Review of Findings and Controversy in the Context of Research Theory," *Deprivation of Maternal Care,* Public Health Paper No. 14 (Geneva: World Health Organization, 1962).
2. Mary K. Bauman and Norman M. Yoder, *Adjustment to Blindness—Re-Viewed* (Springfield, Illinois: Charles C Thomas, 1966).
3. F. Cerulli and Estelle E. Sugarman, "Emotional Disturbance—Infancy: Counseling the Family," *New Outlook for the Blind* (1961), 55.
4. Jerome Cohen, "The Effects of Blindness on Children's Development," *New Outlook for the Blind* (1966), 60.
5. Pauline C. Cohen, "The Impact of the Handicapped Child on the Family," *New Outlook for the Blind* (1964), 58.
6. W. Dennis, ed., *Readings in Child Psychology* (2d ed.; Englewood Cliffs, New Jersey: Prentice-Hall, 1963).
7. Ann S. Elonen and Sarah B. Zwarensteyn, "Appraisal of Developmental Lag in Certain Blind Children," *Journal of Pediatrics* (1964), 65, 599–610.
8. W. Goldfarb, "Emotional and Intellectual Consequences of Psychologic Deprivation in Infancy: a Re-evaluation," in *Psychopathology of Childhood,* ed. by P. H. Hoch, and J. Zubin (New York: Grune and Stratton, 1955).
9. H. F. Harlow, "The Nature of Love," *American Psychologist* (1958), 13, 673–685.
10. H. R. Kent, *The Effect of Repeated Praise or Blame on the Work Achievement of Blind Children* (Unpublished Doctoral thesis, Columbia University, 1956).
11. Ada Kozier, "Casework with Parents of Blind Children," *Social Casework* (1962), 43.
12. Shirley L. Land and Shalom E. Vineberg, "Locus of Control in Blind Children," *Exceptional Children* (1965), 31.
13. Elizabeth Langley, "Self-Image: The Formative Years," *New Outlook for the Blind* (1961), 55.
14. Berthold Lowenfeld, *Our Blind Children—Growing and Learning with Them* (Springfield, Illinois: Charles C Thomas, 1956).
15. ———, "The Blind Child as an Integral Part of the Family and Community," *New Outlook for the Blind* (1965), 59.
16. Elizabeth Maloney, "Direct Intervention on Behalf of the Blind Child," *Social Casework* (1962), 43.
17. Kathryn E. Maxfield and Harriet A. Fjeld, "The Social Maturity of the Visually Handicapped Preschool Child," *Child Development,* 13.
18. Mariam Norris, Patricia J. Spaulding and Fern H. Brodie, *Blindness in Children* (Chicago: The University of Chicago Press, 1957).
19. Lynn Ourth and Kenneth B. Brown, "Inadequate Mothering and Disturbance in the Neonatal Period," *Child Development* (1961), 32, 287–295.

20. Arthur H. Parmelee, Jr., "Developmental Studies of Blind Children," *New Outlook for the Blind* (1966), 60.
21. Dane Prugh, Elizabeth Staub, Harriet Sands, Ruth Kirschbaum and Ellenora Lenihan, "A Study of the Emotional Reactions of Children and Families to Hospitalization and Illness," *American Journal of Orthopsychiatry* (1953), 23, 70–106.
22. Robert A. Scott, "Introduction to the West Coast Regional Conference on Research Related to Blind and Severely Visually Impaired Children." *Proceedings of the West Coast Regional Conference on Research Related to Blind and Severely Visually Impaired Children* (New York, December, 1965).
23. Vita S. Somers, *The Influence of Parental Attitudes and Social Environment on the Personality of the Adolescent Blind* (New York: American Foundation for the Blind, 1944).
24. Luciana Visentini Steinzor, "Siblings of Visually Handicapped Children," *New Outlook for the Blind* (1967), 61.
25. ———, "Visually Handicapped Children: Their Attitudes Toward Blindness," *New Outlook for the Blind* (1966), 60.
26. Marvin B. Sussman, "Family Structure, Parent-Child Relationships and Disability," Paper presented at The Pennsylvania State University, April 9–12, 1967, Conference on Needed Research in the Behavioral Sciences and the Humanities with Reference to Problems Related to Blindness.
27. Sara Telson, "Parent Counseling," *New Outlook for the Blind* (1965), 59.
28. R. T. Verrillo, *A Study of Adjustment and the Relationship Between Parental Attitudes and Adjustment in Visually Impaired and Sighted Adolescents* (Unpublished Doctoral thesis, University of Rochester, 1958).
29. N. Westlund and Adelaide Palumbo, "Parental Rejection of Crippled Children," *American Journal of Orthopsychiatry* (1946), 16.
30. J. R. Wittenborn, "A Study of Adoptive Children," *Psychological Monographs,* 70; Nos. 1, 2, and 3 (1956).
31. L. J. Yarrow, "Maternal Deprivation: Toward an Empirical and Conceptual Re-evaluation," *Psychological Bulletin* (1961), 58.

SESSION REPORT

Peter Kratcoski

Dr. Marvin B. Sussman asserted that future research on the family in which there lives a visually handicapped child should use the total family system as the unit of analysis. In the past, research has concentrated on the handicapped child in abstraction. Now it is recognized that the handicapped child must be considered in the context of being a member of a family unit which constitutes a system. The reciprocal role relationships and the costs and rewards for each family member who adheres to a particular role must be taken into account.

The needs of the non-handicapped members of the family must be taken into account in any consideration of the visually handicapped child. Research should consider the mechanisms available for the visually handicapped child to achieve excellence in one or two roles (physical or social) in which he will be superior to normal individuals. This excellence could serve as a bargaining basis for status, recognition, and rewards, as well as a way for the visually handicapped child to re-evaluate his worth and improve his self-conception.

Less emphasis should be placed, Dr. Sussman decided, on individual psychological development and more consideration should be given to the child's place in the larger society (that is, the family, the school, and the community).

Dr. H. Robert Blank cited, as ripe for research, the area of reciprocity of rewards for all those involved with the visually handicapped child. It would be useful to understand, in other words, what give-and-take is involved in relationships between the visually handicapped child and his parents, his siblings, and agency personnel.

Research could discover ways to attract good professional staff members to work with agencies for the visually handicapped. Today there is evidence that the best people in the field drift toward positions with high status and psychological rewards, and so the most competent people, according to Dr. Blank, are found in academic circles and medical centers. Meanwhile, those working in agencies give most attention and service to those visually handicapped children who reward them in return. Consequently the multi-handicapped child is liable to be the one who is neglected. Programs might be developed to reallocate roles and rewards so that everyone in need of services receives them.

It is Dr. Sussman's view that the visually handicapped person today has many more opportunities to move freely in the community, and he has more alternatives open to him than in the past. In fact, in most instances he has the potential to operate almost as a normal human being. However, research is needed to determine how parental care and interaction with the child help or hinder the child's opportunities to develop his potentials. Is overprotection and dependence upon parents an aid or hindrance in the child's quest for normality? What are the consequences of parental overprotection? Is the desire or motivation for free movement of the blind person increased or decreased by overprotection and excessive concern?

The suggestion was made for research into the ways basic theories and research in the social and medical sciences can and should be incorporated and applied by family members and agency personnel working with the visually handicapped child. Dr. Winona L. Morgan expressed the need for developing programs which will test the effectiveness of existing programs and at the same time possess facilities and encourage possibilities for further research.

Dr. Tamara Dembo posed an additional question: What is the physical and psychological process of development which the blind child experiences in his quest to comprehend the unknown and feel security in his world? Dr. Sussman suggested that research is needed into the roles of siblings in the socialization of the visually handicapped child.

Dr. Blank pointed out that research into the relationship between the cause of the child's blindness and the parents' feelings of responsibility, guilt, and inadequacy should be conducted. There is some evidence that, if the first child is normal, the parents will feel less responsible or inadequate if a second child is handicapped or not normal. If blindness is due to accident, the parents may feel they could have averted it and therefore may experience feelings of guilt.

Dr. Morgan offered the idea that research into the family's relationships with a visually handicapped child could be conducted by installing an observer in the home to view the interaction process or by bringing the mother and child to the laboratory for observation.

A comparison of the underlying values and beliefs of parents who are over-protective with their unsighted child and the values and beliefs of parents who allow freedom and opportunities for the blind child to experiment on his own, represents a possibly rewarding challenge to research according to Dr. Dembo.

Since there are indications that a blind person is not able to make distinctions between self and others as easily as a sighted person, Dr. Robert A. Scott emphasized that research is needed into the perception the blind person has about the world of others and the world of self. Research into the reasons why some blind people are independent and others are not, and how this fact reflects upon their earlier training and relationships with parents, family members, and other community acquaintances is equally important, according to Dr. Scott.

Dr. Marvin B. Sussman offered a final list of research ideas:

1. Much more research is needed which is concerned with the role of the father in homes where there is a visually handicapped child. There is some evidence that the father takes on most of the instrumental duties of caring for the handicapped child, while the mother continues and intensifies her duties and relationships with the normal children.

2. Research is needed for investigating ways in which the medical profession can be persuaded to bring the father into the therapy situation. Doctors and counselors assume that the mother is going to handle most of the responsibilities of caring for the child, though this may not be true.

3. Other areas to be considered are the ways a visually handicapped child affects the marital relationship between husband and wife and how the economic position of the family is affected. The question of whether a visually handicapped child generally creates disequilibrium in the family unit or helps to build stronger family cohesion by uniting the family toward resolving a common problem should be considered. If disequilibrium is the result, steps to try to re-establish balance and harmony should be considered.

4. There is a need for research into the development of methodological techniques which can be used to pursue objective research on the visually handicapped.

5. Any systematic research conducted on the visually handicapped should include a control group of non-disabled persons so that it

can be determined more clearly what effects are the result of the disability and what effects are the result of some other factor.

Dr. Morgan adjourned the session after propounding two questions: (1) How can parents help themselves solve their problems with their visually handicapped child without utilizing the resources of a professional or agency; and (2) how can one persuade parents to become involved in groups which have a self-help purpose?

OLD AGE

RESEARCH NEEDS AND DEVELOPMENTS IN GERONTOLOGY

Elias S. Cohen

On January 23, 1967, President Johnson sent the first of a series of special messages to the Ninetieth Congress. This message was a "review of measures taken to aid the older Americans and recommendations for legislation to provide further aid." The President's message reflected the national interest in aging and old age.[1] For example: (1) the last eight Housing Acts contain special public housing provisions for the elderly and special assistance for them when they rent, buy, or modernize their own homes; (2) the Hill-Burton hospital program seeks to expand and improve nursing homes and other long-term care facilities; (3) public welfare provides programs to help restore older people to self-support and self-care; (4) the manpower development and training programs direct special efforts at the problems of the middle-aged and older Americans; and (5) the National Institutes of Health have established programs of research on aging.

In 1965, the Congress enacted, and the President signed into law, two landmark measures for older Americans: (1) *Medicare,* to ease the burden of hospital and doctor bills; and (2) *The Older Americans Act,* to develop community services to put more meaning into the lives of the senior citizens.

Some of the new proposals stem directly from research findings generated by the Bureau of the Census and the Social Security Administration, while others are offered without a solid grounding in the facts; but, in no less than six places in his address, the President called for studies, research, or demonstrations:

> I am directing the Secretary of Health, Education and Welfare to undertake immediately a comprehensive study of the problems of the aged including the cost of prescription drugs under Medicare.
>
> I propose to . . . launch special pilot projects to bring comprehensive medical and rehabilitation services to the aged.

> I propose to . . . begin an extensive research effort to develop thc best means of organizing, delivering, and financing health services needed by the aged.
>
> I am requesting funds for . . . intensive research to find new approaches in the design and operation of hospitals, nursing homes, extended care facilities, and other health institutions.
>
> I recommend that . . . educational and *research programs* on age discrimination be strengthened.
>
> I recommend that . . . a pilot program be started to provide nutritional meals in senior citizen centers.

During the fiscal year 1966 it is estimated that federal benefits and services for persons age 65 and over amounted to more than $2 billion, in addition to the $2.1 billion which accrues to the elderly through tax benefits.[2]

POPULATION TRENDS IN AGING

The demographic revolution has had its greatest effect among the elderly. Probably no other group has been affected as radically by the shifts in population, in wealth, in retirement age, and, of course, in increased longevity.

Rosow points out that our affluent society's values and institutions undermine the position of the old. The shifts in property control; the diminution of the importance of older people in passing on strategic knowledge; the "peculiarly sacred links to ancestors" or to tradition; the weakened kinship of family ties; increasing urbanization; the high productivity of our economy, together with the relatively low participation of the aged; and the lack of need to rely on older workers to contribute to the economy—all of these factors are part of the demographic revolution.[3]

What are some of the environmental changes in store for older people?

1. The numbers of the aged will continue to grow. Today there are 19 million elderly persons in the United States, and it is estimated by the year 2000 there will be 28.2 million.[4]

2. The numbers of the very old—that is, those 75 years of age and more—will continue to increase at about twice the rate of the over 65 group as a whole and at more than twice the rate of the total population. As of May 1966, there were an estimated 13,000 persons in the United States 100 years of age and over, and more than a million people whose age exceeded 85.[5]

3. Widowhood may be regarded as normally accompanying a woman's old age. By the year 2000 there may be as many as nine million aged widows.[6]

4. The aged of tomorrow will be better educated, although for the Negro there is a lag of a full generation, and any catching up may have to be planned for over a period of at least 50 years.[7]

5. Virtually all persons 65 and over will receive old age survivor and disability insurance. The Social Security benefit system will be substantially improved and smaller numbers of old people will rely on public assistance.[8]

6. While private pensions will cover more old people by 1975, no more than 25 or 30 per cent of the aged will be able to count on this source of added income. Indeed, by the end of the century, it is estimated that virtually no one 65 and over will be in the labor force. Thus, sometime in the next 30 years we must envision a situation where old people will rely entirely upon unearned income.[9]

7. The elderly currently live in circumstances of diminished income or poverty. In 1965, half of the 6.9 million families with heads of household aged 65 and over had incomes of less than $3,460. This median was less than half of the median of families with heads of household aged under 65. Almost a quarter (23.4 per cent) of older families had 1965 incomes of less than $2,000. More than 40 per cent of the older families had incomes of less than $3,000.[10]

8. Almost five million older people living alone or with non-relatives in 1965 were in even worse circumstances. Half of the 4.7 million older people in this group had incomes of less than $1,348. This median was about 40 per cent of the median for the under 65 individuals not living in families. A third of the older individuals living alone had incomes of less than $1,000, and about 60 per cent had incomes of less than $1,500.[11]

9. Retirement will probably come earlier for most older people, but it will be accompanied by reduced Social Security and pension benefits. There is a growing emphasis on company-initiated early retirement. Nearly one-fifth of company pension plans now use involuntary early retirement, and the practice is expected to increase. Early retirement provisions may be beneficial or they

may create a new class of poor. Current trends indicate that fewer and fewer older persons will be included in the labor force until, by the year 2000, national production will depend entirely upon persons under 65.[12]

10. The improvement of mortality rates among non-whites may not be accompanied by commensurate improved socio-economic status. The Negro at all ages suffers far greater deprivation than his white counterpart. A lifetime of discrimination exacts a special toll from the aged and this problem alone may necessitate two generations of carefully planned programs.[13]

11. Today persons over 65 have one chance in 7 of requiring short-term hospital care and one chance in 25 of needing long-term care, and these chances increase with age. While only one in 50 of those between 65 and 72 require long-term care, one in 15 of those 73 and over require this care. The implications for an older population, which becomes more heavily weighted in the upper age ranges, are clear.[14]

12. We will continue to limp along, adding something under 40,000 public housing units for the elderly each year. However, in 1960, of the housing units with heads of household 60 years and over, 20.4 per cent (or 2.7 million) were dilapidated or inadequate. For non-whites, more than 50 per cent of such housing units were classified as inadequate or as lacking facilities.[15]

13. The political power of the elderly will steadily increase. Whereas the aged represent about 15 per cent of those eligible to vote today, in the future they will begin to approximate 25 per cent.

14. The shift of our population to the cities will continue until 75 to 85 per cent of our total population lives in urban sprawls. There will be increasing reliance on automobiles or other systems of transportation. Living arrangements in the new super-cities may produce special problems for those who cannot afford, or, because of physical limitation, cannot manage transportation.[16]

15. About 1.3 million (or just under 10 per cent) of the farm population in the United States is 65 and over. Older people are forming a growing proportion of the farm population because young persons leave the farm more quickly than older persons. However, the elderly will probably form a growing proportion

of those living in cities—not so much because of convenience as because the central city will become more and more the locus for the poor.[17]

16. The increase in the number of persons 65 years and older taken together with the increase in the number of persons under age 18 indicates an increase in the dependency ratio of persons under 18 and of those 65 and over compared to those between 18 and 65. This particular trend may be of some interest to economists who view this increase in the dependency ratio in terms of increases in productivity.[18]

MAJOR QUESTIONS IN GERONTOLOGICAL RESEARCH

Shock points out that solutions to the complex problems in gerontology will require the application of the research techniques of practically every scientific discipline.

> Effective research must be directed toward a specific question. Research is a technical operation, and not all questions can be answered in the form asked. Many broad and general questions of great social importance must be broken down into simpler and more specific questions before they can be adequately attacked by research methods. . . . It is unfortunately true that the greater the social significance of the question, the less apt it is to be answerable in terms of tightly designed experiments. However, many of these broad important questions can be broken down into a series of more sharply focused questions which can be studied. . . . We are being asked the broad important questions before we have built up much of a backlog of answers to the small, specific detailed questions.[19]

Gerontology is concerned with the development of life, the adjustment of human beings to their environment in the years between maturity and death, and the reaction of society to the elderly. Understanding the aging process will give us answers about increased probabilities of death that come with advancing years, changes in human relationships, changes in human capacity, psychological and physiological changes which occur with the passing of time, as well as important clues on how to compensate for physiological, psychological, and economically utilitarian decrements.

Full understanding of the impact of aging requires observations made over a life span. Shock maintains that "the essence of gerontological research is that comparisons must be made between organisms at least at two points in their life span after the attainment of maturity." Aging as such, he points out, "cannot be studied where observations are made only on older animals or people." [20]

While a good many competent investigators have identified some of the research questions, there is no research policy either at a governmental or nongovernmental level that has the same single-minded purpose that we had when we attacked poliomyelitis, and we do not have a research policy that compares with our current concerns for heart disease and cancer.

Shock [21] poses four basic goals of research in aging:

1. What are aging people like, and why do they behave the way they do?

2. Why is it that the probability of death increases with age?

3. What conditions influence this probability? Are they genetic in character or environmental in origin?

4. What are the time sequences in interrelationships of changes in different characteristics?

There is still a great deal of work to be done on the question of what aging really is. Anderson[22] raises a series of theoretical questions which impinge on the basic nature of aging and its biological, psychological, and environmental aspects. Is aging the result of a general factor operating throughout the entire human system to change particular structures and functions, or is it the cumulative effect of many factors specific to particular structures and functions? If there is a general factor, is it nervous, hormonal, metabolic, or circulatory in nature? If there is a unitary principle in terms of a biochemical substance, physical state, or psychological process, is aging monolithic, or is it a matter of losses of small parts or units, a matter of decline in homeostatic functions and controls—"a matter of deterioration in behavioral adjustments"—or a combination of the three?

Kastenbaum furnishes an excellent description of theories of human aging in which he reviews the somatic mutation theory and the immunological theory. He proceeds from the cellular level to a review of a theory of aging concerned with changes in the central nervous system and changes in the central control mechanisms of the organism. He points up the distinction between biologists and the psychologist-sociologists. "Biologists tend to regard aging as a sequence of events that essentially is unfavorable to the individual organism, but differ among themselves concerning which sequences of change are most 'fundamental' or most 'intrinsic.' The notion that aging might be a 'normal' process that is not entirely detrimental to the individual seems to receive more support in the psycho-social than in the biological realm." [23]

He discusses the disengagement theory which has captured the attention of many investigators. "Briefly, the theory proposes that . . . normal aging is a mutual withdrawal or 'disengagement' between the aging person and others in the social system to which he belongs—a withdrawal initiated by the individual himself, or by others in the system. When disengagement is complete, the equilibrium that existed in middle life between the individual and society has given way to a new equilibrium characterized by greater distance and a changed basis for solidarity." [24]

Much of the research in social gerontology has been descriptive, and often the findings are difficult to apply because they have been unrelated to any theoretical construct. A case for the broad view of research needs has been made out by Tibbitts.[25] He defines the objects of social gerontology, first, understanding the manner in which time-related biological and psychological changes and environmental and cultural factors influence the development of personality and behavior of older adults and their role status and collective behavior and, second, understanding aging as a phenomenon of society and social change.

As some major areas for study Tibbitts suggests the examination of the impact of the evolving economies and the transition from handwork to automation and cybernation on the place of elderly people in society and states that these factors may be even more important than the demographic factors of birth rates, migrations, distributions, and comparisons of population components. He also points out that we have yet to develop sophisticated criteria for determining the onset of aging and for distinguishing between the old and the very old.

Finally, Tibbitts raises the general question about the impact of large numbers of older people in retirement status on structured institutions of our society. What is the meaning of retirement to the elderly and to the young? He suggests that rising numbers of the old and the very old with their concomitant decrements in physical and mental health must raise questions about the differential abilities of this population, and, hence, about the above differential solutions to meet problems. Elsewhere, Tibbitts[26] raises the following questions:

1. What is the position of old people in advanced society?

2. What is the role for old people, and can acceptable roles be found?

3. Can old people respond to efforts to integrate them into a society characterized by rapid advances in knowledge and social technological change?

Kent asks, "how much do we really know about old people, and how much do we know about the supposed solutions to their problems?" [27] He raises questions about the impact of early retirement on the elderly—whether it is "good" or "bad." Also is independence a basic goal of older people? He points out that, for many, security is more important than independence.

What is the impact, Kent inquires, of the aged population? Between now and the end of this century, 65 million people will celebrate their 60th birthday, and 20 million will grow from early old age into advanced age.

Because the role of older people and their adjustment to society is so much a function of cultural values and the status accorded to the aged by society at large, some investigators have given high priority to inquiry on the issue of the value system. Accordingly, Rosow[28] raises some interesting questions for research. He suggests that we must first begin to identify the components of the value system. How do values change and how are they influenced?

The same question was raised at a symposium on the aged at an American Orthopsychiatric Association meeting, where it was suggested that we "acquire accurate information concerning why we dislike and reject our older citizens as we do. . . . We must perform, underwrite, and encourage research projects to discover the underlying causes of this social phenomenon. Motivational research has come into great vogue in the commercial arena and there is no reason why we should not make use of its possibilities and techniques in solving the problems of aging." [29]

Approaching this issue from another perspective, Arnold Rose suggests that sociologists might examine the growing group consciousness phenomenon among the elderly. "Because most of the change associated with the acquisition of the role of self-conception of the elderly are negatively evaluated in American culture, and because there is no compensatory attribution of prestige as in other societies, the first reaction of most old people is some kind of disengagement and depression. The disengagement is by no means completely voluntary; the older person is pushed out of his occupation and even out of leadership roles in many kinds of nonoccupational associations." [30]

Citing some evidence in recent political activity, Rose suggests that sociologists "now need to go beyond casual observation and engage in systematic studies of the formation of group identification, of this transformation of a social category into a social group. The whole area of the subculture of the aging needs objective investigation in the same manner sociologists have already studied ethnic, regional, and occupational subcultures."

As critical as these needs are, however, it is my belief—and that of Richard Williams—that the most urgent need for sociological research is in the area of epidemiology. While the field of public health has long pursued this approach, there has been less attention given to it in the area of social disorder. Reichert has discussed those aspects of public health epidemiology which are applicable to the field of social welfare. He points out that the approach proceeds by determining "the distribution of a disease or a condition in a population unit, and by examining factors that influence distribution such as age, sex, occupation, climate, and many more." Assessment in public health, he points out, "tends to be based on epidemiological analysis [involving] the use of classified, measured and counted data regarding the distribution of a disorder in a population unit and regarding factors affecting the distribution." [31]

In the study of aging, I suggest the application of epidemiological approaches through: (1) the definition of conditions and events affecting the individuals; (2) the development of systems for determining prevalence or incidence; and (3) the determination of gross characteristics of those affected, including age, sex, marital status, economic status and geographic location.

Although some data is being gathered, we have not investigated with much sophistication those populations readily available to us. Old age assistance loads and OASDI loads are logical starting places. We have available to us patient populations in mental hospitals and nursing homes. We have little information about the incidences of specific problems of old persons and/or about the nature of those problems. Likewise there is little information about the combinations of problems which are likely to occur, and under what circumstances problems of older people are liable to result in social or physical disabilities. Such analyses may lead us to examine not only the aged, but also younger groups, as Rosow[32] points out, so that we may obtain information on prevention or early identification of problem-prone populations.

Ethel Shanas,[33] an investigator who has surveyed large numbers of the elderly, makes essentially the same point. Elsewhere Dr. Shanas explains as an example that "the number of old people bedfast at home are about the same as the number of old people resident in all our long-term hospitals and nursing homes. Further, there are twice as many old persons bedfast and housebound in the community. . . . as live in institutions of all kinds including homes for the aged together with hospitals and nursing homes." She then raises the following questions: "Who is taking care of these bedfast and housebound old people who live at home? What services are needed by these persons? What services are needed by their families? What proportion of these bedfast and housebound persons would be in nursing homes or domiciliary homes, if such housing were readily available to them? What about the staffing of service program for this special group of the elderly? Is it feasible to train other older people to work specifically with the bedfast and housebound aged living at home?"

In the area of psychology, Shock [34] poses some basic questions: What are the factors that influence personal adjustment in older people, and, further, how do the personality and emotional characteristics of people change with age?

Anderson [35] raises fundamental questions about whether the behavioral adjustment which may accompany old age arises from the destruction of or the survival of tissues and structures struggling to meet the exigencies of life. A related question he suggests for research, is a fundamental one: Does active participation and intellectual activity preserve intelligence and, further, does an active concern with learning increase the capacity of the individual to learn at older ages? Presumably, if we have enough data, particularly from longitudinal studies, we might discover the proper time to intervene.

In a Presidential address before the American Psychological Association, Botwinick [36] outlined a variety of areas in which considerable problems still remain as hope for psychological studies:

1. Creativity and achievement
2. Intelligence
3. Speed of response
4. Rigidity
5. Motivation and capacity

6. Cautiousness

7. Certainty and expectancy

8. Attention ego functioning and reactivity

(Botwinick readily acknowledged that these areas are most decidedly selective and he gave no attention to problems and concepts of longevity, correlates of impending death, cultural influences, social problems such as retirement and loneliness, and such physiological concerns as brain damage.)

Williams [37] suggests an analysis of the gap between social requirements and psychological capacity as a promising avenue of research, and inquires whether intergenerational differences become critical and appear as psychological deficits in the face of the growing complexity and increased demands of society.

Though no attempt has been made in this paper to review the work being done in geriatrics, Van Zonnerveld [38] raises the following questions for research in the area he calls *social* geriatrics ("that part of geriatrics that studies the relationship between health and disease in the aged and the environment in its widest sense"):

1. What happens to the health of the elderly population in the course of time?

2. What are the dimensions and distribution of ill health among aging and old people in terms of incidence, prevalence, mortality, and health needs?

3. Can we clarify the practical application and effects on the health of the aging and aged of all our efforts in the fields of medical and social care?

4. What is the natural history of chronic and disabling diseases so prevalent in old people?

5. Can we clarify the combination of clinical phenomena in the aged, compared to those in the young?

He notes a dearth of analytical epidemiological research in gerontology and states that few attempts have been made to register the results of sociomedical research.

In the medical area, Geill [39] makes some suggestions as to what the future of geriatrics will be. Efforts will be directed at preventing diseases from becoming chronic, accompanying people into old age. This will lead to research in methods of early detection of diseases and analysis of factors which predispose one toward diseases. Geill further suggests that radiological and genetic studies on the significance of internal and external age and disease factors must constitute an essential portion of this work. It should be noted that here the questions and issues are more precise than they are in the social field.

There will be special interests attached to studies of the paraproteins; and because there are some biological theories which suggest that aging represents hyperactivity of the autoimmune processes, problems of immunization will consume interest. Studies of the side effects of drugs have particular importance in geriatrics because of the effect on the organism of long-term ingestion. Little is known about the possibility of drug damage to organs such as the heart and the brain as a result of long-term ingestion of drugs. Those interested in this particular phase of the future of research may want to refer to this article for the identification of some of the medical and molecular biological issues that Geill provides.

Within the area of social gerontology, research questions are raised about housing; retirement plans and the institution of retirement; the utility of certain social services and programs; and the impact of publicly supported programs of recreation, income maintenance, institutional and other living arrangements, welfare services, community organization. Tibbitts and Shmelzer [40] have suggested a number of problems which require study. Does special housing for the elderly add to or detract from social and community participation, satisfactory self-expression in life, good health, and independence? (A corollary to this question is: Can we identify the special characteristics of individuals which require support through special housing arrangements; and, if so, can we develop instruments for assessing the needs of elderly people precisely?) Can socially deprived, mildly confused, or physically marginal people be absorbed in so-called normal housing for the elderly, and if so, in what proportions?

The entire issue of institutional arrangements is open to research, and it, too, relates to the questions as to what kinds of decrements can best be served and supported by different types of institutional services. Can we, for example, devise adequate criteria for measuring the impact and quality of institutional services? What effect do government programs of payments, mortgage insurance, and direct loans have on the kind of care which people seek for themselves or for other elderly parents or friends?

Tibbitts and Shmelzer go on to raise questions about the impact of services. For example, do community services really lessen the need for institutionalization? To what extent will various services be utilized only during periods of crisis, and to what extent will the utilization be continued? What governmental and nongovernmental devices are effective in improving the quality of life of the elderly? Is it possible or desirable in a so-called pluralistic society to achieve systematic approaches and efficiency in meeting total community needs through an integration of voluntary, secular, and church-related organizations serving needs of specific groups?

With regard to retirement they ask: What are practical and appropriate roles for retired people? What are the variations in life styles in retirement among the aged in terms of age, sex, physical status, education, social class, and income? Do activity centers or educational programs have an impact on the well-being of the elderly, or is the impact selective?

In the area of social services, some of the same questions begin to arise: What specific services are needed in order to meet needs and how can we identify the needs with precision? In this connection, worth citing is a gross method of measuring need utilized in a survey of old-age assistance grants to elderly people in 20 county public assistance agencies in six states.[41]

Finally, one should reiterate the plea made by virtually all writers concerned with the future of research: We need more longitudinal research on a broad population base. Similarly, we need longitudinal studies on stratified samples followed from the time of selection until death, with detailed studies made of age changes and cross-comparisons between strata (for example, studies of aged low income, middle income, and high income groups over a number of years in order to examine adjustment to stresses and crises of aging). We also need longitudinal studies of samples selected on categorical bases in terms of disease patterns, inherited characteristics, and educational levels. Hopefully, longitudinal studies may be able to give us clues to the factors predisposing toward success or failure in retirement in terms of social adjustment and contentment.

Longitudinal research, however, is not without its problems. These projects consume time and money. The interest of the subjects may flag. Some subjects may leave the area or investigators may leave the institution carrying out the research. While in many areas this may not be too important, in others corrections for the personal element may be required. Changes in methods of examining subjects, even when unproved, make the data obtained in different years incommensurable. These differences have an effect on the analysis of age trends. Because of these problems there are relatively few such studies completed or in process. Nevertheless, despite the difficulties, longitudinal research on human beings offers the only possible answer to a great many of the questions that have been posed here.[42]

SOME EXAMPLES OF STUDIES IN PROCESS OR RECENTLY COMPLETED

At Duke University a longitudinal study was initiated about ten years ago with a community sample of 260 individuals falling in the age range of 60 to 94—the median age being 70.[43] The aims were to identify social, psychological, and physiological factors influencing the behavior of the elderly, and to relate these changes to intellectual functioning, personality, and social competence. Subsidiary aims had to do with methodology, and maintenance of a stimulating research atmosphere in order to attract personnel. At the time of the published report, about 52 per cent of the original sample were participating. Of those who were not, 30 per cent had died, 6 per cent refused to continue or participate or had otherwise been lost, and the remaining 12 per cent were too ill or disabled to continue.

A multidisciplinary approach to the study has permitted the findings of workers in two or more disciplines to be integrated in complex statistical models. For example, physical and social data have been studied to examine certain activities and interests in relation to the state of physical functioning. Disengagement has been examined in relation to selected health, psychiatric, and sociological indices. It has been possible to compare the findings of ophthalmological, audiometric, and physiological examinations made with subjects controlled for intelligence to determine the effects of visual and auditory loss on cognitive functioning.

Some of the findings already indicate that in terms of this particular group there is little support for the disengagement theory. Social activity "has been found to be a significant correlate of life's satisfaction except among the very old. . . ." When studied longitudinally, a minority of the elderly have been found to display a persistent pattern of low activity and high life satisfaction. Busse[43] suggests, therefore, that relatively active elderly people are more likely to maintain morale than those who are inactive. Another important finding he offers is that self-evaluations of health are not reliable among the elderly.

In Minnesota, a study of initially healthy business and professional men has been underway for 19 years. The study, which concentrates on cardiovascular and/or respiratory disorders[44] is expected to continue for another six years until the men have been covered for 25 years with examinations repeated at intervals of approximately one year, covering the span from middle age to early old age. The objective of this particular study is to contribute answers on predisease characteristics.

Both Busse and Brozek are unequivocal in their assertions that it is only through longitudinal research that we can secure information on the effect of age on the functioning in an individual.

Finally, it is pertinent to mention three projects being carried on at the University of California.[45] The growth study in Berkeley began with a sample of infants and is now following 60 subjects in their late 30's. Second, the guidance study has followed some 200 subjects from infancy until their mid 30's in an investigation of physical, mental, and personality development and their interrelationships. Third, the Oakland growth study followed children from the age of 11 through high school with several adult follow-up studies. These studies have produced a sample of more than a hundred people now in their mid 40's on whom considerable material has been collected.

The remainder of this paper's review of research in the field is a selective approach and will attempt to describe some of the more significant work recently done or still in process.

There have been some useful reviews of research in process recently produced through the Department of Health, Education and Welfare. Other "round-ups" may be found elsewhere.[46] The most recent survey of research in the social welfare field offered a review of 35 projects relating to the chronically ill and aged funded by various federal agencies.[47] The review is not an exhaustive report but rather an illustrative one. Some of the projects described in that report are summarized below with additional material secured from another more detailed federal report on six studies.[48]

At the University of Michigan, a study is underway to develop materials and methods for preretirement programs for industrial workers. Another, extending over a period of three years, studies the effects of pre-retirement education on adjustment in retirement of hourly-rated workers. The purpose of the project is to test the hypothesis that a group of hourly-rated automobile workers who participated in a group-discussion type of preretirement education adjusted better in retirement than a similar group which did not participate. Another study sought to examine the influence of anticipated levels of retirement income on spending and saving decisions before retirement in order to assess the impact of private pension plans on preretirement behavior of participants. This was a national sample survey conducted initially in 1962 with 1,300 families. The study indicated that the amount contributed to private pension plans did not have much effect on the amount of money that families saved. What was of greater significance was whether or not families tended to be savings-oriented.

A study at Iowa State University examines the process of withdrawing from active participation in employment and seeks to determine how plans for and actual retirement from work vary among occupational groups. This is a three year study being done in small towns. Approximately 500 persons are being interviewed in each occupational category with some supplemental mail questionnaires to determine how retirement plans were actually implemented.

Studies at Cornell University have been performed to measure the value of preretirement counseling programs. Eight plants with preretirement counseling programs were reviewed closely following mail surveys. These plants and their employees and retirees were interviewed and contrasted with workers and retirees in plants that have no counseling programs. Those employees who had counseling knew more about retirement policies than those who had had none.

A national sample of about 4,000 persons (not representative) of retirees was interviewed in 1952, 1954, 1956, and 1958–59. This study sought to index changes which "normal" older persons undergo and to determine the correlates of such changes in order to understand better the retirement process and what it is that makes it easier or more difficult to accept. Single women appeared to have more favorable attitudes toward retirement than those who were married or widowed. Reluctance to retire, it was found, seemed to be less related to negative feelings toward the new activities associated with retirement (or lack of activities) than with the feelings of apprehension concerning economic well-being after retirement. Seventy-eight per cent of the sample of retired men felt that if one can afford it, one should retire and take it easy. This might appear to support the disengagement theory of aging as opposed to the activist theory of aging.

The University of New Hampshire conducted a study examining early retirement as a means of work force control. One of the major concerns of this study was the use and evaluation of early retirement provisions to control the size of the work force at plants when technological improvements, mergers, production cutbacks, and so on required a reduction in work force. One of the objects of this study was to assess the impact of such early retirement practices on the company, the retiree, and public income maintenance programs such as public assistance.

Irving Rosow's landmark study, "The Aged, Family and Friends,"[49] examines the relation between two sets of older people's social ties—with their adult children and with their neighbors or friends. The study was undertaken on the assumption that these different sets of relations might be connected. Among the factors about which Rosow gathered data were kin and friendship interaction, emotional dependence, role loss, and changes, including those in marital status, health, living arrangements, and household composition, proximity of children, and socio-economic status.

Rosow had hypothesized that the aged having limited contact with children would show a compensating tendency to interact more frequently with neighbors than those who had frequent contact with their children. His findings did not confirm this hypothesis; however, there was a tendency toward increased contact with neighbors when low contact with children was accompanied by a high role loss.

Rosow's study in many ways related to his earlier work in which he suggested that acceptance of the cliche "old people want to be wholly integrated into the mainstream of community life" may not entirely square with the facts. Actually, what old people want, he found, is to be segregated but close to what is going on in the community among younger groups; what they do not want is to be isolated and completely away—in colonies. As he points out, the isolated pattern concentrates older people together but separates them from surrounding social life. The segregated pattern concentrates older people but insulates rather than isolates them from a larger community environment. His findings indicate that segregated retirement housing arrangements concentrate rather than diffuse the field of potential friends and support. This, he suggests, assists rather than detracts from improved social integration.[50]

According to the studies at Cornell University, children tend to furnish help to their aged parents, although the most likely flow of assistance in the areas of health and economics is from the aged parents to their adult children. About one-half of those surveyed indicated that parents took care of their children when they were ill, and about 40 per cent of the children presumably would furnish the same help to the elderly. However, the difference between the two groups was not great.

Where financial assistance was concerned, more than 40 per cent of the elderly parents were reported to have given financial assistance to their children; however, only 10 per cent of the adult children were reported to have given financial assistance to their parents. But 80 per cent of the parents said they never required financial help, and about one in seven said that while they occasionally needed help, they never asked their children to furnish it.

An important finding in this study deals with the relationship between affectional and financial ties. It indicates that "the maintenance of close affectional ties is of paramount importance to the older generation; that they are unwilling to jeopardize these ties with their children by expecting financial assistance from them." This finding would seem to have important significance in considering regulations and laws on filial responsibility. Many older people probably deprive themselves severely and forego public assistance grants rather than go through with the necessary business of seeking support payments from their adult children.

One of the important studies now reaching a conclusion, the protective services project in Cleveland, examines the impact of these services on persons whose behavior indicates mental incapability ". . . of adequately caring for [themselves] and [their] interests without serious consequences to [themselves] or others," and where no other source of help to meet needs is available.

A control and an experimental group were set up. Several measures on the impact of service were applied, the most important being the measurement of sheer survival. "Will there be any difference in the survival rate of the two populations, the one benefiting from protective services?" The second measure was that of contentment: How does the individual feel? Others were measurements of physical and mental functioning, physical symptoms experienced by the subject, and the degree of stress experienced by their closest friends.

Early findings reveal that there are few and insubstantial differences between the service and control populations on any of the measures of effectiveness of protective services. No difference is detected in survival rates. There is some difference in the contentment score for the service group. Measures of physical functioning show no difference. Reid's conclusions on the studies he surveyed have general applicability:

1. The meaning of aging is contingent upon a variety of things. Old age can mean different things to different people.

2. Economic condition and health condition are the most significant variables in terms of personal meaning of old age. It is significant that the elderly, unlike the young, cannot look toward things getting better. The best they can hope for is that they will maintain their health and economic condition at some kind of reasonable level.

3. Social arrangements are important. While interaction with neighbors or persons other than children or spouse is good, the absence of such interaction is not necessarily bad.

4. Planning ahead for retirement is most likely to enhance retirement status. However, this is not just a matter of individual decision. It seems to be a measure of the function of ability to plan ahead and convert plans into arrangements that can influence the future. People who are poor when they are young cannot do that. Failure to plan may also be a function of inadequate knowledge. Providing people with knowledge does seem to be of benefit, although the protective services project seems to indicate that we are very far from understanding what we can do to help the almost helpless.

5. The studies reviewed indicate that more precision is needed in our understanding about the intergenerational relationships and what we can do to implement social policy to strengthen rather than weaken those ties. Reid suggests it might be more realistic to recognize that not only have many relatives severed emotional ties with the elderly but that they have a right to do so.

A final group of research studies are those which have just gotten underway as a result of grants for research by the Administration on Aging of the Department of Health, Education and Welfare. The projects approved so far are concerned with community organization, problems of retirement, factors in adjustment to aging, and the special needs of certain groups among the elderly.[51]

The New York State College of Agriculture at Ithaca (Cornell University), for example, is undertaking a long-range comparative study of community structure and its effect on the happiness, well-being, and community participation of older people. It will seek to determine those factors in the community which account for variations in success or failure of community services for the aged. The study will review some 90 communities in New York State, rating them on services and opportunities provided to older people.

The second research study in community organization will be an analysis of older people's needs in the Boston area, compared to the existence of suitable services and the extent of use or reasons for non-use. Particular attention will be given to utilization of services and the impact of geographical mobility and social integration on social functioning and well-being of the elderly. The analysis will be based on earlier findings of studies which included interviews with 1,500 men and women over 65 and some 600 younger people discussing their aged parents.

A somewhat related study is one which will be carried out by the Los Angeles County Federation of Labor (AFL-CIO) to determine the economic and social situation and unmet needs of retired union members and to study the potential for expanding services and developing new ones through both union and community agencies and the use of leadership skills of retired union members.

Two studies have to do with the place of women among the senior citizen population. Roosevelt University in Chicago has undertaken a study of two groups of widows—those who lost their husbands between the ages of 50 and 64 and those widowed from 65 on. The study will examine the changes which take place in finances, living arrangements, daily activities, and social life, and will determine, if possible, what programs are most effective in helping widows through the time of crisis and into a purposeful and satisfying life.

A study at Miami University, Oxford, Ohio, concerns the adjustment of women who retire from the labor market. This investigation it is hoped, will yield clues about the needs for roles among this growing group of women.

The Department of Rural Sociology of the University of Wisconsin is studying the motivation and adjustment of older people who move upon retirement, with special reference to health and welfare problems associated with moves to retirement communities outside the home state.

Finally, in this group of research projects I want to give special attention to one which is examining the needs and use of services among Negro and white aged persons. The objectives are as follows:

> It is the specific objective of this project to conduct research into the correspondence of social, economic and health services with the conditions, needs, and utilization patterns of *aged, non-institutionalized residents* of *urban neighborhoods of low socio-economic status.* We intend to determine what condition, need, and utilization differences exist between Negro and white aged which may affect the kinds of welfare services consumed and the ways in which these services are secured and consumed by members of each group. We also intend to identify selected and social factors which may affect both differences between the groups in the areas specified and their consumption of service. The use of public assistance programs will be given particular attention in the analysis of data to determine both the extent to which these programs reach those aged in the community who, in the course of this study, are found to be eligible for service and the social, economic, and health characteristics of recipients and non-recipients. These objectives will be accom-

plished in surveys of both a representative sample of the total non-institutionalized aged population of low socio-economic central city neighborhoods and of all public and voluntary agencies serving those neighborhoods.

Comparisons of the aged Negro with his white counterpart are essential to determining whether conditions, need and utilization patterns, and attitudes described are unique to aged Negroes or whether the findings can be generalized to the entire aged population resident in neighborhoods of comparable socio-economic levels. Similarly, comparisons will be made between non-recipients of public assistance and recipients, within both the Negro and white populations, to determine whether conditions described are unique to recipients or whether the findings can be generalized to the aged Negro and white populations of low socio-economic central city neighborhoods.

The general approach in this design comes under what Wolins has called a "multi-focal" approach. First, through survey research on a sample of non-institutionalized community residents we will secure information on their social, health and economic conditions and needs; their use of services; their feelings about utilization and service; and factors which may influence both the existence of needs, reflecting negative conditions, and the use of services. Second, through a survey of the formal agencies serving the community we will determine both the content, methods of delivery and availability of service programs and their present utilization rates as compared to their maximum rates.

It is not felt that public or voluntary agencies serving aged residents of low income areas can plan service programs on the basis of data on one racial group. However, it is suggested that many agencies could plan service programs for the total aged population in the geographical area served by the agency with an awareness of and provision for existing differences in conditions, needs and attitudes between members of the two predominant racial groups in the city. It is the specific goal of this study to provide information on such differences to agencies, both public and voluntary, serving the community to be studied. It is expected that findings from this study will facilitate the adjustment of present service programs under the State Office of Public Assistance so as to insure the most efficient delivery of services to the aged and so that the aged may be able to make fullest use of present opportunities. It is also expected that findings from this study will make possible new programs under public assistance which may, in turn, enable the aged to function at an optimum level.[52]

OBSTACLES IN APPLYING RESEARCH FINDINGS TO SOCIAL POLICY DECISION-MAKING

Despite the proliferation of reports and investigations, and despite the increasing availability of funds for research, it is apparent that we lack a policy about what it is we want researched. Elsewhere I have described the cultural and organization factors involved in this issue.[53]

The current state of disorganization in social research is due to the tendency for research to be directed primarily by personal interest rather than by a centralized goal formulation from the social policy makers and the program operators. Some of the disorganization is related to highly valued feelings about academic and scientific freedom, and some to lack of experience in operations research. There is also a lack of communication between the policy makers and the research investigators.

A second group of obstacles, related to the first, arises from the relatively low value social agencies place upon planning as an appropriate and integral function of agency operation. Despite a host of new programs for the elderly we cannot discern coordinated planning machinery which can assess the condition of the older American and can take into consideration alternative approaches to problems, various solutions within some kind of cost-benefit framework, and suggested instructions for policy makers and program operators.

Research funds are being consumed by universities and private groups whose relationship to the policy makers is at best tenuous. The public agencies have not yet made the proper kinds of connections to the research centers and the research centers are not getting the right kind of feedback from those dealing with the ultimate consumers of service, and these factors which are adversely affecting the use of research findings are used to change the value scheme and to justify the introduction of new machinery into government.

One of the first things that we need to learn more about is how political social policy decisions are reached and what value systems operate to influence policy. Understanding more about political decision-making tends to make planning both within and without and program-deciding program-operating units more relevant.

In 1961, Sheppard attempted to stimulate interest in research on aging and political behavior. Unfortunately, few political sociologists have responded to his effort. He asks, among other things, what differences exist among states in voting trends, election outcomes, and legislative behavior that can be traced directly and indirectly to differences in the age distribution of their populations. He asks similar questions about changes in political behavior and characteristics among those states experiencing different rates of increase or decrease in the proportions of older voters. Conscious efforts must also be made to change cultural attitudes toward the elderly. This implies analysis of those attitudes, determination of their sources, determination of those elements which are susceptible to change and then the establishment of programs to produce the change.

Finally, public agencies must develop machinery for social goal formulation. This means that there must be staffs within the operating agencies capable of formulating the specific researchable questions and indicating the areas which require assessment and development of resources to achieve a given goal.

NOTES

1. Lyndon B. Johnson, "Message from the President of the United States on Older Americans to the 90th Congress, First Session," *Document No. 40* (Washington: Government Printing Office, January 23, 1967).
2. U.S. Department of Health, Education and Welfare, Administration on Aging, "Federal Benefits and Services for the FY 1965 and 1966," Memorandum, Supplement to *Useful Facts #10* (Washington: Government Printing Office, January 6, 1967).
3. I. Rosow, "Old Age: One Moral Dilemma of an Affluent Society," *The Gerontologist,* Vol. 2, No. 4, 1962, 184–185.
4. U.S. Department of Health, Education and Welfare, Administration on Aging, "Charts on Population Trends, Marital Status, and Income," *Memorandum, Useful Facts #12* (Washington: Government Printing Office, December 7, 1966).
5. ———, "National Population Trends As of July 1, 1966 (Analytical Tables), Table 1" *Memorandum, Useful Facts #15* (Washington: Government Printing Office, January 5, 1967).
6. ———, "Year-end Statistical Round-up," *Memorandum, Useful Facts # 15, op. cit.;* and *Memorandum, Useful Facts #16* (Washington: Government Printing Office, January 6, 1967).
7. U.S. Department of Commerce, Bureau of the Census, "Current Population Reports," *Memorandum, Useful Facts #16, op. cit.; and Educational Change in a Generation, Series P-20, No 132* (Washington: Government Printing Office, September 22, 1964).
8. Lyndon B. Johnson, "Message," *op. cit.*
9. L. Epstein, "Income of the Aged in 1962: First Findings of the 1963 Survey of the Aged," *Social Security Bulletin,* Vol. 27, No. 3 (Washington: U.S. Department of Health, Education and Welfare, 1963).
10. U.S. Department of Health, Education and Welfare, *Useful Facts #16, op. cit.*
11. *Ibid.*
12. E. Palmore, "Retirement Patterns Among Aged Men: Findings of the 1963 Survey of the Aged, Report on Study of Retirement Policies and Practices in Industry," in *Social Security Bulletin,* Vol. 27, No. 8 (Washington: U.S. Department of Health, Education and Welfare, 1963).
13. M. Orshansky, "The Aged Negro and His Income," *Social Security Bulletin,* Vol. 27, No. 2 (Washington: U.S. Department of Health, Education and Welfare, 1963).
14. D. Rice, *Health Insurance Coverage of the Aged and Their Hospital Utilization in 1962,* Findings of the 1963 Survey of the Aged, *Social Security Bulletin,* Vol. 27, No. 7 (Washington: U.S. Department of Health, Education and Welfare, 1963).

15. U.S. Bureau of the Census, "Housing of Senior Citizens, Table J," *U.S. Census of Housing: 1960,* Vol. VII (Washington: Government Printing Office, 1962), xv.
16. G. Grier, "Goals and Objectives in Aging," Paper presented before the Annual Conference of State Executives on Aging (Washington, D.C., April 24, 1964) (multilith).
17. *Useful Facts No. 16, op. cit.*
18. *Useful Facts No. 15, op. cit.*
19. N. Shock, *Trends in Geronotology,* (2d ed.; Palo Alto, California: Stanford University Press, 1957), 114–115.
20. *Ibid.,* 116.
21. N. Shock, *Trends in Gerontology, op. cit.,* 114–115.
22. J. E. Anderson, "Research Problems in Aging," *Psychological Aspects in Aging,* ed. J. E. Anderson (Washington: American Psychological Association, Inc., 1956).
23. R. Kastenbaum, "Theories of Human Aging: Search for a Conceptual Framework," *Journal of Social Issues,* Vol. 21, No. 4, October, 1965.
24. M. Elaine Cumming, "New Thoughts on the Theory of Disengagement," *New Thoughts on Old Age,* ed. R. Kastenbaum (New York: Springer, 1964), 3–18.
25. C. Tibbitts, "The Future of Research in Social Gerontology," *Age with a Future,* ed. P. From Hansen (Copenhagen, 1964), 139–145.
26. ———, *Middle Aged and Older People in American Society,* Pamphlet OA, No. 227 (Washington: Government Printing Office, 1965).
27. D. P. Kent, *Aging Fact and Fancy,* Pamphlet OA, No. 224 (Washington: Government Printing Office, 1965).
28. I. Rosow, "Old Age," *op. cit.,* 184–185.
29. E. Cohen, "Cultural Attitudes Toward Aging and Their Implications for Public Planning," *Journal of the American Geriatrics Society,* May, 1960.
30. A. Rose, "The Subculture of the Aging: A Topic for Sociological Research," *The Gerontologist,* Vol. 2, No. 3, September, 1962.
31. K. Reichert, "In Program Planning, What Can Social Work Adapt from Public Health?," Paper presented at the Institute for Social Workers in Public Health (California, 1959) (mimeo).
32. I. Rosow, "Old Age," *op. cit.,* 184–185.
33. Ethel Shanas, "Viewpoint and Interview with Ethel Shanas, Ph.D.," *Geriatrics,* Vol. 21, No. 4, April, 1966, 110; and Ethel Shanas, "Social Research in Aging and Its Programmatic Implications," Paper prepared for the Institute for State Executives in Aging, Brandeis University, Waltham, Massachusetts, March 19–25, 1967.
34. N. Shock, *Trends in Gerontology, op. cit.,* 114–115.
35. J. E. Anderson, "Research Problems," *op. cit.*
36. J. Botwinick, "Research Problems in Concepts in the Study of Aging," *The Gerontologist,* Vol. 4, No. 3, September, 1964.
37. Richard H. Williams, *Implications for Future Research, Processes of Aging,* Vol. 1 (New York: Atherton Press, 1963).
38. Van Zonnerveld, "Forefront: Social Geriatrics," *Geriatrics,* Vol. 21, No. 11, November, 1966.
39. T. Geill, M.D., "The Future of Geriatric Research," *The Gerontologist,* Vol. 5, No. 2, June, 1965, 57.
40. C. Tibbitts and J. L. Shmelzer, "New Directions in Aging and Their Research Implications," *Welfare in Review,* February, 1965.
41. C. Kellam and C. O'Reilly, "Measuring the Needs of Older People" (University of Wisconsin, 1964) (Monograph-mimeo).
42. J. Brozek, A. Keys, H. L. Taylor, "Longitudinal Research: The Minnesota

Study," *Proceedings Seventh International Congress on Gerontology,* Vol. 1 (Vienna, 1966), 269.

43. E. W. Busse, M.D., "Longitudinal Research: The Duke Study," *Proceedings Seventh International Congress of Gerontology,* Vol. 1 (Vienna, 1966), 283.
44. J. Brozek, et al., "Longitudinal Research," *op. cit.,* 269.
45. M. C. Jones, "Longitudinal Studies at the University of California," *Proceedings Seventh International Congress on Gerontology,* Vol. 1 (Vienna, 1966), 275.
46. Two examples are: I. Bader and A. Hoffman, "Research in Aging, Adding Life to Years," *Bulletin of the Institute of Gerontology,* Vol. 13, supplements Nos. 2 and 3; D. Dickins, "Research in Gerontology: Its Status and Needs," *Agricultural Science Review,* Fall, 1964; U.S. Department of Health, Education and Welfare, *Aging: A Review of Research and Training Grants Supported by the National Institutes of Health* (Washington: Government Printing Office, 1958); and, of course, Shock's landmark volume.
47. U.S. Department of Health, Education and Welfare, *Abstracts of Research and Demonstration Projects in Social Welfare and Related Fields* (Washington: Government Printing Office, no date).
48. O. M. Reid, *Aging Americans, Welfare in Review,* U.S. Department of Health, Education and Welfare Bulletin, Vol. 4, No. 5 (Washington: Government Printing Office, May, 1966).
49. I. Rosow, "The Aged, Family and Friends," *Social Security Bulletin,* Vol. 28, No. 11 (Washington: Government Printing Office, November, 1965).
50. ———, "Retirement Housing and Social Integration," *The Gerontologist,* Vol. 1, No. 2, June, 1961.
51. U.S. Department of Health, Education and Welfare, Administration on Aging, "Press Releases," Nos. L-23, L-51, L-89, unnumbered release dated November 3, 1966.
52. ———, "Needs and Use of Services Among Negro and White Aged," (Project Grant No. AA4-67-027-01).
53. Elias S. Cohen, "Cultural and Organizational Factors Affecting the Use of Research Findings in Setting Social Policy for the Aging in the United States," *Proceedings Seventh International Congress on Gerontology,* Vol. 6 (Vienna, 1966), 363.
54. H. L. Sheppard, "Implications of An Aging Population for Political Sociology," *Politics of Age,* Proceedings of the University of Michigan 14th Annual Conference on Aging, Ann Arbor, Michigan, June 19–20, 1961, ed. by W. Donahue, and C. Tibbitts and published by Division of Gerontology, The University of Michigan, Ann Arbor, 1962.

DEVELOPMENTS AND RESEARCH NEEDS IN WORK WITH THE AGED BLIND

Melvin E. Saterbak

I believe that in work for the blind we have been operating on past experience and many times on the basis of "hunches," supposedly with sufficient data to justify existing and planned programs. All research conducted for other segments of our population could and should include the blind population. Research methodology would have to include some specific structuring to include variables pertinent to visually impaired people. It is conceivable that in a longitudinal study, blindness would probably not be a variable until the later years with most of the population in the test group. This to me would be a good basis of comparing variables regarding the loss of vision with the normal factors of aging.

Eisenberg[1] states, "fundamental to the existence of all human beings is shelter. Blind people no less than any other group need and have the right to adequate shelter. Thus, many citizens have given specific attention to the problems of housing for blind, chronically ill, and aged persons, early in the development of social organization." Within the last half century many homes for the blind have either closed or changed in character. Confronted with the changing social welfare concepts and practices, new techniques in rehabilitation and protective services, many workers for the blind have become aware of the lessening need for specialized residental facilities. The younger blind people today have been able to avail themselves of increased opportunities within their own communities. Eisenberg continues, "At the same time, as longevity in the United States has continued to increase, blindness has become an increasing characteristic of old age, and simultaneously with improved preventive methods, especially among young people, the blind population has become, to a significant degree, characterized by advanced age. It cannot be repeated too often that more than 50 per cent of blind people are over 55 with an estimate of some 200,000 total in this category. About 2,000 blind people live in homes for the blind."

On January 1, 1966, The Minneapolis Society for the Blind implemented a Vocational Rehabilitation Administration Project staffed to assist in "phasing out" a home for the blind. This staff (social worker, orientation-mobility specialist, home teacher, recreation therapist, occupational therapist, and Project director) coordinated the relocation of 60 blind people into 18 community facilities (board and care, foster care, and nursing homes) as well as apartments and board and room resources. As a result of contracting these facilities, we identified another 59 visually impaired individuals who had no previous contact with an agency for the blind.

Mr. Eisenberg[2] goes on to say, "one cannot exhaust the list of hypothetical statements, such as: (1) blind people prefer to be with other people; (2) blind people benefit from association with other blind people; (3) integration into the sighted community and social relationships with sighted people are enriching experiences for blind people; (4) elderly people prefer to remain in their own neighborhoods and familiar surroundings." We know our society has some very definite prejudices about blindness and this appears to be amplified with elderly blind persons.

Froistad[3] says:

> Housing is particularly significant to the general well-being of individuals tied to their immediate surroundings; that is, the very elderly, individuals with crippling conditions which limit mobility and blind persons who cannot travel independently. Many such individuals, who also have limited incomes, are literally captives of their immediate surroundings. Travel training may free the physically active blind person but there are also many who cannot benefit to any great degree from such instruction. When the environment in which individuals must pass their lives is particularly uncongenial, their lives may truly be hardly worth living.

Froistad goes on to say that some of the things that workers for the blind (as well as volunteers, board members, and the general public) should be concerned about regarding our cultural concept of services to the blind in the community are such facts as these:

1. Elderly blind and visually handicapped persons have mainly become blind in later years. Their interests are identical with interests of other contemporaries who have sight, but who probably have some other disability. They do not want to be separated from people of similar interests and taste.

2. The dependency of elderly visually impaired persons varies greatly. They may be far less dependent and require considerably less care than a contemporary, for example, who is badly crippled, has a severe bladder problem, has lost his memory, or is a chronic complainer.

3. Housing blind persons separately aggravates their disability because they have the same problem—they can't see. When housed with elderly sighted persons among homes, they will normally number less than one out of ten and there will always be someone who is happy to serve as the blind person's eyes. A blind person may have more physical strength, better hearing, or better memory than his friends and will be able to share these assets with his sighted contemporaries.

In Minneapolis we have found that services must be available to the staff of facilities where elderly visually impaired people are residing. If services to these persons are not available plus followup training for staff in the facilities, one of two things usually happens. (1) The blind person is not permitted to participate in activities because the staff is fearful of working with visually impaired people or unsure of how they can involve them; or (2) The blind person is given so much assistance and overprotection that his participation is very artificial and of no benefit to him.

In Cincinnati, at the Clovernook Home and School for the Blind, Froistad[4] identified a reversal of the trend away from a combined sheltered shop and residence; and he noted that, in two years, the workshop doubled the number of persons employed. The home no longer accepts elderly persons for residential care but limits its service to those who are employable and gives preference to individuals with multiple handicaps. In cooperation with the Cincinnati Association for the Blind, which provides social casework services for the blind in the greater Cincinnati area, elderly blind persons are given help in finding suitable housing in the community.

In 1961, Berg and Burchslag[5] conducted a health study of the residents in the Parkview Home, Rose Eisenberg Memorial, in Chicago.

> The population consisted of 134 men and women with an average age of 80 years. Through their diagnostic program they estimated about one-third of their residents, about 44 in number, had some problem with sight, varying in degree of severity. In this group there are 29 women and 15 men, about eight of whom could be considered legally blind. All these residents consider themselves limited visually

> and for this reason they restrict their activities. It is more important that we identify that the entire pattern of the Parkview Home was fashioned for sighted people—the staff as well as the residents, expect people to see, and they function on this assumption. Visual problems are regarded as isolated phenomena. We see more and more that this is a fallacy. Visual impairment often accompanies and is part of general physical deterioration and to understand this is basic to any ongoing program.

Berg and Burchslag found that their diagnostic acuity was inaccurate because they lacked knowledge and understanding of the refinements of the problem. They asked these questions:

1. What are the differences, if any, of which we must be aware, and in what areas do they lie?

2. Do we sufficiently understand the significance of the great loss sustained by a person with diminishing vision complicated with aging?

3. What are the attitudes that prevail now and how can they be classified?

4. Are there changes in the relationship with other people? How are these changes manifested?

5. What is meant by "adjustment" of these people to their handicap?

I would add: where do we need the most emphasis for services to the family, the peer group, or the client? Is there a greater problem of the sighted peer group in society adjusting to visual loss than the adjustment of the individual himself?

Berg and Burchslag[6] report that they believe older blind people can live adequately and become an integrated part of the program of nursing homes, with more effective planning indicated in the following areas:

1. A precise medical diagnosis of visual disability with specific recommendations for physical and social planning at time of admission is a basic requirement.

2. A continuing program of staff training and orientation at all levels, from maintenance to professional, is needed to help the staff understand the nature of the problem and how they can most helpfully interact with the residents in every phase of the daily routine.

3. There is a need to strengthen and utilize all techniques in all departments so that the resident with the visual problem can be included in normal activity programming in the home.

Regarding longitudinal studies varying from 20 to 40 years in duration for the aging person as well as the blind, I think Doctor Fromm's[7] reply to aging is most interesting: "I must admit if someone called me an old fool I wouldn't mind so much; half of the statement is a fact, the other half is at least debatable. However, if you would call me a *senior citizen,* I would feel quite uneasy because it is one of those terms which seem to cover up something very embarrassing and shameful." As one talks about the psychological problems of aging, this is the first question we have to answer: Is old age something embarrassing? Is it a painful stage on the way out which should be sugar-coated with all sorts of words, or is it just a stage of life like adolescence, like infancy, like middle-age, and is the problem not the same as it is with all stages of living; namely, how do we live and how are we most alive in that particular stage?

I believe we can give every opportunity to the visually impaired aging individual that is available to the sighted aging individual, but we should emphasize those services that are necessary to permit maximum participation and independence within their environment. In Minneapolis we are attempting to demonstrate how a specialized community services staff operating out of an agency for the blind can meet the needs of blind people through (1) client services, (2) family services, and (3) agency or staff inservice training sessions structured to meet the needs of the aging blind person living in community facilities (training facility staff in such things as personal management, crafts, recreation, self-care, and basic orientation-mobility concepts), enabling them to provide ongoing service. In an effort to determine the major disability before considering the amount and type of services the aging blind person can benefit from, we also evaluate the impairment as it relates to other disabilities.

According to Doctor Gilbert,[8]

> research on aging shows that there is a gradual physical deterioration of all organs and systems of the body. The result is a decline in efficient functioning of the body—organs become sluggish in their activity, reactions slow down, and endurance lessens. Due to changes in the sensory organs, arteriosclerosis, and perhaps also some changes in the brain and nervous system, losses occur in hearing, and in the senses of taste, touch, smell and balance. Although the eye is one of the most efficient organs of the body, changes occur here also.
>
> Normally, with advancing age, there is a loss of orbital fat and

of water in the tissues. The eyelids become thinner and lose their elasticity; the color of the iris fades, the pupil becomes smaller, and the pupillary reaction slower, the cornea loses its transparency and luster, and the fibers thicken. Increasing amounts of inert, desiccated tissue become concentrated in the center of the lenses and the rate of growth declines, leading to decreased accommodation. The retina becomes thinner and denser, and often atrophy occurs in the periphery and optic nerve. The sclera becomes desiccated, thinner and denser, and loses elasticity which results in increased ocular rigidity. Increased interstitial tissues and thickening of the arteries are common; calcification and thickening of blood vessels may cause far-sightedness and cataracts. These degenerative changes increase as age advances and lead to a gradual decline of all measurable visual functions. Because of the decreased accommodation, it becomes more and more difficult to focus at near points; the visual field narrows; critical foveal flicker decreases; visual acuity is lessened; speed of adaptation decreases; and color matching becomes more difficult.

What are the variables that would decrease the rate of deterioration? What effect do insults suffered through life—the accidents, the injuries, the illnesses—have upon the organs, the systems, and the individual himself? When sight is lost, either at an early age or later in life, what happens to the remaining sensory functions in the periods of later maturity and old age? Does the older blind person retain his auditory acuity better than the older sighted person, or maintain better his ability to interpret auditory clues because of his continued enforced use of this mode of communication? Or does he find the effort too great and tend to withdraw into himself thus accelerating his normally expected decline?

Does the loss of sight accelerate or retard the normally expected deterioration with age in the sensory functions areas? In his study of tactual perception in younger and older, sighted and blind subjects, Frank Catalano attempted "to determine first whether stereognosis is more acute in younger persons than older persons; second, to learn whether this faculty is better developed in blind than in sighted subjects; and finally, to determine specifically whether those older blind subjects, who in the absence of vision have been necessarily forced to use their tactual perception, would show less decline in this area than the older sighted subjects who have never needed to exercise this function."

Results showed that although the individuals differed widely, older persons, on the whole, performed significantly less well on tasks of tactual perception than younger persons, regardless of whether they were blind or sighted. There was no significant difference between the performances of male and female subjects, regardless of whether they were blind or sighted or between performances with the right and left hands. Younger sighted and blind subjects performed similarly on these tasks. Older blind subjects tended to do less well on tasks of tactual perception than older sighted subjects. However, further analysis of these differences suggests that the relative inferiority of the older blind group was due primarily to poor performances of those who were institutionalized. These differences were not evident when the non-institutionalized older blind persons were compared with the older sighted group, none of whom were institutionalized. As well as could be determined, all of these subjects had cutaneous and proprioceptive sensations so that we must assume that much of the loss is probably central in origin. While we have no certain knowledge of any definite brain lesion, there are here sufficient indications of brain changes to suggest that more astereognosis* exists among older people than among younger persons, regardless of whether they are blind or sighted. Probably some of this astereognosis is the result of normal aging process, some of it is the acceleration of deterioration by disease and also by the decline of opportunity, interest, and effort. This last was most evident in the institutionalized group which is necessarily a more protected group, with more limited opportunity for development of initiative.

The institutional variable is parallel with the findings in Minneapolis. Of the 60 blind people relocated from an institution for the blind (44 of the 60 were more than 50 years of age), the following observations were made:

1. Fifty-five per cent, or 33 persons, moved into more independent living situations upon relocation. Thirty-three per cent, or 20 persons, remained at the same level of independence; and 12 per cent, or 11 persons, moved into a less independent setting.

2. Fifty per cent of the former blind residents are now living in more independent situations than either the board and care or nursing care classification.

3. Thirty-five per cent of the group over 65 had moved into more independent living situations. However, 50 per cent of this group over 65 moved into less independent living situations.

The conclusions were:

These people had the potential for more independent living, but functioned at a less independent level as a result of segregation into a

* "Stereognosis" is the faculty of perceiving and understanding the form and nature of an object by touch; astereognosis is the loss of this faculty. Astereognosis is the result of a lesion in the brain and is diagnosable only when cutaneous and proprioceptive sensations are intact.

housing situation for the blind. When faced with the necessity of moving, they chose a more independent situation either as a result of motivation through counseling services, or because they did not choose to live in existing community facilities providing similar care.

Upon leaving the home, half of the residents over 65 seemed to decrease in independence. Is this simply due to the process of aging, or is it the result of emotional hardship of such a change in an older person's life after living at one location for between five and ten years? At the same time many individuals in this age group are now living happy, active lives.

How much can the other senses cooperate and reinforce each other to compensate for the loss of sight? Is this more evident in those who remain in the community and lead active lives than in those who live in institutional environments where they are looked after, sheltered, and protected? What kind of work can older blind persons do? What factors do other diseases play, such as arteriosclerosis, which may have caused blindness and which also affects other organs and systems of the body in such a way as to intensify and accelerate the total process of deterioration? Is there a loss of important means of orientation that will affect the functioning of the brain of the older person? How does the lack of communication and orientation further weaken the already declining memory and learning ability? Are senile disorders more prevalent among blind persons than among sighted persons? In providing services such as psychotherapy or group counseling, will the older blind individual respond better in a group composed solely of blind and sighted persons; in a group of the same sex; in a group of both men and women; or in a group just of the blind? [9]

Although emphasis in society is on an early retirement age, it was our observation while phasing out a home for the blind in Minneapolis during the last year, that six people between the ages of 50 and 65 improved their status through homebound employment. Two people over 65 are employed in active homebound employment. Those people who improved their employment status did so because:

1. They had the potential but needed some specialized services.

2. They were functioning at a less independent level because fewer demands were placed on them in a segregated housing situation.

All of the residents that have increased their status in both employment and housing have taken advantage of some part of the community services offered through the Vocational Rehabilitation Administration Project.

Before launching into future set programs, we must attempt to answer some important questions either through demonstration or research.

In his paper prepared for this Consultation, Cohen cites Kent who raises the question, "Is independence indeed a goal of older people?" If independence is not indeed a goal of older people, then we would think the amplification of dependence would result when blindness is present. However, if the opposite is true, then older blind persons would benefit from structured services in the same amount and quality as anyone else. As Kent continues: "because the role of older people and their adjustment to society is so much a factor of cultural values and the status accorded to the aged, by the society at large, some investigators have given high priority to the inquiry of the issue of the value system." It would seem even more important in dealing with the stereotyped concepts that society has about blindness and its implications. I believe we must consider the same basic considerations in the aging sighted person, as suggested by Cohen:

1. Definition of conditions and events affecting the individual.

2. Developing systems for determining prevalence or incidence.

3. Determination of gross characteristics of those affected—including sex, marital status, economic status, geographical location, and so on.

If it is true that planned segregated facilities, such as housing developments with various types of physical care accommodations, are meeting the needs of the aging population, then, with some evaluation and addition of special services, the aging blind person, I believe, could well benefit from these same facilities in our communities. Is an institutional setting or a rehabilitation facility necessary for the multiply-handicapped older blind persons, or can these services be administered through community services, specialized staff, and inservice training of existing staff in community facilities? I think even more important with the aging blind person than with the aging person, is the conscious effort to change the cultural attitude toward this group. As Cohen observes, this implies the analysis of those attitudes, determination of their sources, determination of those elements which are susceptible to change, and then the establishment of programs that produce the change.

I have implied numerous research possibilities in this paper but would suggest the following examples for a starting point.

1. There exist in the aged blind population (at least) three distinct groups: (1) those who are congenitally blind; (2) those who lost sight in teenage years or before the age of 50; (3) those who lost their sight after age 50.

Groups could be differentiated by comparing them as to a number of different variables (that is, IQ, education, length of active employment, personality measures, degree of "independence"—this would have to be operationally defined) at which people are currently operating, number and kind of other physical disabilities, type of housing, and extent of rehabilitation services received in the past.

2. Assuming the differences as stated in (1) above, a study to determine if the needs of the aging blind really differ significantly from those of the sighted geriatric population.

3. A study to determine where the major emphasis of services should be found: (1) client, (2) family, (3) peer group, (4) staff in local community agencies and facilities, or (5) a combination of all, with increased emphasis on (3) and (4) rather than on (1) and (2).

NOTES

1. Arthur Eisenberg, "Perspectives on Living Arrangements for Blind People," *New Outlook for the Blind,* Vol. 58, October, 1964, 233–235.
2. *Ibid.*
3. William M. Froistad, "Housing and Aspects of Services to the Blind," *New Outlook for the Blind,* Vol. 58, October, 1964, 239–243.
4. *Ibid.*
5. Mary Berg and Betty Burchslag, "Observations on Visually Handicapped Residents in a Geriatric Setting," *New Outlook for the Blind,* Vol. 58, October, 1964, 243–245.
6. *Ibid.*
7. Erich Fromm, "Psychological Problems of Aging," *Journal of Rehabilitation,* Vol. 32, September–October, 1966, 10–13.
8. Jeanne Gilbert, "Old Age and Blindness—Research Needs," *New Outlook for the Blind,* Vol. 59, February, 1965, 49–51.
9. *Ibid.*

SESSION REPORT

Gian Sarup

After the reading of the analyst paper, Commissioner Elias Cohen made a number of specific recommendations for research into the problems of the aged blind. In view of the striking fact that approximately half of the blind population is in the age category of 50+ years, he expressed belief that the problem of blindness in old age could be profitably studied through an epidemiological approach. Numerical data regarding distribution of an impairment are a prerequisite to the planning of service delivery systems. In agreeing with Melvin E. Saterbak's suggestion, Commissioner Cohen proposed longitudinal and comparative studies on characteristic problems of different segments of the blind population, such as the congenitally blind, the persons who became blind during childhood or adolescence, and the visually handicapped during old age.

The impact of visual impairment on old age adjustment needs to be investigated, along with the interrelated effects of multiple handicaps. Another area that merits attention for research is the realm of social values and attitudes towards blindness that render the afflicted person non-productive in a utility-oriented culture. Research efforts should also be directed towards identifying the psychological meaning of old age among the blind and of blindness among the elderly. In the direction of these (and other) recommended areas of research concerning the aged blind, Commissioner Cohen drew attention to the availability, for research purposes, of a captive population in health and care institutions.

Charles Gallozzi pointed out the misuse of the word "blindness" for the partial loss of vision among the aged, and cautioned researchers to be conscious of the differences in the problem and need patterns of those who have been totally and incurably blind among the aged and those suffering from partial disabilities of vision in old age. Accordingly, J. O. Murphy stressed the need for a differential adjustment of welfare services for the blind and the visually handicapped sections of the aged population; and Dr. Norman M. Yoder pointed out that the adjustment problems of the person with residual vision can often be more acute than the ones faced by the totally blind. A related observation on this point was offered by Dr. Donald P. Kent to the effect that in identifying primary disability in a person, there is a tendency to ignore the other handicaps, and he wanted service delivery systems to take cognizance of this widespread practice while dispensing services to the handicapped.

Mr. Saterbak mentioned the often encountered resistance among the visually handicapped elderly people to becoming identified with the blind population, and their resulting disinclination to avail themselves of the services offered by agencies for the blind. Dr. Douglas C. MacFarland, therefore, underlined the need for an action program geared to educate the public on blindness and, thus, to remove the stigma associated with blindness in the public mind. He suggested that the emotional blockage towards blindness might be appreciably reduced through an educational (public relations) effort such as that done by workers in the area of mental sickness. Mr. Gallozzi offered the semantic solution of dropping the emotionally charged word, "blindness," in favor of a relatively neutral term like "visually handicapped" to describe persons who have suffered only a partial loss of visual capacity, but at this stage in the discussion various participants pointed out practical difficulties in fund raising if the descriptive label were changed.

Referring to Dr. Robert J. Teare's enquiry about the possible problems that welfare departments would like to see researched, Commissioner Cohen referred to the need for information on differential utilization of services by various segments of the handicapped population, especially the underprivileged sections, so as to adjust service delivery systems to population needs. Systematic information concerning incidence and prevalence of blindness and visual disorders and disabilities among the institutionalized sick, and about the extent and quality of facilities available to the visually impaired, could also be of use to welfare departments.

Mr. Gallozzi raised the problem of determining the special reading needs of the blind, a subject which deserves research effort. He regarded the method of acquiring reading material in the libraries on the basis of requests received from a few articulate blind persons as essentially inadequate to cater to the needs of the entire category of the aged blind.

Dr. Elena D. Gall recommended interdisciplinary collaboration to understand the problems of the aged blind. She also underscored the desirability of first-hand experience on the part of researchers with the population they seek to study. Dr. Clayton Morgan recommended the desired role of empathic insights by the researcher into the problems of the blind; and he, additionally, advocated the necessity of bringing into the research enterprise the techniques and experiential insights of some of the knowlegeable people from the aged blind population. The visually handicapped having the necessary skills should be associated actively with research.

Commissioner Cohen observed that generational differences among the aged blind are likely to be increasingly marked, and need to be carefully studied. Shanas' observation that a sizable portion of the aged population is fairly well adjusted, in contrast to the dismal picture of their lot painted in current gerontology, gave rise to a number of points concerning the nature of subjective and environmental factors that facilitate satisfactory adjustment of some individuals in the face of aging and gradual physical impairment including visual losses. Research should be directed to the dynamics of adjustment among the aged blind.

Joseph Kohn wanted the needs of the aged blind to be more fully researched especially since the concentration of services was currently on the younger age groups among the blind. This emphasis would, in his view, bring the service programs in contact with a relatively neglected segment of the blind population.

Dr. Kent made the concluding recommendation for a functional definition of the blind and for the necessity of a multidisciplinary perspective and experimental involvement in future research into problems related to the aged blind.

CHILDHOOD AND ADOLESCENCE

NEEDED RESEARCH ON ADOLESCENTS: SEEING AND BLIND

Carolyn W. Sherif

This article treats problems of research on human beings during a crucial period of their lives, roughly between the ages of eleven or twelve years and nineteen or so. With reference to problems of blindness, its implications are restricted, therefore, to those individuals whose sight is impaired before or during those years. Because the author is a social psychologist, the focus is on problems of social behavior and motivation.

In a world whose views of the human condition are already fragmented by academic and practical specialties, additional slicing into age periods may seem needless butchery. On the contrary, integrated accounts of a period in human development must of necessity utilize concepts and research methods from the several academic disciplines. The adolescent period is a particularly fertile field for interdisciplinary integration in theory and research.

Adolescence is a period of singular significance in human development. True, the child is father of the man. But in modern societies, physiological maturation after childhood is accompanied by a period of social transition with profound consequences for the remaining decades of life. Whether the individual reaches this period advantaged or disadvantaged, sighted or blind, secure or insecure, he still must cope with the challenge and the obstacles produced by his changing body in a world reluctant to grant adult status.

The ways in which the transition is accomplished are significant for the individual's future, at least on a par with events during childhood. The currently renewed interest in the significance of early childhood, particularly in intellectual development, should not obscure the decisive importance of the adolescent period, especially in motivational-emotional spheres and decision-making that affects the way in which intellectual achievements will be utilized.

THE TRANSITION FROM CHILDHOOD TO ADULTHOOD IN MODERN SOCIETIES

With a decade or so of life behind, and five or six more years to go, the growing child starts to develop physically into an adult. Society recognizes the physical changes by according the individual a new standing vis-à-vis his fellow humans. While puberty marks its onset, *adolescence* is defined, even in the dictionary, as a period of social change—a transition period from boyhood or girlhood to adulthood.

The events and problems of adolescence vary enormously in different cultural and socio-economic settings. In nearly all societies, however, there are two sets of universals: (1) A more rapid pace of growth toward adult physique accompanied by pronounced hormonal and metabolic changes associated with sexual maturation. (2) Changes in the individual's position relative to others with accompanying shifts in responsibilities, activities, and behavior in the direction of adult autonomy as it is defined in the particular social milieu.

The adolescent's body tells him that he is changing, and others notice it, also. Expectations of his family, his teachers, his friends, and even the compelling images from the mass media depicting his age group begin to change. He is expected to be more responsible, at least in the conduct of routine activities and self care.

The adolescent is not expected to be as dependent upon parents and other adults as he was in childhood but is expected to start acting more "grownup." These changes require that the individual redefine his relationship to his world. If he did not, despite adult appearance, his behavior would retain the dependency on adults.

In short, the adolescent period in modern societies presents the individual with the problem of reformulating the relationships between self and significant other people. This is the fundamental psychological problem of adolescence and it is a problem of general importance in theories of human behavior: the formation and change of the self concept.[1]

Fortunately, the physiological changes and the new social demands of adolescence occur when cognitive and intellectual development are well advanced. Although by no means consistent in all areas, the adolescent who has achieved secondary school status has shifted from the predominantly concrete to a more abstract mode of cognitive functioning.[2] At least in those domains where he has a working body of higher-order, "inclusive" concepts, the adolescent is equipped to learn more rapidly, more intensively and in greater quantity through verbal means rather than drill, practice, and concrete experiences.

Thus equipped intellectually and affectively, the adolescent begins the process of reforming his conceptions of himself relative to parents and other adults, the opposite sex, and to many groups and institutions. The process does not occur overnight. First one, then other sets of attitudes defining what he is and is not are called to question: how he relates to others, what he is expected to do and not to do, where he belongs as a person. Many of these self attitudes project him toward the future, embodying goals that he wants to pursue.

Shaken and moved by profound biochemical and structural changes in his own body, what does the adolescent learn about who he is from the adults around him? In most industrialized societies, the growing youth faces a period of years during which he is neither child nor adult. Socially and economically, he is defined as preparing for adulthood, but he is actually betwixt-and-between for a prolonged period. Adult treatments are contradictory from time to time, first approaching the young person as an adult, then reverting to restrictions and protectiveness more appropriate for a child.

The adolescent period produces a dilemma for the individual to the extent that it is a prolonged transition with unclear or unsatisfactory procedures for progressing to adult status, privilege, and responsibility. In modern societies, adolescence has been aptly called a period of "psychological weaning" from dependence on parents and adults. Yet how rapidly and in what areas such weaning is to occur are seldom clear.

Adolescents can, and do, turn to adults for guidance. But there is a rift between the generations, produced by social change and by the enormous complexity of modern social life. The rift is more marked than a gradual weaning from dependence on adults, even though it need not involve overt conflict between the generations. The perspective of adulthood is different. The problems of adolescence do not seem as urgent to adults as they do to youth themselves. Their counsel to plan for the future, work and wait is no solution to what is so pressing here and now.

If their environment holds no solution to their predicament, psychological relief may be sought in fantasy, day dreams, and retreat to private worlds. Such retreats were so typical half a century ago that the diary and the religious conversion furnished the student of adolescence in this country with a rich source of data. But in modern societies, the schemes for school, community, and social life have changed. The adolescent moves and is exposed to a great deal of information about them. Soon, he finds that he is not alone: his age-mates are in much the same boat.

Thus the adolescent moves toward his age-mates, more intensely, more frequently and more significantly than in childhood.[3] The actual movement toward age-mates is symptomatic of a general shift from the strong ties of dependence upon adults in childhood to intense concern with how one stacks up with other adolescents.

Problems of being accepted, of belonging, of being recognized or being ignored by age-mates become major concerns. To be neglected, rejected, or scorned at a time when one's self identity is changing is a painful experience that the adolescent will go to great lengths to avoid. When coupled with an earlier history of insecure ties with family and other groups, the experience may impel an almost frantic search for belongingness some place with someone, and at almost any price.[4]

Adolescence in modern societies, then, involves an important shift in the person's self and identification with others toward more intense and more significant involvement with his own generation. For the time being, the youth's conception of self is linked firmly in the domain of other adolescents. *Their* standards and guidelines become more salient in defining how *I-as-a-person* stack up. *They* become the reference set providing standards for deciding whether *I* am normal, average, superior, or inferior.

Implications of the General Picture

The challenge of adolescence and the dilemmas it presents resemble those facing a person blinded at any age: changing important aspects of one's self conception relative to others, gaining and accepting responsibility for self, shifting from dependence toward independence, increasing mobility without direct supervisory care, gaining skills for future use. The blind adolescent faces problems associated with blindness concurrently with similar problems of transition to adult status. Lest we leap to the conclusion that the blind adolescent is, therefore, necessarily confronted by crushing problems, let us look again at the general picture of adolescence.

The physiological and social changes of adolescence shake the individual's self identity as formed in childhood, but this very flux produces a willingness, even eagerness for change, for establishing new bearings. It is a time ripe for new activities, new efforts, the formation of new attitudes, and the setting of new goals. Further, the level of cognitive and intellectual functioning attained by and during adolescence permits more rapid acquisition of skills and concepts, some theorists believe much more rapid and extensive than current educational practices encourage.[5] Finally, the deep concern and interest in age-mates widens the possible arenas for independent and autonomous activity.

Thus, if he has not already learned too well from people in his surroundings that a blind person must forever be totally dependent on others for care and support, the blind child entering adolescence begins a period that can be conducive to attaining special skills and experiences needed to compensate for his undeniable handicap in becoming an independent adult man or woman.

At the same time, he enters adolescence classed by most people around him as a special kind of person, socially defined as helpless and dependent, apparently by many rehabilitation workers as well as by other adults and peers.[6] Very probably he requires assistance in many activities considered normal for his age. He faces a future in which the "opportunity structure" in work and many other areas of living[7] differs from that for a sighted person in the same social setting. The probability for heterosexual attachment and eventual marriage differs, particularly if the blind person is a girl.[8] A blind adolescent faces a special set of problems with great significance for his transition to adulthood. His sensory deficiency is only one side of the coin, for the expectations of adults and age-mates with whom he interacts daily may impose even more rigid handicaps.

SOME PITFALLS IN THEORY AND RESEARCH ON ADOLESCENTS

Traditionally, academic fashions have tended to center around one factor or set of factors made prominent by an influential theorist or research program. Especially in recent years, such fads and fashions in academic and research circles have reflected the availability of research funds on behavior problems of social concern. Utilization of the "opportunity structure" for research support by psychologists and social scientists has had many salutary effects. It has also produced theoretical confusion and a good deal of research hastily conceived and executed. In some ways, therefore, a problem area stands a better chance of receiving integrated treatment if it does *not* become a popular topic for specialized inquiry, particularly if that popularity defines the problem area as unique and unrelated to previous research of general import. For example, it would be most unfortunate if problems of blindness for adolescents were to be treated as entirely new problems, unrelated to problems of adolescence or of blindness in general.

Forty years ago, the study of adolescent behavior and the adolescent period focused on growth and the I.Q., undeniably important concepts for research. However, these concepts are not adequate alone to deal with the problems of social behavior during adolescence, as shown by Harold and Mary Cover Jones and their associates[9] in their documentation of social interaction among adolescents studied longitudinally in the California growth studies. The popularity of psychodynamic concepts focused interest on the disturbed adolescent and on the family, an area of traditional interest among sociologists as well. For a time, one could easily conclude that the vicissitudes of family life and child rearing practices of early childhood were the only key to unlock problems of adolescent behavior.

This emphasizes the following points: The behavioral and social sciences are new and unevenly developed. Any adequate theory, hence research on human behavior during adolescence, has to include the multiple influences that are known from previous research to affect development and to exert their effects *interdependently,* not in one-step causation. This means that theory and research must view the individual within his sociocultural environment and specific locations, in relation to the groups of people who *count* for him (family, teachers, age-mates), and in terms of his own particular background and personal tendencies—as all of these relate to one another.

For years, there have been prominent theorists on social behavior and development who have emphasized that individual behavior has to be studied within its concrete social milieu which, in turn, is related to a larger sociocultural setting. Here it is sufficient to mention the names of Charles H. Cooley, G. H. Mead, W. I. Thomas, and Robert Park in sociology, and of James M. Baldwin, F. C. Bartlett, Kurt Lewin, Gardner Murphy, and Muzafer Sherif in social psychology.

What is needed are concepts, research procedures, and measurements capable of integrating the character of the individual's day-to-day interaction with others in matters related to his desires and cherished goals with the values and images of success or failure prevailing among those people, and their circumstances within the larger social scheme. Anything less than the attempt to meet this research challenge will yield partial or distorted pictures of the factors affecting adolescent development and behavior.

Guidelines from Recent Research Trends

Recent research on adolescents has exhibited certain trends that are conducive to an integrated approach to adolescent behavior and that are applicable in study of the blind.[10] These trends will be stated briefly, then illustrated in more detail with specific examples.

1. There is a trend away from the study of particular attitudes, interests, and personality characteristics as discrete elements determining behavior, and toward the study of significant clusters as parts of the individual's self system that are subject to change and are manifest in concrete reactions to and interactions in definite social environments.[11]

2. Correspondingly, self–other attitudes and goals have been explicitly related to sociocultural values, socio-economic level, and institutional arrangements that affect both the nature and the content of interaction involving adolescents and adults. In recognition of the multiple environmental influences on adolescents, the developing research trend is toward identifying the particular pattern of influences through multivariate analysis and through various combinations of data gathering procedures.[12]

3. Renewed interest and actual research operations have been applied to specific study of adolescent behavior as it occurs in interaction situations within institutional settings[13] and in the company of age-mates constituting reference groups, that is, groups to which the adolescent belongs or aspires to belong.[14]

By far the most needed research on adolescent behavior is that focused upon the specific interaction episodes over a period of time among adolescents and with adults. A few examples will suffice to illustrate the possible reward, as well as the problems of such research.

In attempting to compare the educational and vocational aspirations of Maori and European youth in New Zealand, Ausubel[15] administered a battery of paper-and-pencil tests to matched samples of Maori and non-Maori adolescents in urban and rural environments. The samples were matched according to school class, ability group in school, and father's occupation. The test battery was designed to tap aspirations, achievement motives, and various supportive personality traits. Ausubel did find differences between rural and urban adolescents. However, unexpectedly, within the rural and urban samples the test results for the Maori and non-Maori youth were remarkably similar, despite the fact that the Maori drop-out rate from school at 15 years of age is high and that few Maoris actually pursue the skilled trades and professions to which his subjects aspired.

By additional study of Maori community life and parent–youth relations, Ausubel was able to spell out the reasons for the apparent contradiction between aspirations and actual performance. Although acculturated to the educational and occupational goals of Europeans in school, Maori youth spend their free time in a context that is not supportive of sustained effort toward those goals. Parents put few pressures on the youth for achievement, and less support or encouragement. Relationship with peers, which is highly valued in Maori culture, requires considerable time and effort for the conduct of interpersonal relations as a group member, with little reward or recognition of individual achievement. Thus, by viewing the adolescent Maori in give-and-take with those who count most in his eyes in community and at school, the apparent contradiction between high goals and low achievement became intelligible. This analysis of the discrepancy between acceptance of goals for achievement and their translation into action is, by the way, remarkably similar to findings on Spanish-speaking youth in the United States.[16]

The family, and especially the parents, once received all credit or blame for the desirable or undesirable behavior patterns and high or low aspirations of their adolescent offspring. Recent research is indicating more and more that family influences are seldom isolated determinants.

For example, Rosenberg reported that self-esteem was lower among adolescents whose parents divorced in Catholic or Jewish families, but not in Protestant families.[18] High parental stress on college attendance is closely related to girls' decisions to attend college, but negatively associated with boys' plans.[19] Effects of working mothers on adolescent attitudes depend on socio-economic class of the family.[20] While occupational choice is related to family status and strivings for mobility, it is also related to choice of age-mate friends.[21] Clearly, research focus on family relationships is important but provides only part of the picture.

Among the influences that become very important in adolescence research are the socio-economic level and facilities of the specific setting in which the individual develops. While the family reflects differences in this respect, the family setting does not exhaust the situations in which the adolescent is exposed to the advantages and limitations of his socio-economic milieu. By the time youths reach adolescence, the level of aspiration for education, in work, and for various aspects of success in life varies according to the socio-economic level of their neighborhoods, of the particular school they attend (whether this be lower or higher than their location of residence), and of the particular age-mates with whom they associate.[22] A reasonable deduction from the large body of research available is that adolescents who pursue high aspirations are typically exposed to family values, neighborhood and community influences, schools and age-mates that are largely congruent with such efforts. Contrary to some popular belief, the aspirations of lower class youth are not uniformly low. However, the best available studies to date indicate that those pursuing high goals through appropriate preparatory steps are more likely to be found attending middle class schools, to have friends who are middle class, and to be exposed to parental influence toward upward mobility.

Experimental work on level of aspiration indicates that when an individual sees a great discrepancy between his ability and the tasks required of him, or between a standard of performance and his past experience in attaining such a standard, he is likely to lower his goals. In cases where ability level is actually too low to achieve the standard, this is a realistic solution. However, there is more to the problem.

We are now aware that many lower class youth performing poorly in school, for example, could attain higher levels of performance if given opportunity and if willing to sustain the necessary effort. We know that a large proportion of youth who drop out of school at the legal age or shortly thereafter are no more deficient on standard tests than many who complete high school and some who continue to college. We are prone to attribute such failures to psychological causation: to lack of character, to "weak ego," to emotional instability.

Such attribution may be correct by the time the final drama is played. But what led to the unfortunate climax, to giving up, to retiring and withdrawing? Surely in relation to problems of blind adolescents, this is the question that calls for answers through research, as it is in general. What engenders the acceptance of high challenge? What sustains persistence in difficult tasks over time? What produces shrinking from difficulty and possible failure, even when improvement and eventual attainment are possible?

Particularly during adolescence, when one's self concept is in flux, contradictions between goals and means to reach them, between what is practiced and what is preached, between encouragement from one source and lack of encouragement from another are keenly experienced. Who and what should he or she believe and make an effort to pursue? Everyone, particularly during adolescence, needs some social support from people who really count for him, in maintaining some self esteem, and even in maintaining a modicum of psychological stability. Never to have had such support or to find it utterly lacking during adolescence leads in many cases to severe psychological disturbance and even to suicide attempts.

Among the important sources affecting the challenges an adolescent will accept, the standards he sets for himself, and his future goals, is his age-mate reference group—those age-mates whose values and opinions and treatments count in his eyes. So powerful is the age-mate climate that at times it can countermand the combined effects of other sources of influence. In a study of *Cottage Six,* a residential unit in a therapeutic milieu designed for delinquent boys, Polsky[23] found that many of the efforts of the psychiatrists, psychologists, and social workers to rehabilitate and educate through regular personal conferences, classes, and other activities were thwarted daily by a system of close interpersonal ties among the boys within the cabin. These ties were based on the principle of rule through toughness and might. They operated informally as a power structure more influential for a boy than his personal therapist. Custodial staff within the cottage, taking their job to be maintenance of order, implicitly cooperated with the adolescent social structure, working through its highest status members and offering small support for the deviant. In subsequent work, Polsky has attempted to contrast different patterns of interaction by the cottage staff as these support or change the boys' relationships within the cottage.[24]

Similarly, in her interviews with institutionalized delinquent girls, conducted only after gaining the girls' confidence, Konopka[25] refers again and again to the importance of age-mate ties with some stability for the maintenance of personal stability. One 17-year-old formed friendships while incarcerated, and sought them out when released. "That is violation of probation rules," she said, "but these are my friends! I know it was a violation but I thought I could get by with it. I *had* to!" The intense emotional significance of her devotion has its obverse in the desolation that Konopka reports of girls who "cease to fight" for some niche with others where they belong. It was they, she noted, who "make suicide attempts or take drugs or start the flight into mental illness."

It seems safe to say that adult treatment and training of adolescents is never more than part of an interaction system, in which the youth's relationships with age-mates represent another major part. This is one implication of the failures in controlled research to demonstrate significant consequences of systematic counseling procedures over fairly long periods, when no concomitant change is made in the day-to-day activities of youths with their peers.[26]

In reporting on the adolescent unit in the psychiatric section of a state hospital, the psychiatrist F. T. Rafferty[27] remarked: "In a relatively tight geographical space with a reasonable staff-patient ratio, it is always a surprise to realize how much behavior is beyond the influence of staff." The boys and girls in this unit were psychologically disturbed and notably lacking in successful experiences with age-mates. Yet, withdrawal from each other or indifference was not characteristic of their behavior. Their preoccupation with one another, translated into rather primitive attempts at domination, is apparent in Rafferty's description of the unit:

> One of the constantly disturbing activities in a unit is the almost continuous testing and shifting of dominance relationships among the youngsters. The aggressive interaction that marks this kind of activity will occur overtly or covertly, depending on staff's reaction to it. . . . A new boy with appropriate dominance equipment can move up the scale and in a matter of a few weeks be challenging the leader. A new girl or a shift in a girl's loyalty will set off a series of changes up and down the ladder. The struggle for dominance at the top of the children's organization flows directly over into the staff. The two or three boys struggling for the number one position will use open challenges to staff as a means of competing. They will usually succeed in acquiring a dominance relationship over a number of staff until they overreach and provoke the staff as a group to make some show of dominance, usually through a disciplinary move.

It is not intended that these descriptions of disturbed and delinquent youth be taken as typical of adolescents and certainly not as comparable to the interaction of blind adolescents with their peers, blind or sighted. They have been included to emphasize the generalization that any research on adolescents that omits specific study of the individual's place among his age-mates and his concrete relationships with them is doomed to give an extremely one-sided view of the influences shaping his conception of himself, the standards he sets for himself, his goals, and his concrete actions related to them.

THE INDIVIDUAL IN THE CONTEXT OF HIS REFERENCE GROUPS

Explicit recognition of the multiple influences on adolescent behavior and the importance of how these influences are patterned led Muzafer Sherif to initiate a research program in 1958 with the aim of developing more adequate research designs and methods for their study.[28] I shall summarize this research in somewhat more detail because it has faced major problems of research method and represents a programmatic attempt to integrate concepts and techniques from several academic disciplines within a single research plan. As a result of this research, we are in a better position than formerly to specify when certain research techniques are useful and when others are required.

The focus of the entire research program was the interaction over a period of time among adolescents who associated informally in activities of their own choosing, that is, small reference groups of agemates. However, the design started with variables quite far removed from these individual adolescents—namely, at the sociocultural level. The neighborhoods where the adolescents lived were assessed and ranked according to socio-economic level, cultural composition, and family status (using the Shevky-Bell analysis). In addition, the character and facilities of the areas were studied and mapped, so that the movements of the youth and the opportunities available in their setting could be specified.

Although far removed conceptually from the concrete behaviors of individuals, this first step proved exceedingly useful. The socio-economic, cultural, and family data provided a basis for understanding many activities of the youths, the moves that had to be made to find a place to meet, and the facilities available. Some of the data on the attitudes and preoccupations of the youth would have been almost unexplainable without this basic sociological and cultural data. For example, one group of Spanish-American boys was entirely uninterested in sports, a phenomenon that made them appear extremely deviant until related to the fact that they came from a neighborhood populated by the newer arrivals from Mexico, the least acculturated to American life. Here, they were not deviant in this respect at all.

Next, within neighborhoods of low, middle, and upper socio-economic rank, representative samples of students were surveyed in schools serving each area. Based on the general finding that during the adolescent period youths are keenly tuned to their own generation, this survey sought to establish the typical values, standards for achievement, and goals prevalent among youths in each area. The instrument designed for this purpose (Self-Radius and Goals Schedule) was a paper-and-pencil questionnaire. In keeping with modern interpretations of the results of such instruments, the findings were viewed as evidence for the conceptions prevailing among youth as to what responses were "socially desirable" in the eyes of adults.[29]

We found that youth's views of the socially desirable did differ according to socio-economic and cultural background, but were not nearly so striking or clear-cut as the theoretical literature on class and subcultural differences might lead one to expect. This important finding is supported in a number of recent studies comparing self-esteem, personal values, goals, and conceptions of acceptable behavior across socio-economic groups.[30] It suggests the hazards in proposing explanations of behavior on the basis of value systems (about blindness, for example) without empirical demonstration that the individual has actually been exposed to such values in give-and-take with others.

The data on prevailing adolescent values and goals, in turn, provided a framework for assessing the attitudes and behaviors of particular small groups of youths who interacted within each neighborhood. They permit answers to such questions as the following: Are these youth representative of the "leading crowd" in their neighborhoods, as Coleman[31] used that phrase in his studies of the social structure in high schools? Are their values and goals representative of the majority of youth with whom they are in contact, or are they highly unrepresentative?

Direct observation of interaction among the youths themselves over periods of from six to nine months was the primary method for data collection on the focal aspect of the research program. The general problem is that they are sophisticated enough to be keenly aware of adults' intentions in studying them and to adapt their behavior to this awareness. When interacting with one another in important or intimate activities, they are highly responsive to even the presence of an outsider, particularly if they know that they are the object of observation.

Accordingly, procedures for data collection were devised to avoid this "research effect." Observers in their early twenties were selected who "fit" into each neighborhood in terms of appearance and background. In brief, their task was to locate a group for study on the basis of their observations of frequent and regular interaction in activities unprogrammed by adults, and without regard to how socially desirable or undesirable these activities might be.

They established a reasonable pretext for being in the neighborhood that would permit contact with the group and provide a basis for establishing rapport at a pace and through means that the group members initiated, not the observer. Despite these precautions, there were some groups so private and so suspicious of outsiders that it was extremely difficult for the observer to secure access.

The observer made regular ratings concerned with the role relationships and prevailing values or norms in the groups. The reliability of these ratings was checked through a combination of other techniques, including ratings by independent observers, sociometric choices, and situational tests introduced naturally after the observer had succeeded in establishing the members' confidence in his integrity or, at least, his harmless intent. These methods demonstrate that significant quantitative data can be collected in natural situations without the artificiality that conventional "tests" and laboratory experiments produce.[32]

Finally, near the conclusion of the study, case history materials were collected on the background of each individual member of the groups. As one might suspect, these materials revealed that the relative importance of an age-mate group to an individual member was a complex interaction of the strength of his ties with family, his success in school and community activities, and his relationships with other groups of age-mates. Competition for status or actual conflict with other groups and pressures from adults typically increased the member's attachment to a group in which he was accepted.

On the basis of intensive study of more than 24 groups in several cities, it is evident that adolescent attitudes and goals are profoundly affected by the interaction process with age-mates. Over a period of time, the informal interaction is patterned into established reciprocities (give-and-take) among the various members and regulated by customs, standards, or norms that all come to share if they are "good" identified members. At times, the consequences were mutually supportive of values promoted by teachers and parents. In other cases, the age-mate group led its members in directions detrimental to the efforts of adults.

IMPLICATIONS FOR NEEDED RESEARCH

The guidelines sketched here are readily applicable to research on problems of blind adolescents. The key to such translation is the study of visually handicapped youth, not in isolation or even as a unique population, but as individuals undergoing the adolescent transition without sight in relation to a world composed largely of the seeing. The research reviewed indicates, first of all, that the socioeconomic and cultural background and the residence of the blind adolescent must be studied as the framework. What are the values and stereotypes about blindness that he encounters in so many concrete instances in his surroundings? What life chances does it offer for a blind adolescent and adult, and how does he view them?

Next, the concrete setting of his training and daily life has to be brought into the picture. What are the values prevailing among staff and students in the residential school he attends or of teachers and students in regular school classes? Specific information on this aspect is sorely needed.

The actual process of building an adult image of self and one's relation to others occurs in the daily give-and-take between youth and adult, between youth and age-mates, between youth as they respond to the concepts of human achievement and success presented through mass media. It is by intensified study of this process *as it takes place over a period of time* that research on adolescents can contribute to problems of the blind and that research on blind adolescents can contribute greatly to our general understanding of adolescent behavior.

With full awareness of obstacles and possible hazards, I propose, however, that the most needed research on adolescent behavior is studies that systematically introduce innovations in the environmental conditions for interaction among adolescents and with adults. Both from naturalistic accounts and from experiments in the field, we know that it is possible to manipulate the environment to produce highly solidaric groups united in cooperative interaction toward common goals.[33] We know that during such interaction, individuals are strongly motivated and mutually supported by their fellow members to attempt and execute highly challenging tasks. We know that during such interactions in cooperative tasks, pre-existing stereotypes and unfavorable attitudes can be changed. Such changes wrought over a period of time through the powerful medium of interaction among blind and sighted adolescents along with concerned adults, might contribute to the re-formation of the self concept in ways beneficial to each. If social agencies charged with responsibility in creating the environments that currently prevail become dissatisfied, the systematic study of controlled changes will become more feasible. In that event, the unfortunate divorce between much current research and current practice can be resolved in common efforts by researchers and practitioners to embark together on viable programs to answer questions significant to each.

NOTES

1. For example see: Muzafer Sherif and Hadley Cantril, *The Psychology of Egoinvolvements* (New York: Wiley, 1966); J. Horrocks, *The Psychology of Adolescence* (Boston: Houghton-Mifflin, 1963); and Muzafer Sherif and Carolyn W. Sherif, *Problems of Youth* (Chicago: Aldine, 1965), chap. 1.
2. Barbel Inhelder and Jean Piaget, *The Growth of Logical Thinking from Childhood to Adolescence* (New York: Basic Books, 1958); and D. P. Ausubel and Pearl Ausubel, "Cognitive Development in Adolescence," *Review of Educational Research,* Vol. 36, No. 4 (1966), chap. 1, 403–413.
3. Pertinent evidence is examined in Muzafer Sherif and Carolyn W. Sherif, *Reference Groups: Exploration into the Conformity and Deviation of Adolescents* (New York: Harper and Row, 1964).
4. Gisella Konopka, *The Adolescent Girl in Conflict* (Englewood Cliffs, New Jersey: Prentice-Hall, 1966).
5. See: Ausubel and Ausubel, "Cognitive Development," *op. cit.*
6. See: R. G. Barker, *Adjustment to Physical Handicap and Illness: A Survey of the Social Psychology of Physique and Disability* (New York: Social Science Research Council, 1953), 277.
7. The term was used in analysis of delinquency, but is equally appropriate for the situation of non-delinquents and the visually handicapped. See: R. H. Cloward and L. E. Ohlin, *Delinquency and Opportunity* (New York: Free Press of Glencoe, 1960).
8. The under-representation of married females in studies of the blind strongly suggests sex differences in opportunity. See: Mary K. Bauman, *Adjustment to Blindness* (Harrisburg: State Council for the Blind, Commonwealth of Pennsylvania, 1954); and Mary K. Bauman, *Characteristics of Blind and Visually Handicapped People in Professional Sales and Managerial Work* (Harrisburg: Pennsylvania Office for the Blind, 1963).
9. For example see: H. E. Jones, *Development in Adolescence* (New York: Appleton-Century, 1943).
10. The following summary of trends is based on the author's survey of research from 1960 to 1965. See: Carolyn W. Sherif, "Adolescence: Motivational Attitudinal and Personality Factors," *Review of Educational Research,* Vol. 36, No. 4 (1966), chap. iv, 437–449.
11. Examples include Sherif and Sherif, *Reference Groups, op. cit.;* and Morris Rosenberg, *Society and the Adolescent Self-Image* (Princeton, New Jersey: Princeton University Press, 1965).
12. Multivariate analysis was used by: Morris Rosenberg, *op. cit.;* Bernice M. Moore and W. H. Holtzman, *Tomorrow's Parents: A Study of Youth and Their Families* (Austin: University of Texas Press, 1965); R. H. Turner, *The Social Context of Ambition* (San Francisco: Chandler, 1964). Combinations of research procedures were used by D. P. Ausubel, *Maori Youth* (Wellington, New Zealand: Price Milburn and Co., 1961); and Sherif and Sherif, *ibid.*
13. For example see: H. W. Polsky, *Cottage Six* (New York: Russell Sage Foundation, 1962); F. T. Rafferty, "Group Organization Theory and the Adolescent Inpatient Unit," Muzafer Sherif and Carolyn W. Sherif, *op. cit.,* chap. 10.
14. See: Sherif and Sherif, *op. cit.;* and J. F. Short and T. L. Strodtbeck, *Group Process and Gang Delinquency* (Chicago: University of Chicago Press, 1965).

15. D. P. Ausubel, *Maori Youth, op. cit.*
16. Sherif and Sherif, *Reference Groups, op. cit.*
17. P. H. Mussen, *et al.*, "The Influence of Father-Son Relationships on Adolescent Personality and Attitudes," *Journal of Child Psychology and Psychiatry,* 4 (April, 1963), 3–16.
18. Morris Rosenberg, *Society and the Adolescent Self-Image, op. cit.*
19. J. D. Bordua, "Educational Aspirations and Parental Stress on College," *Social Forces,* 38 (March, 1960), 262–269.
20. Moore and Holtzman, *Tomorrow's Parents, op. cit.*
21. For example see: A. O. Haller and C. E. Butterworth, "Peer Influences on Levels of Occupational and Educational Aspiration," *Social Forces,* 38 (May, 1960), 289–295; R. L. Simpson, "Parental Influence, Anticipatory Socialization, and Social Mobility," *American Sociological Review,* 27 (August, 1962), 517–522; and G. D. Bell, "Processes in the Formation of Adolescents' Aspirations," *Social Forces,* 42 (December, 1963), 179–195.
22. See: Sherif and Sherif, *Reference Groups, op. cit.;* and R. H. Turner, *The Social Context of Ambition, op. cit.*
23. H. W. Polsky, *Cottage Six, op. cit.*
24. H. W. Polsky and D. S. Claster, "The Structure and Functions of Adult-Youth Systems," Sherif and Sherif, *Problems of Youth, op. cit.,* chap. ix.
25. Gisella Konopka, *The Adolescent Girl, op. cit.,* p. 88.
26. For example see: H. J. Meyer, E. F. Borgatta, and W. C. Jones, *Girls at Vocational High* (New York: Russell Sage Foundation, 1965).
27. F. T. Rafferty, "Group Organization Theory," *op. cit.,* p. 223.
28. The program is summarized along with background literature in Sherif and Sherif, *Reference Groups, op. cit.* More recent findings are Sherif and Sherif, *Problems of Youth* (1965), chapters 12 and 13.
29. A. L. Edwards, *The Social Desirability Variable in Attitude and Personality Assessment* (New York: Dryden, 1957).
30. Works previously cited by Rosenberg, Turner and Sherif and Sherif included such findings.
31. S. J. Coleman, *The Adolescent Society* (New York: Free Press of Glencoe, 1961).
32. Cf. J. F. Short and T. L. Strodtbeck, *Group Process, op. cit.;* Muzafer Sherif and Carolyn W. Sherif, "Group Processes and Collective Interaction," *Journal of Research in Crime and Delinquency* (1967) (in press).
33. See: Muzafer Sherif, *In Common Predicament: Social Psychology of Intergroup Conflict and Cooperation* (Boston: Houghton-Mifflin International Series, 1966).

ADJUSTMENT OF THE BLIND ADOLESCENT

Carl J. Davis

The analysis of the basic paper, "Needed Research on Adolescents," has been a comfortable task. My paper is directed toward exposition and support of the basic paper via reference to experience in personality counseling with blind adolescents and reference to former research conducted with blind adolescents.

Over the period of the past three decades a number of studies of "adolescent adjustment" (the purpose for placing this term in quotes will be explained later) and/or studies of the personality characteristics of visually handicapped adolescents have been reported. Many of these reports have been criticized by other persons when reporting on their own research. Many of the criticisms are valid, particularly when one considers the weaknesses in experimental design and methodology. Typical errors of this order appear in the lack of sampling control in the reports by Brown,[1] Hubbard,[2] and Hastings.[3] Less gross, but significant errors of sampling were made by Brieland [4] and Morgan.[5] Morgan and Bauman considered only blind subjects, while Brieland,[4] Cowen *et al.*,[7] Jervis and Haslerud,[8] and others compared blind and seeing or blind, partially-seeing, and seeing subjects. Some of the blind adolescents were compared with the seeing on the basis of normative data for pencil-and-paper tests standardized on and published for use with the seeing (Morgan, Kahn and Wood [9]). Most of the studies ignore age of onset of blindness.

Many observers have felt no need to consider degree of vision. Yet the few that have paid attention to this variable consistently indicate the appropriateness of differentiating such groups. Age-grade levels are too frequently not considered and the socio-economic level of groups has been rarely thought worthy of inclusion in a research design. As a consequence, such research reported prior to the late 50's has produced a clouded picture of a blind adolescent who at one time and place is as well adjusted as his seeing peers while in another temporal-geographic location he is less well adjusted than his sighted age-mate. The confusion is compounded by the sampling errors that make generalization impossible.

On the other hand, Jervis[10] and Cowen and his associates[7] recently reported more sophisticated studies that applied more stringently the accepted precepts for experimental design. (Perhaps Bauman[6] should have been included in this group, because she has always been sensitive to the process of experimental design. However, in the instance of reporting on the development of the *Adolescent Emotional Factors Inventory,* the design of the project was not described.) Both of these studies are very acceptable projects, and most professionals who are acquainted with the Rochester undertaking consider it the most creditable research program that has been conducted with visually-handicapped subjects.

In spite of the quality of the experimental design, both Jervis[10] and Cowen[7] suggest that statistical analysis of data does not present a complete description of their subjects. Jervis points out that, although the statistical difference between his groups of subjects on a card-sort was not significant, the blind subjects tended to cluster at the ends of the continuum while the seeing subjects distributed themselves in a more normal fashion. In addition, he points out that handling interview stimuli in terms of groups rather than individuals led to a tendency for extreme responses to cancel. Cowen's summary contains suggestions that the study of cases beyond the degree of statistical significance would lead to better descriptions of his groups. It appears that qualitative analysis of the available data would produce more descriptive information on the groups studied.

At this point the writer suggests that the development of computer machinery has made it *too easy* to collect and process data. Simultaneously, the availability of data processing devices may restrict investigation in depth because of the limitations of the machines available to a particular research worker. Several years ago a doctoral candidate at a nearby university consulted with the writer about a particular braille testing device with which he was having difficulty. Discussion brought forth quite conclusively that the concept was excellent but the mode of presentation was illogical. A logical presentation was suggested and acknowledged by the candidate. Yet the logical mode was rejected because it could not be programmed for the computer then available to the candidate. How many research projects are restricted in scope and product because of the limitations of machinery available to the worker, or because of the worker's limited knowledge of equipment available to him? How many projects are limited in scope because of the relative ease of processing easily collected, easily quantified data in preference to descriptive information that is difficult, and sometimes impossible, to codify for machine processing?

What type of information do we want to collect in order to study adolescent adjustment? At the beginning of this paper the term "adolescent adjustment" was placed within quotation marks for a specific reason. All of the reports that have been mentioned have claimed to present information describing the "adjustment" of blind adolescents. Yet each project has based its claim on a sampling of behavior at *one* period of each subject's life span. Thus each study contains within it the implication that its sampling is measuring an end product.

Understanding of the process of development cannot be obtained by the procedures that have been used to date. Dr. Sherif has provided a model that has considerable merit. Systematic observations over an extended period of time can be the source of very valid, useful descriptions of the process of adjustment. Yet, as described in the basic paper, such projects would provide us with information on what is merely a segment of the process. Should it be assumed that the process between ages 12 and 13 is the same as the process between ages 15 and 16? Is it necessary that each stage of the process be studied and related appropriately to other stages of the developmental sequence? These questions are posed because too much reliance on case histories can obscure important subtleties in interpersonal relationships. Every person who has worked with adolescents in intensive counseling or psychotherapy is aware that all too frequently, in spite of excellently compiled case histories, the counselor will have a validly established conceptual framework shattered by the introduction of new material that produces an entirely new perspective. Thus it is suggested that the basic model that has been submitted be applied for all age groups in the period of adolescence. In addition, the recommendation is made that validating studies that are designed as longitudinal projects be made a part of the total plan.

The person who has worked as a counselor to blind adolescents will probably say that the problems of adjustment for this group are no different than they would be for a group of seeing adolescents, only that they differ in intensity. It is not the purpose of this paper to debate that point. It is more important to expand upon the accurate statement by Dr. Sherif "that a blind adolescent faces a special set of problems with great significance for his transition to adulthood."

Probably the most significant problem for the congenitally blind child is his concept of his own body image and his concept of the body image of the opposite sex. From preschool days the seeing adolescent has been able to compare his own body structure with that of others of his own and the opposite sex. He is thereby able to verify his adequacy, or lack of it, in a variety of situations. On the other hand, the blind adolescent has suffered from all the prohibitions that society imposes upon tactual observation of one's own, or a friend's physique. The prohibitions are compounded when exploration of the physique of a member of the opposite sex is considered.[11] Thus it is readily seen that an area of great concern to all adolescents is considerably more intense for the blind youth.

Another area of major concern, referred to by Dr. Sherif, is the blind adolescent's dependency status. It was correctly stated that society may view the blind person as permanently dependent. All too frequently the family of the blind adolescent intensifies this attitude in a manner that, at best, inhibits his movement toward independence. More important is the fact that the blind adolescent lives in a world of seeing adolescents who move rapidly toward independence, particularly the independence of mobility. Mobility in the community, the use of or ownership of an automobile or motorbike, are key status goals for adolescents. These specific goals are denied to the blind adolescent, but he has status needs. Does he repress these drives, or does he sublimate them?

Concern about heterosexual activity is probably much more intense for the blind adolescent than it is for the adolescent who sees. His anxieties are similar to those that trouble the seeing adolescent, that is, adult expectancy, feelings of inadequacy, contact, communication, mobility; but his lack of perception leaves him with a lot less freedom than his seeing age-mates (Lowenfeld [12]). These factors tend to make the blind adolescent react in this area, as in some other areas, by moving toward either of the ends of the adjustmental continuum as Jervis[10] has suggested. He becomes either strongly self-deprecatory or vigorously self-assertive. The counselor who works with these adolescents is aware of the strength of the defenses that are used to protect the exposure of true feelings. Considerable time must be expended before these youths are able to communicate their true feelings, because it appears that such defenses are somewhat different from the defensive mechanisms of the seeing youth. It seems that the seeing youth has less need to defend himself against his environment before he reaches adolescence than does the blind youth. Consequently, the blind youth reaches adolescence with an established pattern of defenses that may be lacking in the seeing. The defenses are then reinforced in adolescents to the point where they may become either extremely difficult to pierce, or so brittle that attempts to penetrate them may shatter the whole defensive constellation. Consequently, care must be taken to approach the blind adolescent with great caution and subtlety in order to understand him and in order to avoid traumatizing him.

In the selection of life goals, particularly vocational objectives, a blind youth is exposed to more stringent demands and more restricted choices than his seeing peers. At the same time he is subject to conflicting expectancies to a greater degree than seeing youth. To a much greater degree than the seeing, the blind youth is confronted all the way through his school career with the projected image concept. Through that process there is applied, by teachers and rehabilitation personnel, continual emphasis on the need to present a positive picture to the "seeing world." Even though the same professional personnel may permit their own children to grow beards, be unwashed, wear tight jeans, sweatshirts, or miniskirts, they constantly reiterate to their blind pupils or clients that they may never relax the effort to present the best image of a blind person. Should the blind youth rebel he is chastised not only by the professional but by his better conditioned age-mates and the blind adults. These are areas wherein the blind youth is criticized or punished for his efforts to become a "normal adolescent."

Conflicting demands relative to vocational choice are made upon many blind youths. Too frequently parents maintain classical, erroneous stereotypes of the blind. It is customary in today's society for the parents of seeing youths to desire a college education for their children. However, with the parent of the blind child there exists a component of this desire that exerts a form of stress upon the blind youth different from the stress parental expectancy places upon seeing youth. The notion that a blind adult is either a genius or a mendicant causes these parents to impose unrealistic educational and vocational goals at the same time that educational personnel are attempting to develop realistic self-appraisal in the adolescent.

I have been attempting to describe some of the areas in which the stress of adolescent adjustment for blind youth may differ in degree or in kind from the stress with which seeing youth are confronted. Up to this point comment has been concerned with the general category of blind adolescents. Yet they are not a unitary group. They divide into a variety of sub-groups with differentiating characteristics of great importance to the person undertaking research. Dr. Sherif suggests that the congenitally blind adolescents face a different set of adjustment problems from that of the child who has been blinded in adolescence. The difference between the two groups is obvious. One has lived and grown with visual impairment while the other has suddenly had his body structure altered in a very significant fashion. Cholden[13] has given us some insight into the process of adjustment to blindness. I suggest that this process may proceed more easily for the adolescent than for the adult because the personality structure of the adolescent, still in an evolving process, is not traumatized to the degree that one finds in the adult personality structure, which in theory is more mature and more stable. Yet the quality of the personality structure before blindness is probably a significant fact in the process of adjustment. Also, we know little about the process of adjustment to adolescence after, or concomitantly with, becoming blind. Age of onset of blindness is a critical variable that must be controlled in all research with blind children and adults. Relative to age of blinding, the role of visual imagery and visual memory may be a significant factor in the adjustment of blind adolescents.

Cowen *et al.*[7] indicate that the partly-sighted may differ in their adjustment to blindness. This is a distinct group which may very probably separate into sub-groupings when adolescent adjustment is concerned. In my counseling experience such differences seem to appear. Somewhere along the gradient of measurable visual acuity between minimal visual perception and the limiting legal definition of blindness there is a place at which a legally blind adolescent cannot conceptualize himself as a blind person. The place on the measurable gradient is a range rather than a point and visual perceptual function plays as important a role in the determination of self-conceptualization as does measurable visual acuity. Nonetheless there are legally blind youths who do not have a concept of themselves as blind persons. On many occasions these partly-seeing youths have told the counselor: "My basic problem is that I am neither fish nor fowl. I'm not blind and I'm not a seeing person." What follows is a description of conflict within, due to variable function in differing situations, and conflict from without, due to variable expectancies from different adults and different seeing age-mates.

The separation for research purposes of blind youth in public schools from blind children in residential schools is an obvious differentiation of subjects. All blind residential school subjects are exposed for at least nine months of the year to middle class levels of educational and socio-economic expectancies while all blind public school pupils are not exposed to similar uniform expectancies. Hence, the application of the socio-economic dimension of Dr. Sherif's model may yield some interesting contrasts. Also, it would be interesting to know whether the residence of blind youth in a middle-class environment has an upgrading effect upon parents of such children when the parents were originally members of a lower socio-economic group. From experience I suggest that some parents of lower status seek the higher level expectancies for their blind children.

On a fairly regular basis as a part of a recreational-social program, I see locally the intermingling of blind and seeing groups. Some of the time there appears to be a spontaneous fusing of the groups, but at other times there is a distance between the groups perceivable to the skilled observer even though they are intermingling and interacting. With the adolescents observed, the key appeared to center around communication or the lack of it. Knowledge of the pluses and minuses of such grouping would indeed make it possible to extend social, recreational, and economic participation of the blind.

CONCLUSION

I suggest that the model in the basic paper be expanded to include its application at various critical age ranges during the entire period from the prepubertal stage to the final stages of adolescent development. In addition I suggest that longitudinal studies be made as a verification of the age-level procedures.

It is hoped that the combined efforts will stimulate research programs so that all may benefit by a better understanding of the adjustment processes of blind adolescents.

NOTES

1. P. A. Brown, "Responses of Blind and Seeing Adolescents to an Introversion-Extroversion Questionnaire," *Journal of Psychology,* 6 (1938), 137–147; and P. A. Brown, "Responses of Blind and Seeing Adolescents to a Neurotic Inventory," *Journal of Psychology,* 7 (1939), 211–221.
2. I. E. Hubbard, "An Objective Study of the Personality of the Blind," (unpublished Master's thesis, Washington University, 1945).
3. H. J. Hastings, "An Investigation of Some Aspects of the Personality of the Blind" (Seminar Study, University of California, Berkeley, 1947).
4. D. M. Brieland, "A Comparative Study of the Speech of Blind and Sighted Children," *Speech Monographs,* 17 (1950), 98–103.
5. D. H. Morgan, "Emotional Adjustment of Visually Handicapped Adolescents," *Journal of Educational Psychology,* 35 (1944), 65–81.
6. Mary K. Bauman, "Group Differences Disclosed by Inventory Items," *International Journal of the Blind,* 13 (1964), 101–106.
7. E. L. Cowen, R. P. Underberg, R. T. Verillo and F. G. Benham, *Adjustment to Visual Disability in Adolescence* (New York: American Foundation for the Blind, 1961).

8. F. M. Jervis and G. M. Haslerud, "Quantitative and Qualitative Difference in Frustration Between Blind and Sighted Adolescents," *Journal of Psychology,* 29 (1950), 67–76.
9. R. Kohn and K. Wood, "An Experimental Investigation of Obstacle Perception and Its Relationship to Personality and Intellectual Factors," (unpublished Master's thesis, Boston University, School of Education, 1957).
10. F. M. Jervis, "A Comparison of Self-concepts of Blind and Sighted Children in Guidance Programs for Blind Children," *Publication No. 20* of the Perkins School for the Blind (Watertown, Mass., 1960).
11. Carl J. Davis, "The Development of the Self-concept in the Blind Child," in the *Proceedings of the 46th Conference of the American Association of Instructors of the Blind,* Miami, Florida (1962).
12. B. Lowenfeld, *Our Blind Children* (Springfield, Illinois: Charles C Thomas, 1964).
13. L. S. Cholden, *A Psychiatrist Works with Blindness* (New York: American Foundation for the Blind, 1958).

SESSION REPORT

Adrienne V. Little and John R. Swinton

During the discussion period, Dr. Carolyn Sherif added the following extemporaneous remarks to her prepared paper:

> I should like to start by saying that when I originally accepted the invitation to prepare a paper on adolescence for this Consultation, I was assured that there would be another one on childhood, on the earlier years of development. Indeed it is difficult to discuss adolescence at all without such background. Fortunately, however, we have an excellent developmental psychologist (Dr. Dale B. Harris) as our chairman.
>
> I have had to confess my ignorance about blind adolescents, or partially seeing adolescents, or adolescents who see with difficulty; and I come here today hopefully to learn from you about it. The only thing that I would call attention to is that in some sense I see a similarity between the problems of the typical adolescent and the adolescent faced with the fact that he has no sight or little sight. These problems have to do, of course, with taking responsibilities in a world that defines one in a way that one may not like and therefore literally deprives one of certain opportunities, to acquire new skills, and to solve the persistent dilemma between being adult—being responsible—and being immature.
>
> In my basic paper I reviewed for you some of the recent research trends in the study of adolescence, of adolescents' attitudes and goals especially. I have noted several cautions there, and I want to explain why. I am continually struck by the communication difficulties between the so-called research people and the so-called applied people. Most of it seems to me unnecessary, and I hope that through my paper it will be possible for us to communicate. That is why the obvious pitfalls of research in the field were pointed out for you in advance.
>
> One of these pitfalls is that in research the single factor research study—the effect of this or that, or *X* is a function of *Y*—can be very deceptive. We groping researchers need to know all we can about the realities of the phenomena we are studying through multivariate analysis—that is, the simultaneous consideration of many sources of influence rather than just one.
>
> Another example of a research pitfall is the practice of using just one research technique. We now have the need to use a variety of

different procedures: observations of what goes on coupled with a test, background information, and socio-cultural information simultaneously converging on the problem of the study.

The other research lesson that I tried to emphasize is one that is becoming prominent in all the social sciences that study behavior today. In psychology it is popularly called the "social psychology of the psychological experiment." In sociology I think they are talking about the research effect. And there are the allied concepts of researcher bias. We are finally all waking up to the fact that our research methods and instruments do have an effect upon the phenomenon we are studying. People do not behave in the same way when they are faced with the problems of answering questions from someone in whose eyes they don't want to appear dumb or uninformed as they do when they are in their natural life situation. In our study of adolescence far more than in the study of childhood, this problem faces us. There are reasons for it. Adolescents are conceptually so much more sophisticated than children; and they know what the adults expect of them. I'm not saying that we discard all the information we get when adolescents know they are specifically being studied; I am saying that in order to check its validity we have to have a means of studying them that permits us to see how life goes on among adolescents (and with adults) when they are not aware that they are the objects of direct inquiry or that their worth as a person is in question.

This need is illustrated in the paper with great emphasis given to studies of the day-to-day interactions and interpersonal relationships among adolescent youth that Muzafer Sherif has conducted for almost ten years now. In addition, examples are given in the paper —examples from studies of delinquent girls and even from an inpatient clinic or a mental hospital—to try to document in some detail the extreme importance that interpersonal relationship with an age-mate is accorded during this period.

Finally, I hope that these kinds of information can be used in research in which agencies are charged with responsibility for remedial training and preparatory work for youngsters lacking sight in some degree and can be conducted by researchers generally interested in the adolescent process, both for the benefit of the general study of adolescence and for the study of the blind.

I cannot emphasize too strongly that I would not like to see research into either childhood or adolescence of the blind become a highly specialized field. I say this because of my profound conviction that to understand the development of the individual with special problems in life we have to come into contact at least with the study of the usual course of development in a given society.

CONCEPTS AND DEFINITIONS

It was then debated whether adolescence is a real experience with a strictly biological basis or partly, as in "old age," a state of mind.

Dr. Elena Gall suggested that it is partly a matter of self image and partly a matter of the expectations of others. Do the blind enter this period at a different time? Dr. Gall suggested this as a possible area for research.

Dr. Sherif feels that biological factors are more important in defining adolescence than in defining old age because biological change during adolescence is so rapid.

Dr. Marvin Sussman remarked that there exists insufficient information about the agents and mechanisms of the socialization process during adolescence, and suggested that this is a source of ambivalence in parents. But Dr. Sherif pointed out that quite a bit is already known about socialization during this period. For example, peer-group relationships are important mediators for all socializing agents in adolescence.

The problem of distinguishing different levels of maturation was raised. The levels of social maturity and of intellectual maturity must be sorted out as they may be quite different from one individual to another. Miss Yvonne Agazarian felt it worth investigating how one differentiates immaturity related to adolescent problems and immaturity related to blindness.

METHODOLOGY

Blind children must be studied in many different environments and situations, and Dr. Sherif emphasized that research in "natural" situations is necessary in order to eliminate the "research effect" which often occurs in observational studies. Some of the different situations mentioned at various times in the discussions were: sex, age, and race of the child; degree and age of onset of blindness; education, socio-economic status, family situation; type of neighborhood; school and peer-group relations.

Miss Agazarian and Dr. Sherif agreed that more blind people should be involved in drawing up research designs. While it was argued that not only "the blind know what is best for the blind," Dr. Douglas MacFarland asserted that sighted investigators do seem to be unaware of the needs of the blind and of what types of prostheses they will accept.

It was brought out that attempts to include the blind on planning committees have failed in the past. Dr. Tamara Dembo joined William F. Gallagher in suggesting that this may be because a fear of embarassing these people inhibits open discussion.

A more subjective, descriptive approach to research was suggested. The analysis of personal experiences with the blind was considered an important preliminary to research on concrete problems. This type of research might take the form of family clinics or round-tables to determine the problems of parents and teachers of blind adolescents, as suggested by Dr. Gall.

The effects of disseminating information concerning misleading ideas about the blind ought to be tested, according to Dr. Sherif, with emphasis upon whether this type of communication has positive or negative effects.

RESEARCH CONTENT

Interactions with Others

How does a blind child choose his age-mates, both sighted and blind? How do such factors as degree of blindness and institutional setting restrict his choice? These were questions suggested by Carl J. Davis. Problems of heterosexual social development were also discussed by Mr. Davis and Miss Agazarian. Studies could be made, they said, to see how both blind and seeing adolescents can open up channels of communication with each other.

Attitudinal studies of parents, teachers, and others in contact with blind adolescents ought to be made, according to Drs. Dembo and Gall; and more research on adult–adolescent interactions is needed, according to Dr. Sherif. What are the expectations of parents for their blind children? How do they hinder maturation processes? What are the sources of conflict between parent and child?

Maturation

Perhaps, as Dr. Sussman suggested, the role-learning process in blind children ought to be studied. Both the blind person and the adolescent are expected to assume the role while learning it (that is, the normal role or the adult role). How is this complicated in the adolescent who is also blind? How do affective relationships in the family complicate role learning?

The maturation rate of blind adolescents was considered an important area for research. Several discussants, principally Drs. MacFarland, Scholl, and Sherif, felt that they are a few years behind normal children in development. Others felt that this gap is narrowing due to higher expectations (Mr. Davis) and increased contact with seeing peers (Stewart E. Armstrong). Examples of very advanced blind adolescents were also given by Don Staley.

Social development was thought to be hindered by the absence of the visual cues and the "unspoken language" which are so important in adolescence. Dr. Sherif encouraged studying how these factors operate. Institutional living was also seen by Dr. Dembo as hindering maturation.

The development of the self concept in the blind as well as the development of independence and responsibility were considered critical areas for study by Drs. Dembo and Scholl.

Motivation and Rewards

The problem of differential rewards for blind and seeing students could be an area for new research. One discussant, Mr. Staley, cited blindness as a motivating factor for some students who go from poor to excellent after the onset of blindness. However, Dr. Robert A. Scott attributed higher grades to over-rewarding by teachers but warned that over-rewarding can also have a negative effect when the child becomes suspicious of excessive rewards.

Lack of punishment for criminal acts was thought to discourage the development of responsibility by L. H. Autry, who thought that an investigation of the crime rate among blind adolescents may be needed. However, some discussants, such as Mrs. Sidney E. Pollack and Mr. Gallagher, felt that delinquency is due less to blindness than to other factors. Delinquency was also thought to take different forms (for example, passive resistance) in blind children due to the increased probability of getting caught.

Teaching Problems

An important area for study is that of how gestures, movements, and facial expressions are learned. Research on how to teach blind children these things might be put to good use, according to Mr. Gallagher. It was suggested that the Laban movement system developed in England could be adapted for teaching to blind children. This approach, said Dr. Scholl, may help improve relationships with seeing children. Dr. Sherif feels, however, that this kind of training should be started well before adolescence. Finally, the teaching of highly abstract concepts (for example, the "right angle") without visual materials was also seen as a problem area by Mr. Gallagher.

SOCIAL PARTICIPATION AND CITIZENSHIP

AN INTERPRETIVE REVIEW OF RESEARCH DEALING WITH SOCIAL PARTICIPATION AND CITIZENSHIP

James H. Copp

The topic to which this paper is devoted is so broad and ill-defined at its boundaries that I am going to exercise an author's license by arbitrarily limiting its scope. I am going to define narrowly "social participation" to include only membership and member activities in the so-called formal organizations and voluntary associations. Social participation, in this paper, will not include such definitely social activities as visiting family and friends, dating, going to the movies, or attending football games. The question as to whether or not such other social activities are "social participation" will be ignored. Such activities are often found correlated with membership in voluntary organizations, but at the same time evidence suggests these primary group behaviors may be somewhat different in kind.[26,27]

INTRODUCTION: THE NATURE OF SOCIAL PARTICIPATION AND CITIZENSHIP

In this paper "citizenship" will include voting in elections, running for and holding office, serving on appointive committees authorized by governing bodies, taking overt action to influence governmental officials on issues dealing with the common welfare, membership in and service to political parties, and all legitimate actions taken in the belief that they promote the general well-being of the body politic. In other words, in this paper "citizenship" will be a matter of actions.

If it is permissible to define "social participation" and "citizenship" in these particular ways, it becomes apparent that the two terms have much in common. Because of the limitations imposed on government and the limited responsibilities accepted by those who govern, many functions assumed by government in other societies are fulfilled by voluntary associations in American society. Citizenship can be viewed as participation in a special kind of association, the body politic. Both voluntary associations and government involve formal roles and sets of rules defining legitimate action. They share ideals of parliamentarianism, democracy, voluntarism, equity (for members). They both evoke only a part of the self, the "public self," rather than the more private self. Postures, manners, and diction at a meeting betray a high degree of image management on the part of the actor. In looking at the research on social participation and citizenship, we should keep this "public self" nature of the participation behavior in mind.

Another thing that can be noted about both social participation and citizenship is that these activities (assuming that one is neither a government official nor an executive secretary of an association) are off-duty or spare time activities. With the exceptions noted, social or civic participation does not enter into explicit job or occupational specifications. Civic activity is a *community* expectation, not an employment requirement (although employers may encourage and support social and civic participation of the "desirable" sort by their employees).[54a]

Thus participation is a leisure, consumption activity rather than a sustenance activity. As a leisure activity, it must compete with family, friends, and personal regenerative activities for the time available after work. The retreat from full participation to a society of "limited liability" [39] may be explained in part by the sheer attractiveness and abundance of leisure alternatives in our civilization ranging all the way from fun with friends to autism before the television screen. Significantly, the personal and social factors that research has found related to social and civic participation are the same factors that have more recently been found related to participation in leisure activities.[22,38,66]

As a consumption activity, social and civic participation involve the allocation of surpluses. If after sustenance requirements have been fulfilled, there is little time, energy, and money to dispose in participation, participation can be expected to be minimal. Studies of social participation and political activity have shown this to be the case.[46,58,67,86,87] Thus the most disadvantaged in our social order are least able to do anything about their condition through group action.[68]

A further aspect of the allocative nature of social and civic participation is the problem of choice. Will it be the Men's Brotherhood or the P.T.A., the Lions or the Kiwanis, the Altar Society or the

Garden Club, the Democrats or the Republicans? In making these choices it would seem that some kind of optimizing takes place in terms of previous socialization, social aspirations, self concept, and perceived attractiveness of the organization's program. With citizenship as well as with the voluntary associations, there is also the choice of how deeply to become involved. Although a few people appear to be active in everything, the great majority are very restrictive in their choices. Thus new organizations in the community may draw from the joiners rather than the unaffiliated.

As this discussion has already hinted, participation is assumed to be a motivated activity, and the various motives that impel behavior in other life sectors[10a] should be operative here. However, gregariousness, or the so-called affiliative motive,[72] would seem to be particularly important. A by-product of all participation activity is fellowship. But this need may also be satisfied in a milieu not involving social participation or citizenship activity, such as in the family or peer group.[26,48] Social participation cannot be explained by gregariousness, although a frustration of fellowship satisfactions in private life might turn the individual to voluntary associations and public life.[23,48,50]

THE ENVIRONMENT OF PARTICIPATION

A factor as important as participation itself is the environment in which it takes place. By "environment" is meant primarily the social structure, the society and the community, as well as ecological and physical factors.

Whether or not participation, as defined in this paper, takes place in a voluntary sense depends to a very large extent on the nature of the parent society. Americans easily lose sight of this fact. Only when the proliferation of voluntary associations in American society is compared with the relative paucity in France, the Soviet Union, and other countries does the importance of the societal milieu become apparent. As Arnold Rose[70] points out, a government may view voluntary associations as rivals for power, as subversive elements, and restrict, outlaw, or destroy associations not under the control of the government.

Another structural feature of American society should be pointed out. American government continues to be minimum government. Many spheres of life are considered none of the Federal or State government's business. Add to this the fact that American citizens are terribly reluctant to extend the powers of public officials, and we find a situation in which many important maintenance activities in a community or society are not performed. As a result, voluntary organizations spring up to build hospitals; to fight cancer, crime, corrupt government, and the consumption of alcoholic beverages; to meet disaster and fire; to propagate the faith; and to promote commerce.

A simple regional illustration will dramatize the importance of social structure for the development of voluntary organizations. The Southern states, unlike the North, do not have a township form of government. As a result many extremely local issues and problems tend to be overlooked by the broader county government. Not surprisingly we find community clubs and the community development movement stronger in the South than anywhere else in the country.[33a] Voluntary effort tends to appear where important maintenance functions are not performed by government. In the North, community or civic improvement associations tend to appear only when local government has been slow to adopt innovations strongly desired by newcomers.[79a]

The character of the local community also seems to be a factor in the relative number of organizations that emerge. It has long been observed that communities that are heterogeneous with respect to class and ethnic composition have more organizations.[47] Exclusiveness may lead to the formation of additional organizations to meet felt needs.[65] There is an in-group response to out-group exclusion.[4]

Some research also suggests that the prevailing degree of organized social activity in a neighborhood affects individual participation. That is, there may be community norms specifying the appropriate amount of organizational activity.[9,10] Depending on the neighborhood, this norm may be high or low.

Another set of environmental factors affecting participation is made up of sheer ecological considerations. Although transportation has been greatly improved, isolation and distance are still retarding factors in rural social participation and citizenship activities.[13,19,6] The same would be true in the urban setting. Distance, the availability of transportation,[20] and safety on the streets at night could conceivably be factors influencing the volume of participation. Although great improvements have been made in transportation and mobility, personal costs of movement from one place to another remain limiting factors in how far and how often we will go to participate in social and civic activities. It is interesting to note that research indicates that participation among suburbanites is less than among central city dwellers.[90]

The final environmental factor affecting participation is extremely local; it is the climate within a given organization.[11] At the local level, the nature of the people who are in an organization often influences the willingness of nonmembers to join. Often, especially in rural areas, the important qualities are relative prestige, morality, and personal warmth. The climate of the group is most strongly represented by the leaders of the association. The style of leadership—laissez-faire, democratic, or autocratic—is very important.

Leaders may subtly indicate to members how much participation is wanted. The life cycle of an organization would also affect the stimulation afforded by the climate of the organization. An organization at rest, with few challenges to meet, other than survival, may not be attractive to potential members and may not provide much stimulation to participation for the individual who is a member.

These same observations about the climate within the organization would hold for citizenship. When there are few issues, the voters stay away.[17] When public officials do not solicit civic responsibility activities, little is forthcoming. Power often shifts from one party to another because entrenched party leaders have been unable to absorb new talent into the party. The climate within labor unions, too, has often promoted apathetic participation.[5]

Therefore, an important consideration influencing the degree of social and civic participation is the nature of the milieu in which the participation is to take place. Participation always takes place within a larger field, and conditions within that field may facilitate or retard the degree to which the individual plays a part in public life.

RESEARCH FINDINGS ON INDIVIDUAL PARTICIPATION

Although the field of social participation research is an old one, research in political participation seems to have developed somewhat more recently, with a flood of research appearing in the 1950's. A steady stream of social participation research can be traced back at least 40 years,[42] with scattered studies appearing in the previous 20 years. Most of this research is highly cumulative, findings are indeed supported by subsequent studies. In fact, with a few exceptions, the repetitive character of social participation research, from the late 20's to the late 50's, has a deadening monotony. Only in the 60's are new variables being tried, and participation is beginning to be viewed from a systemic context larger than the individual actor. This section will briefly summarize findings on *individual* social and civic participation.

The Extent of Participation in American Society

Although Americans have the reputation of being joiners and this reputation can be documented in the literature from de Tocqueville, to Lord Bryce, to the Beards,[36,48] research has failed to support this caricature of American people. If we only look at the so-called middle classes, the portrayal is somewhat more accurate, but survey after survey has shown that, if we exclude church and union membership, most Americans are unaffiliated with *any* organization.[3,16,33,34,38,48,73,87]

Thus, only in comparison with the state of affairs in other countries does the proliferation of voluntary associations seem striking and does the organizational participation of individuals seem excessive. That the mass of Americans are relatively unaffiliated and passive participants suggests to Scott Greer that Americans have opted for a "society of limited liability" wherein the member sits back and exercises an occasional veto to what he regards as too much or too little, legitimate or illegitimate, on the part of the leaders.[39]

Some political scientists have tended to view the low level of organizational activity as evidence of "massification" and a cause for alarm.[49] It is pointed out that the opposition defeating positive social measures such as school bond issues and fluoridation of water often comes from the unaffiliated exercising their veto.[79] Thus the low degree of participation in organizations in American society has been viewed as either a hedonistic adjustment in everyday living or as a threat to our democratic institutions and even a harbinger of authoritarian trends in the social order.

Given the fact that participation is unequal and generally low among individuals and that various implications have been attributed to this inequality, the following paragraphs will be devoted to findings regarding the variables that have been found associated with variations in social participation. These findings are based on the adult non-institutionalized population in rural and urban areas of this country.

Age

Participation in organization varies with age in a curvilinear non-monotonic fashion.[33,59] One low point is in the early 20's, the other occurs as the person approaches retirement. The peak intensity of participation occurs in the 40's and 50's. The low rate in the youth has been attributed to the distractions of courtship, marriage, and subsequent family formation. The high point in middle age has been explained by the freedom from the responsibilities of caring for young children. The low period in the 60's is undoubtedly related to retirement. It is interesting to note that the decline takes place *before* age 65, and that subsequently there is a slight increase in participation. Eventually, social and civic participation decline in response to the infirmities and social deprivations of old age. The decline and recovery in the 60's is especially interesting because it seems to reflect self attitudes and community expectations in addition to mere physical decline. Altered opportunities for social interaction because of loss of spouse have been noted in the literature.[10b]

It should be noted that explanations for changes in social participation over the life cycle, although plausible, tend to be post hoc. Furthermore, these changes have not been recorded for a cohort of individuals over a period of time, but for individuals of various ages, with quite different life histories, at a given point in time.

Except for infants and the elderly, age does not impose severe limits on social participation and citizenship. Rather, people at certain ages are found in rather similar life situations which either enlarge or constrain the ease of participation. Significantly, wealth or income seems to do very nicely in offsetting the negative influence of age on participation.[32,83]

Sex

In American society, differences in participation between the sexes are noticeable, but not large.[6,63,75] Whether the sexes participate equally or unequally is based in part on sub-cultural variations in the definitions of the woman's role. Voting turnout, holding public office, and political activity are somewhat lower for women,[45] again reflecting cultural expectations that females will be nurtural and supportive rather than power-seeking. On the other hand, women are more frequently involved in church activities than men.[6,22a,38] This undoubtedly reflects role expectations as well as the fact that women still comprise an oppressed minority group in our society. It is well established that lower class women are much less active in formal organizations than lower class men.[48,75] This finding is generally assumed to reflect subcultural variations in expectations. The mother of infant children obviously has special handicaps to participation. Other than for these reasons—conceptions of femininity, motherhood, and social class—there are only minor differences in the participation patterns between the sexes.

Socio-Economic Factors

In practically all studies in which the relationship is examined, socio-economic differences are found to be one of the greatest sources of variation in participation. [6,12,13,19,27,33,34,38,45,67,73,75,86,87] The degree of association (correlations as high as 0.50 are reported) between participation and social class and the pervasiveness of this relationship among the various kinds of organizations studied and the various indicators of social class utilized are nothing short of remarkable. Here is not a casual relationship, but one piercing to the core of participation. The strong correlations hold for church as well as union participation, for expressive as well as instrumental organizations, for voting as well as office holding. Let us examine various socio-economic indicators serially.

EDUCATION Educational attainment is one of the strongest predictors of participation, frequently found more highly associated than either income or occupation.[32] As has been pointed out, the educated person has more resources, is more valuable to an organization. Consequently, practically all groups attempt to exploit the resources of the educated person. By virtue of his education, he is generally more skillful in the manipulation of symbols and images and thus feels less threatened as an actor in an organization. Education is assumed to confer certain qualities on the individual and is taken as a mark of qualification for responsibility or office. Degrees supposedly confer a charisma on the individual. In other words, the educated person does have an advantage because of his training, but he has an even greater advantage in that members of the community assume that education confers somewhat magical qualities as well. Hence the great pressure on the educated person to participate.[12,14]

INCOME Money, the great facilitator, whether represented by wealth or income is characteristically related to participation.[58, also 3,10,13,27,32, 33,34,38,46,48,55a,67,86,87] In a way, participation is for those with surpluses, for those who have exceeded a minimum standard of consumption. The active participant often must be in a position to afford a replacement in his occupational responsibilities. It might also be pointed out that the person with wealth has more to be concerned about, more to protect, and therefore needs organizations and a stable civic system more than the person without wealth.[51]

There is another reason for the association between wealth and participation. The phenomenon is best illustrated among millionaires' descendants who enter social service, civic activities, and politics. Participation in social and civic activities is a way of finding meaning, of testing oneself, and of validating one's high status. Prestige comes not from money, but from the use which this resource permits one to make of his life.

OCCUPATION That participation is generally found related to occupational status[3,10,13,27,67,73,87] is easily understandable. Educational attainment is commonly a qualification for occupational placement. Occupation, in turn, is to some degree related to income. Occupations themselves confer skills that are useful in civic and social affairs.[51] The high status jobholder may have access to plant facilities, equipment, personnel, and funds that are useful to the organization. He also has business or professional contacts who are very helpful in getting things done.[84] On the other hand, at high status levels in business, one's club activities and civic participation are often thought of as indirect ways of advancement. Beyond these rather selfish motivations there also seems in American society to be a culturally imposed sense of obligation to serve the community, or what Campbell *et al.* call "citizen duty." [17]

Finally, in addition to the foregoing considerations, it should be pointed out that persons at the higher occupational levels are able to participate with more ease and confidence in social and civic life because of the greater amount of information about community affairs[30,76] and nationwide trends[44] acquired by virtue of their positions. In a word, it is much *easier* for the person at the higher occupational levels than the lower occupational strata to participate; the costs and the risks are relatively lower, and the self-confidence greater.[30]

STATUS CRYSTALLIZATION Lenski made a significant contribution to participation research when he examined the relationship between social participation and "status crystallization," [53] which is the degree to which an individual's various status characteristics are congruent (at the same level). An example of incomplete status crystallization would be the high school graduate bus driver living in an upper middle class residential area. Lenski found that people with incongruent status characteristics had fewer memberships and more lapsed memberships; and that when they joined organizations, they joined for nonsociable reasons. He explains these findings in terms of the disturbing social interaction experiences that these incongruities are likely to elicit.

RACE Considering their generally lower income, educational, and occupational attainment, Negroes appear to participate in social organization more than might be expected.[4,47] This has been explained in terms of the Negro's restriction in many phases of life, frequently including rather restricted living conditions and resulting in release through associational activity.[65] It is known that exclusion from white-dominated organizations has led to the development of a parallel set of social organizations for colored people. Until recently, the major emphasis in Negro participation has been in expressive rather than instrumental types of organizations. This, no doubt, has been due to the emotional frustrations of being black in a white society. Up to this time, the Negro's participation in citizenship activities has been lower than the corresponding rate for whites. Part of the reason would be the depressed social class position of Negroes. The rest of the reason would lie in the white community's expectation and the Negro's self-concept of his citizenship responsibilities, a self concept developed in a discriminating society.

CONCLUSION ABOUT SOCIO-ECONOMIC FACTORS A question has been raised regarding the association of socio-economic factors and participation in social and civic activities. The question is whether the socio-economic characteristics themselves impel participation or whether the community expects higher participation from the upper classes. The evidence that there are strong community expectations about participation levels has been well documented,[12,14] both among community members and among high status position holders who confess this strong community pressure. Thus, the high status person who does not participate or serve would experience guilt about violating community expectations.

Yet it must be noted that the community is not very well armed with sanctions to impose on the high status resident. It is true that such a resident can reduce patronage with the person in business, but evidence also suggests that unpopular decisions by public servants may be bad for business.

It appears that the high participation generally found among high status people cannot be explained by guilt or pressure of economic sanctions, valid though they may be. Earlier, it was observed that the advantages of high status position make participation less costly and more rewarding for the upper class person.[46] There is very little change and role stress involved as the professional or managerial person moves from his occupational life to his social and civic life (assuming his various status characteristics have a high degree of crystallization). Often these two aspects of his life are closely intermingled throughout the day.[55]

The strong association between social class and social and civic participation has a very important implication for social structure. The fact that the actives are drawn disproportionately from the upper socio-economic strata means that our voluntary associations for our civic leadership and political life are dominated by the upper classes;[67] that there are strong aristocratic tendencies in our society that are at variance with equalitarian and democratic assumptions underlying American society. It also means that voluntary, as well as governmental undertakings tend to be phrased from the perspective of the "haves" rather than of the "have-nots." At the worst, this leads to programs treating symptoms and solving non-existent problems.

Family

A most significant finding that has not been given sufficient emphasis in participation research is the strong similarity among family members in their participation.[2,11,20,26,35a,41a] Part of the reason is social class, whose influence has just been reviewed. But equally important are internal standards of appropriateness established within the family. Families may support or oppose social and civic participation as a leisure activity. Cynics suggest that social participation ensues from strained family relationships.[23] Evidence supports this, but the degree of association is low. More important, as an agency of socialization, the family imparts a sense of duty or a sense of apathy to its members regarding civic participation. Studies of political participation indicate the strong influence of family involvement in political affairs and political interest on subsequent political participation in the individual.[11]

Social Mobility and Migration

Migration appears to have a temporary depressing effect on participation,[89] especially for farm-to-urban migrants without college training.[88] It should be added that migrants tend to be at the age at which participation is lowest and that residential requirements for voting are such that migrants are temporarily disenfranchised for varying lengths of time. On the other hand, social mobility seems to have relatively little, or a positive, effect on participation rates.[24,34]

Personality

It is naïvely assumed by the casual observer that active participants in organizations must differ in personality from nonparticipants. The joiner is described as energetic, extroverted, dominant, or gregarious. Yet few areas of participation research have yielded such disappointing results.[11,12] Part of the reason for this is that a person can exercise his energy, extroversion, dominance, and gregariousness outside of social and civic organizations.

Certain personality characteristics do seem relevant for participation. Among these are optimism, that witch's brew placed under the rubric of "alienation," and various attitudinal correlates which may be either causes or effects of participation. One of the strongest cases for the importance of personality traits and attitude is presented in a paper by Smith.[75a]

OPTIMISM That personality trait about which research findings are most consistent may be labeled "optimism." [11,12,13,18,34,68,69] Characteristically, the high participant is positive in his views about the world in which he lives. The low participator tends to take a negative, skeptical view of his situation. This finding seems to be just as true of voters as it is of joiners. Evidence also suggests that active participants are stable and balanced in their views, while nonparticipants are more easily attracted to extremist positions when they do become involved in issues.[49]

ORIENTATION TO THE COMMUNITY Merton popularized the distinction between "cosmopolitans and locals." [60] Several studies suggest that those who are favorably oriented to the local community, who do not plan to move, have higher rates of participation[13,34,86] and higher levels of knowledge about the community.[76]

ALIENATION Alienation has tended to become a catch-all term for explaining everything that is out of joint in our society. Careful studies arrive at five, seven, or more different meanings for the concept, not all of which are highly interrelated.[25,63a,73a] Alienation has included isolation, powerlessness, and anomie (as measured by the

Srole scale). If, for simplicity, we take alienation to denote a sense of separation and lack of relation to the social order, it is easy to see why alienation should be negatively correlated with participation.[62,78] In a sense, alienation becomes negative participation. This is consistent with the views of McClosky and Schaar, who after a careful review of this evidence, conclude that anomie is a sign of impaired socialization.[59a]

Undoubtedly, this is an oversimplification, yet Erbe found that when he controlled on organizational involvement and socio-economic status, the relationship between alienation and political activity became negligible.[29] In Erbe's analysis alienation appears to be a by-product attitude rather than an independent variable. It would seem that a final verdict on the role of alienation in participation awaits further theoretical analysis, clarified by empirical research, on the notion of alienation.

ATTITUDINAL CORRELATES Active participants in a given organization are found to be more closely identified with the organization, to have more influence, to express more satisfactions, to have stronger ideological interests, and to be better informed in terms of factual knowledge about the association.[7,11,17,20,21,41,46,74] It has frequently been assumed that manipulation of these attitudes would lead to increased participation,[7] but evidence supporting this assumption has not yet been produced. This approach suggests symptom treatment rather than systemic alteration. For instance, greater factual knowledge about an organization could conceivably lead to withdrawal of membership.[21] Advertising campaigns designed to improve the image of an organization could lead to a higher level of expectation about organization performance that could not be met, eventuating in disenchantment and cynicism.

NEW RESEARCH DEPARTURES

The experience of reviewing participation research has led to the feeling that too much of it has been rather cut-and-dried. Much research has involved the earnest rediscovery of prior findings. Recently some new perspectives have been presented which promise to lead to more sophisticated approaches to the understanding of participation. Examples would be the "triggering" phenomenon, the benefit contingency, Greer's notion of "plebiscitary membership," and Wilensky's study of career histories. But the experience of reviewing the research has also revealed deficiencies in approach and areas of ignorance. The theoretical status of the concept of participation is weak. We cannot explain (except for *post hoc* explanation) why social class is related to participation. We lack an adequate taxonomy of organizations. We do not know to what extent participation in different kinds of organizations has differential significance.

New Approaches to Participation

THE "TRIGGERING" PHENOMENON Bowman and Boynton have pointed out that two individuals may be matched in socioeconomic characteristics and family interest in politics, and yet only one will be active in political affairs. Further analysis reveals that something happened in the experience of one that did not occur in the other. Sometimes it is as simple as being asked to participate; other times it is a personal crisis, a dissonant experience, or a glaring inequity that "triggers" the inactive person into activity.[11,60a] Although the triggering phenomenon can hardly be dignified with variable status, it does remind us that people have to be invited and encouraged. Triggering is a stochastic event, only partly controllable.

THE BENEFIT CONTINGENCY Warner, among others, has asked whether members participate more if benefits received are contingent on participation in the organization.[81] The answer to this reasonable question is yes. But Warner found that the answer is not as clear-cut as he anticipated and that other conditions must be introduced into this relationship.[80]

"PLEBISCITARY MEMBERSHIP" Greer is one of the more sanguine commentators on the low level of participation in American society. He argues that contemporary Americans, in their "communities of limited liability," are quite willing to let the active minority direct community affairs, so long as everything proceeds smoothly.[39] Only when the minority gets out of touch with the passive majority do they get feedback in veto form. Though recognizing the mass society implications of such participation, Greer suggests that the plebiscites might exert sufficient check on leadership "to represent a modest achievement of democratic participation and control through consent." Barber's approach to mass apathy would be congruent with this view.[5]

DETERMINANTS OF POLITICAL APATHY Rosenberg, in a very appropriate essay,[71] reminds us that as members of primary groups and economic networks we are not as free to participate as we might wish and that there are serious risks and costs to ego and occupational success in political controversy. He also cites alienation type themes of futility and then goes on to point out that in political affairs there may be long periods where there is an absence of stimuli to act (for example, elections are scheduled at long intervals). Rosenberg's analysis effectively demonstrates that political nonparticipation is a natural rather than pathological phenomenon. For too long low participation has been regarded as a moral failing which must be corrected; his essay is a valuable antidote. Dotson[26] and Foskett[31] take a similar position on the nonpathology of nonparticipation.

CAREER STABILITY In one of the most creative recent analyses, Wilensky has shown that a logical progression of jobs in one's work career leads to a higher level of participation.[85] ". . . chaotic experience in the economic order fosters a retreat from both work and the larger communal life." The reasons for this relationship are not developed in detail, but there are obvious connections here with the alienation and optimism themes. Wilensky points out that the direction of causation is difficult to infer, but presents arguments suggesting the direction is from career to participation. The larger implication of this finding is that in understanding individual participation we must look at the total man in all his aspects and history for clues to his characteristic stance in social and civic life. Too often we fail to view the individual life history as a system.[84]

Unfinished Business

NEED FOR THEORETICAL DEVELOPMENT Operationally (as was done at the beginning of this paper) we can point to behaviors that comprise participation, but what is participation at the theoretical level? Is it merely conforming to role prescriptions? How about participation by the same individual in several associations? Perhaps social participation is the wrong way to conceptualize the phenomenon. In the present state of affairs it is obvious that we have a concept before we have a theory.

One possible direction for theoretical work is hinted broadly in the literature. The suggestion is offered that we view participation as a reflection of the social order. V. O. Key, Jr. puts it this way: "Examination of popular participation in the political process may suggest crucial insights into the nature of the political order. Variations in the nature of the act of voting may serve as fundamental characteristics of the state as may qualitative differences in voting." [45] Fosket remarks that ". . . this marked skewness in the distribution of participation may be less a matter of 'lethargy' and more a matter of social structure." [31] At least two observers have noted that high participation occurs in "tight little island" situations. Minnis[61] reviewing Goldhamer's dissertation notes, "Goldhamer points out that the voluntary . . . association tends to flourish in a setting in which the community can function as an all-inclusive group." Greer observes that "only where [high] functional interdependence occurs is participation strong: constraint is, in this sense, the key to community." [39] These quotations suggest that the place to begin theoretically is with social structure. If participation is to be understood, greater knowledge of our social system may be a prerequisite. To observe the system function, heed participation.

This position has already been well stated by Fred Katz, who suggests that social participation might be approached from a network perspective. Katz's basic position is that ". . . ego's social networks indicate the scope of his participation in his society. And, conversely, that existing social networks provide a clue to the strands which actually hold society together." [44a] Here we have the bedrock on which future sound theoretical work on social participation is likely to build.

No doubt the troubling set of concepts in the alienation sphere is involved in the same theoretical solution. The alienated seem to be those who cannot fit into niches of the social structure, who see themselves as losers,[46] or who will not play the game. Thus alienation symbolizes a faulty match of the social system and the personality system.

TAXONOMY OF ORGANIZATIONS Present classifications are excessively primitive. One useful classification is on the basis of task orientation of the group. Those aimed primarily at fellowship and personal satisfactions have been labeled "expressive" and those directed basically for accomplishment of some goal beyond its immediate membership have been labeled "instrumental." [37,43] Another customary classification is according to function—religious, occupational, fraternal, economic, political, recreational.[15] Membership in some types of organizations is mutually exclusive: it is rather difficult to be a Catholic and a Methodist or a Democrat and a Republican at the same time; but one can belong to both the Odd Fellows and the Eagles, the Grange and the Farm Bureau. Most associations also appear to be stratified socio-economically (churches) or with respect to prestige (service clubs).[61] Despite these commonly recognized distinctions we have no good classification systems for organizations.

The lack of a recognized taxonomy makes it extremely difficult to talk with confidence about different kinds of participation. For instance, I do not really know if I have been on safe ground in dealing with citizenship in the same breath as social participation; intuitively, these forms seem alike. We do not know if participation in purely social clubs should be lumped with civic participation. We do not know with much certainty whether a measure which aggregates participation in several groups is defensible.[77a]

I have taken the liberty of dealing with within-group participation (*member* participation) and among-group participation (*social* participation) as if the two kinds were interchangeable in their relationships with other variables. This *appears* to be the case, but it is largely unexplored.

LEISURE AND SOCIAL PARTICIPATION Are social and civic participation to be regarded as leisure activities? As a sociologist of leisure, I have been somewhat surprised to meet the same set of variables correlated at about the same degree with social participation and voting behavior.[22] The family resemblance is so strong that kinship must be inferred between leisure and participation. In both instances the upper socio-economic strata are the most active. "For to every one who has more will be given." These analogies are surely clues to the adequate theoretical development of social participation theory.

NOTES*

1. Robert E. Agger and Vincent Ostrom, "Political Participation in a Small Community," *Political Behavior,* eds. Heinz Eulau, Samuel J. Eldersveld, and Morris Janowitz (Glencoe, Illinois: The Free Press, 1956), 138–148.
2. W. A. Anderson, "The Family and Individual Social Participation," *ASR,* 8 (August, 1943), 420–424.

* The following abbreviations are used for journals:
AJS—American Journal of Sociology
APSR—American Political Science Review
ASR—American Sociological Review
POQ—Public Opinion Quarterly
RS—Rural Sociology
SF—Social Forces

3. Morris Axelrod, "Urban Structure and Social Participation," *ASR,* 21 (February, 1956), 13–18.
4. Nicholas Babchuk and Ralph V. Thompson, "The Voluntary Associations of Negroes," *ASR,* 27 (October, 1962), 647–655.
5. Bernard Barber, "Participation and Mass Apathy in Associations," *Studies in Leadership,* ed. Alvin W. Gouldner (New York: Harper and Bros., 1950), 477–504.
6. Ward W. Bauder, "Social Participation in Rural Society," *Rural Sociology: An Analysis of Contemporary Rural Life,* ed. Alvin L. Bertrand (New York: McGraw-Hill Co., 1958), 142–158.
7. George M. Beal, "Additional Hypotheses in Participation Research," *RS,* 21 (September–December, 1956), 249–256.
8. Howard Beers, "Social Participation Studies," *RS,* 8 (September, 1943), 294–295.
9. Wendell Bell and Maryanne T. Force, "Social Structure and Participation in Different Types of Formal Associations," *SF,* 34 (May, 1956), 345–350.
10. ——— and Maryanne T. Force, "Urban Neighborhood Types and Participation in Formal Associations," *ASR,* 21 (February, 1956), 25–34.
10*a*. Bernard Berelson and Gary A. Steiner, *Human Behavior: An Inventory of Scientific Findings* (New York: Harcourt, Brace and World, Inc., 1964), 239–295.
10*b*. Zena Smith Blau, "Structural Constraints on Friendships in Old Age," *ASR,* 26 (June, 1961), 429–439.
11. Lewis Bowman and G. R. Boynton, "Recruitment Patterns Among Local Party Officials: A Model and Some Preliminary Findings in Selected Locales," *APSR,* 60 (September, 1966), 667–676.
12. Urie Bronfenbrenner, "Personality and Participation: The Case of the Vanishing Variables," *Journal of Social Issues,* Vol. 16, No. 4 (1960), 54–63.
13. Emory J. Brown, *Elements Associated with Activity and Inactivity in Rural Organizations, Pennsylvania Agricultural Experiment Station Bulletin* 574 (University Park, 1954).
14. ———, "The Self as Related to Formal Participation in Three Pennsylvania Rural Communities," *RS,* 18 (December, 1953), 313–321.
15. Roy C. Buck and Baden P. Mudge, *Formal Participation Patterns in a Central Pennsylvania Rural Community, Pennsylvania Agricultural Experiment Station Progress Report* 129 (University Park, 1955).
16. Frederick A. Bushee, "Social Organization in a Small City," *AJS,* 51 (November, 1945), 217–226.
17. Angus Campbell, Philip E. Converse, Warren E. Miller and Donald E. Stokes, *The American Voter* (New York: John Wiley, 1960).
18. John R. Christiansen and Therel R. Black, "Group Participation and Personality Adjustment," *RS,* 19 (June, 1954), 183–185.
19. Gordon M. Connelly and Harry H. Field, "The Non-Voter—Who He Is, What He Thinks," *POQ,* 8 (Summer, 1944), 175–187.
20. James H. Copp, *Factors Associated with Reenrollment in 4-H Clubs, Wisconsin Agricultural Experiment Station Research Bulletin* 195 (Madison, 1956).
21. ———, "Perceptual Influences on Loyalty in a Farmer Cooperative," *RS,* 29 (June, 1964), 168–180.
22. ———, "Theoretical Perspectives on Outdoor Recreation," (Paper read at the 1964 annual meeting of the Rural Sociological Society, Macdonald College, Quebec).
22*a*. ———, *Three Decades of Change in a Stable Rural Community, Penn-*

sylvania Agricultural Experiment Station Progress Report 261 (University Park, 1965).

23. John Cuber with Peggy B. Haroff, *The Significant Americans: A Study of Sexual Behavior Among the Affluent* (New York: Appleton-Century, 1965), 126–129.
24. Richard F. Curtis, "Occupation Mobility and Membership in Formal Voluntary Associations: A Note on Research," *ASR,* 24 (December, 1959), 846–848.
25. Dwight G. Dean, "Alienation: Its Meaning and Measurement," *ASR,* 26 (October, 1961), 753–758.
26. Floyd Kotson, "Patterns of Voluntary Associations Among Urban Working-Class Families," *ASR,* 16 (October, 1951), 687–693.
27. Otis Dudley Duncan and Jay W. Artis, *Social Stratification in a Pennsylvania Rural Community. Pennsylvania Agricultural Experiment Station Bulletin* 543, (University Park, 1951) pp. 38–41.
28. Samuel J. Eldersveld, *Political Parties: A Behavioral Analysis* (Chicago: Rand McNally and Company, 1964).
29. William Erbe, "Social Involvement and Political Activity: A Replication and Elaboration," *ASR,* 29 (April, 1964), 198–215.
30. A. Alexander Fanelli, "Extensiveness of Communication Contacts and Perceptions of the Community," *ASR,* 21 (August, 1956), 439–445.
31. John M. Foskett, "The Influence of Social Participation on Community Programs and Activities," *Community Structure and Analysis,* ed. Marvin B. Sussman (New York: Thomas Y. Crowell Co., 1959), 311–330.
32. ———, "Social Structure and Social Participation," *ASR,* 20 (August, 1955), 431–438.
33. Ronald Freedman and Morris Axelrod, "Who Belongs to What in a Great Metropolis?" *Adult Leadership,* Vol. 1, No. 6 (November, 1952), 6–9.

33*a*. Charles Freeman, "Two Approaches to Community Development: A Situational Analysis" (Paper read at the 1960 Annual Meeting of the Rural Sociological Society, University Park, Pennsylvania).

34. Howard Freeman, Edwin Novak, and Leo Reeder, "Correlates of Membership in Voluntary Associations," *ASR,* 22 (October, 1957), 528–533.
35. R. Oliver Gibson, "Toward a Conceptualization of Absence Behavior of Personnel in Organizations," *Administrative Science Quarterly,* 11 (June, 1966), 107–133.

35*a*. William A. Glaser, "The Family and Voting Turnout," *POQ,* 23 (Winter, 1959), 563–570.

36. Herbert Goldhamer, "Voluntary Associations in the United States," in Paul K. Hatt and Albert J. Reiss, Jr., eds., *Cities and Society: The Revised Reader in Urban Sociology* (Glencoe, Illinois: The Free Press, 1957), 591–596.
37. C. Wayne Gordon and Nicholas Babchuk, "A Typology of Voluntary Associations," *ASR,* 24 (February, 1959), 22–29.
38. Saxon Graham, "Social Correlates of Adult Leisure-Time Behavior," in Marvin B. Sussman, ed., *Community Structure and Analysis* (New York: Thomas Y. Crowell Co., 1959), 331–354.
39. Scott Greer, "Individual Participation in Mass Society," in Roland Young, ed., *Approaches to the Study of Politics* (Evanston, Illinois: Northwestern University Press, 1958), 329–342.
40. ——— and Peter Orleans, "The Mass Society and the Parapolitical Structure," *ASR,* 27 (October, 1962), 643–646.
41. John Harp, "A General Theory of Social Participation," *RS,* 24 (September, 1959), 280–284.

41*a*. Herbert H. Hyman, *Political Socialization: A Study in the Psychology of Political Behavior* (Glencoe, Illinois: The Free Press, 1959).
42. J. L. Hypes, *Social Participation in a Rural New England Town* (New York: Bureau of Publications, Teacher's College, Columbia University, 1927).
43. Arthur P. Jacoby and Nicholas Babchuk, "Instrumental and Expressive Voluntary Associations," *Sociology and Social Research,* 47 (July, 1963), 461–471.
44. Elihu Katz and Paul F. Lazarsfeld, *Personal Influence* (Glencoe, Illinois: The Free Press, 1955), 271–295.
44*a*. Fred E. Katz, "Social Participation and Social Structure," *SF*, 45 (December, 1966), 199–210.
45. V. O. Key, Jr., Politics, Parties, and Pressure Groups (5th ed.; New York: Thomas Y. Crowell Co., 1964), 575.
46. Genevieve Knupfer, "Portrait of an Underdog," *POQ*, 12 (Spring, 1947), 103–114.
47. Mirra Komarovsky, "A Comparative Study of Voluntary Organization of Two Suburban Communities," *Publications of The American Sociological Society: Papers* (May, 1933), 83–93.
48. ———, "The Voluntary Associations of Urban Dwellers," *ASR,* 11 (December, 1946), 686–698.
49. William Kornhauser, *The Politics of Mass Society* (Glencoe, Illinois: The Free Press, 1959).
50. Toimi Kyllonen, "Social Characteristics of Union Activists," *AJS*, 56 (May, 1951), 528–533.
51. Robert E. Lame, *Political Life: Why People Get Involved in Politics* (Glencoe, Illinois: The Free Press, 1959).
52. Bernard Lazerwitz, "Some Factors Associated with Church Attendance," *SF*, 39 (May, 1961), 301–309.
53. Gerhard Lenski, "Social Participation and Status Crystallization," *ASR,* 21 (August, 1956), 458–464.
54. Seymour M. Lipset, Paul F. Lazarsfeld, Allen H. Barton and Juan Linz, "The Psychology of Voting: An Analysis of Political Behavior," *Handbook of Social Psychology,* ed. Gardner Lindzey, Vol. II (Cambridge, Massachusetts: Addison-Wesley Publishing Co., Inc., 1954), 1124–1175.
54*a*. Eugene Litwak, "Voluntary Associations and Neighborhood Cohesion," *ASR*, 26 (April, 1961), 258–271.
55. Norton E. Long, "The Local Community as an Ecology of Games," *AJS*, 64 (November, 1958), 251–261.
55*a*. George A. Lundberg, Mirra Komarovsky and Mary Alice McInery, *Leisure: A Suburban Study* (New York: Columbia University Press, 1934).
56. Herbert Maccoby, "The Differental Political Activity of Participants in a Voluntary Association," *ASR*, 23 (October, 1958), 524–532.
57. Walter T. Martin, "A Consideration of Differences in the Extent and Location of the Formal Associational Activities of Rural Urban Fringe Residents," *ASR*, 17 (December, 1952), 687–694.
58. William G. Mather, "Income and Social Participation," *ASR*, 6 (June, 1941), 380–384.
59. Selz C. Mayo, "Age Profiles of Social Participation in Rural Areas of Wake County, North Carolina," *RS*, 15 (1950), 242–251.
59*a*. Herbert McClosky and John H. Schaar, "Psychological Dimension of Anomy," *ASR*, 30 (February, 1965), 14–40.
60. Robert K. Merton, "Patterns of Influence: Local and Cosmopolitan Influentials," in Robert K. Merton, *Social Theory and Social Structure* (rev. ed.; Glencoe, Illinois: The Free Press, 1957), 387–420.

60*a*. Lester W. Milbrath, *Political Participation* (Chicago: Rand McNally and Co., 1965).
61. Mhyra S. Minnis, "The Patterns of Women's Organizations: Significance, Types, Social Prestige Ranks, and Activities," *Community Structure and Analysis,* ed. Marvin B. Sussman (New York: Thomas Y. Crowell Co., 1959), 269–287.
62. Ephraim Harold Mizruchi, "Social Structure and Anomie in a Small City," *ASR,* 25 (October, 1960), 645–654.
63. Joan W. Moore, "Patterns of Women's Participation in Voluntary Associations," *AJS,* 66 (May, 1961), 592–598.
63*a*. Arthur G. Neal and Salomon Rettig, "Dimensions of Alienation Among Manual and Non-Manual Workers," *ASR,* 28 (August, 1963), 599–608.
64. ——— and Melvin Seeman, "Organizations and Powerlessness: A Test of the Mediation Hypothesis," *ASR,* 29 (April, 1964), 216–226.
65. Anthony M. Orum, "Reappraisal of the Social and Political Participation of Negroes," *AJS,* 72 (July, 1966), 32–46.
66. Outdoor Recreation Resources Review Commission, *Participation in Outdoor Recreation: Factors Affecting Demand Among American Adults, ORRRC Study Report* 20 (Washington, D.C.: U.S. Government Printing Office, 1962).
67. Leonard Reissman, "Class, Leisure, and Social Participation," *ASR,* 19 (February, 1954), 76–84.
68. Arnold M. Rose, "Alienation and Participation: A Comparison of Group Leaders and the 'Mass,'" *ASR,* 27 (December, 1962), 834–838.
69. ———, "Attitudinal Correlates of Social Participation," *SF,* 37 (March, 1959), 202–206.
70. ———, "Voluntary Associations in France," *Theory and Method in the Social Sciences* (Minneapolis: University of Minnesota Press, 1954), 72–115.
71. Morris Rosenberg, "Some Determinants of Political Apathy," *POQ,* 18 (Winter, 1954), 349–366.
72. Stanley Schachter, *The Psychology of Affiliation: Experimental Studies of the Sources of Gregariousness* (Stanford, California: Stanford University Press, 1959).
73. John Scott, Jr., "Membership and Participation in Voluntary Associations," *ASR,* 22 (June, 1957), 315–326.
73*a*. Melvin Seeman, "On the Meaning of Alienation," *ASR,* 24 (December, 1959), 783–791.
74. William Spinard, "Correlates of Trade Union Participation: A Summary of the Literature," *ASR,* 25 (April, 1960), 237–244.
75. Carol Slater, "Class Differences in Definition of Role and Membership in Voluntary Associations Among Urban Married Women," *AJS,* 65 (May, 1960), 616–619.
75*a*. David Horton Smith, "A Psychological Model of Individual Participation in Formal Voluntary Organizations: Applications to Some Chilean Data," *AJS,* 72 (November, 1966), 249–266.
76. Gresham M. Sykes, "The Differential Distribution of Community Knowledge," *SF* (May, 1951), 376–382.
77. James E. Teele, "Measures of Social Participation," *Social Problems,* 10 (Summer, 1962), 31–39.
77*a*. ———, "An Appraisal of Research on Social Participation," *Sociological Quarterly,* 6 (Summer, 1965), 257–267.
78. Frederic Templeton, "Alienation and Political Participation: Some Research Findings," *POQ,* 30 (Summer, 1966), 249–261.
79. Wayne E. Thompson and John E. Horton, "Political Alienation as a Force in Political Action," *SF,* 38 (March, 1960), 190–195.

79*a*. Arthur J. Vidich and Joseph Bensman, *Small Town in Mass Society* (Princeton: Princeton University Press, 1958).
80. W. Keith Warner and William D. Heffernan, "The Benefit-Participation Contingency in Voluntary Farm Organizations" (Paper read at the 1966 Annual Meeting of the Rural Sociological Society, Miami Beach, Florida).
81. ———, "The Benefit-Participation Relationship in Voluntary Organizations" (Madison: Department of Rural Sociology, University of Wisconsin, 1964) (mimeographed).
82. ———, "Problems of Participation," *Journal of Cooperative Extension,* 3 (Winter, 1965), 219–228.
83. Irving L. Webber, "The Organized Social Life of the Retired in Two Florida Communities," *AJS,* 59 (January, 1954), 340–346.
84. Harold L. Wilensky, "Life Cycle, Work, Situation, and Participation in Formal Associations," *Aging and Leisure* (New York: Oxford University Press, 1961), 213–242.
85. ———, "Orderly Careers and Social Participation: The Impact of Work History on Social Integration in the Middle Mass," *ASR,* 26 (August, 1961), 521–539.
86. Julian L. Woodward and Elmo Roper, "Political Activity of American Citizens," *APSR,* 44 (December, 1950), 872–885.
87. Charles R. Wright and Herbert H. Hyman, "Voluntary Association Memberships of American Adults: Evidence from National Sample Surveys," *ASR,* 23 (June, 1958), 284–294.
88. Basil G. Zimmer, "Farm Background and Urban Participation," *AJS,* 6 (March, 1956), 470–475.
89. ———, "Participation of Migrants in Urban Structures," *ASR,* 20 (April, 1955), 218–224.
90. ——— and Amos Hawley, "The Significance of Membership in Associations," *AJS,* 65 (September, 1959), 196–201.
91. ——— and Amos Hawley, "Suburbanization and Church Participation," *SF,* 37 (May, 1959), 348–354.

SOCIAL PARTICIPATION, CITIZENSHIP, AND THE VISUALLY HANDICAPPED

S. C. Ashcroft

The purpose of this paper is to provide an analysis of research on social participation and citizenship as it relates to visually handicapped individuals and to those who work with and for such individuals.

INTRODUCTION

It should be remembered that the prevalence in the general population of persons who are blind as defined for legal purposes is just more than one fifth of one per cent (0.214%) or about two per 1,000. Probably only one in four of these, or about one in 2,000 (96,000) of the general population, is totally blind or does not retain some useful vision. It must also be remembered that probably more than half of these legally blind individuals are 65 or more years of age, and that another approximate 10 per cent are 20 years of age or less and are therefore largely school-aged children and youths. For these groups, social participation and citizenship are conditioned in very significant ways which are different from those of the 20 to 65 age group. In terms of these considerations, less than 40,000 individuals comprise the focal group if severe loss of vision and age are treated as critical variables for research on social participation and citizenship. For a variety of reasons to be considered, I maintain that conventional research approaches for these persons as a special group are not likely to be fruitful.

I hold the view that handicapped individuals do not comprise a special social group by virtue of physical or sensory impairments. Rather, they are members of a larger society much the same as any other individuals. In this paper, the term "individuals who are visually handicapped" or a comparable term, is used rather than "the blind," "the visually handicapped," and so on. Though less convenient, this usage is intended to emphasize the point that visual impairments do not produce a homogeneous group on any dimension crucial for research on social participation and citizenship.

I also share the view—expressed so well by Thomas Cutsforth[8]—that the individual with an impairment is organized and that he is organized to the fullest extent which existing conditions permit. He is thus a whole person organized in terms of what he has and is, rather than what he lacks or is not.

There is, of course, a critical paradox here. Considered briefly later in this paper is the impact of institutional-environmental influences in defining and identifying deviance that vests or tends to vest a group with unique and differentiating characteristics. Such influences, much like an environmental constant such as Chevigny and Braverman[6] have proposed, can produce deviance of equal or greater significance than visual impairment in and of itself.

REVIEW OF RESEARCH ON PARTICIPATION AND CITIZENSHIP

For purposes of his interpretive review of research in the previous paper,[7] Professor Copp has defined his terms narrowly and treated social participation and citizenship as closely related or identical. Social participation and citizenship were defined in operational terms as membership or membership activities in formal organizations and voluntary associations, and citizenship is taken as a matter of *actions* rather than altruistic beliefs and attitudes.

The basic paper provides a consideration of research on the environment of participation ranging from the macrocosm of government to the microcosm of the neighborhood, and including the climate in a given organization and individual participation. With respect to the individual, research is reviewed dealing with the extent of participation in American society along with the factors of age, sex, socioeconomic status, education, income, occupation, and race. Family factors, social mobility, migration, and personality factors are also examined. Of particular interest are the new research approaches to participation.

In turning to *New Research Departures* in his paper, Professor Copp lists problems he has identified through his review: . . . *cut and dried research . . . research involving the earnest rediscovery of prior findings . . . the need for theoretical development . . .*

the need for a taxonomy . . . personality factors difficult to specify precisely . . . repetitive character . . . relabeling of our ignorance . . . confusion of effect for cause.

In discussing research findings on individual participation, Professor Copp says, ". . . with few exceptions, the repetitive character of social participation research . . . has a deadening monotony. Only in the 60's have fresh departures become apparent. New variables are being tried and participation is beginning to be viewed from a systematic context larger than the individual actor."

RELATED ANALYSES AND RESEARCH

Turning to an analysis and application of research in social participation and citizenship in terms of those who are visually handicapped, it will be useful to consider several points of view. One is the "Analysis of What Is Lost" and "Restoration" after the manner of Reverend Thomas J. Carroll in *Blindness.*[5] Carroll lists seven categories of losses, including concomitant losses entailed by blindness. His categories are losses; (1) to psychological security; (2) in basic skills; (3) in communication; (4) in appreciation; (5) concerning occupation and financial status; (6) to the whole personality; and (7) concomitant losses. These concomitant losses include under "occupation and financial status," recreation; career, vocational goals; and job opportunity. Under "personality" they include personal independence, social adequacy, obscurity, self-esteem, and personality organization. These losses seem particularly relevant to the topic at hand.

It must be recognized that Reverend Carroll has focused on the adventitiously blinded person and implies emphasis on those who have sustained severe vision loss. Further, he has derived his analyses from experience and the literature, but has seldom had access to research for his derivations.

Mary K. Bauman[2,3,4] and Pennsylvania have been responsible for providing some very useful research. In concluding the report on *Adjustment to Blindness,* Mrs. Bauman wrote, "There is considerable evidence that individuals without useful vision are more likely to become members of organized groups than are persons who retain some vision, and they are very much more likely to take a leadership part in them. An attitude of suspicion toward others, a sense of being at a disadvantage in dealing with seeing persons, and even the feeling that blindness may be a punishment, are related, not to amount of vision, but to characteristics which can be measured by the personality inventory."

And, most important, Mrs. Bauman said, "Indeed, if it were necessary to summarize all the findings of this study in a single thought, that thought would be that no quality of vision, health, education, or family and social interaction has so much to do with adjustment as have the qualities measured by the intelligence quotient and personality inventory scores."

Mrs. Bauman reported in her 1963 study that 72 per cent of the study population had memberships in professional organizations, 40 per cent had memberships in community groups, 34 per cent had memberships in organizations for the blind. Ten per cent reported no memberships.

In considering group membership, Mrs. Bauman indicated, "Those who seem least likely to join any group are the mathematicians and engineers, and when they do indicate any membership it is only in their own special scientific groups. None indicates any interests in groups for the blind and in general they do not seem to think of themselves as blind people."

Mrs. Bauman also said:

> We also find no relationship between age of visual loss and group membership. We had guessed that those who lost their vision early in life might be more inclined to join organizations for the blind, while those who reached adult life as seeing people might, instead, cling chiefly to regular community groups. Our data do not support this hypothesis. Of the 213 people who were blind before the age of ten, 72 belong to community organizations and 71 to organizations for the blind. Only among the rather small number in this study who lost their vision after they were 40 years of age do we find an apparent lack of interest in organizations for the blind.
>
> The city and small town groups show no significant differences in membership in professional and community groups. The city dwellers do, however, belong to organizations for the blind in significantly greater numbers . . . This may, of course, merely mean that those in small or rural communities do not have such specialized groups available.

Though incidental to another objective, Mary Bauman's research provides information on variables involved in research reviewed by Professor Copp. Bauman's findings raise serious questions regarding the value of replicating participation research with individuals who are visually handicapped.

For another aspect of the issues germane to the present topic, it is interesting to examine a concept developed in sociology of rehabilitation. Freidson[9] lists four activities of rehabilitation agencies.

"First, they specify what personal attributes shall be called handicaps. Second, they seek to identify who conforms to their specifications. Third, they attempt to gain access to those whom they call handicapped. And fourth, they try to get those to whom they gain access to change their behavior so as to conform more closely to what the institutions believe are their potentialities."

The same four activities are inherent in research approaches and research thus falls heir to the same detrimental effects of the population under study. Freidson continues:

> In the course of defining and classifying the universe which they claim needs their services, all control agencies in effect become responsible for drawing clearer lines than in fact exist either in everyday life or in the processes by which people were originally led into their services, and agencies may come to define people as deviant who would not ordinarily have been so defined. Both professionalism and bureaucratization objectify deviance and reify diagnostic categories. In this sense, while such agencies may not actually *create* deviant roles, they do by the nature of their activities refine and clarify their boundaries and, by assuming responsibility for their control, add elements to the roles that may not have existed previously, and so encourage pulling new people into them.
>
> . . . if public labeling or visible segregation from which a labeling conclusion can be drawn occurs, the process may be said to be deviance-producing in that, by labeling the individual, it may organize the responses of the community toward him as a stereotyped deviant. Whereas those around him might never have attained any consensus about his behavior before, each responding to him according to his individual relationship, public labeling establishes a common focus for uniform community responses that carve out a role for him . . .

It should be clear that the management of deviance is quite capable of organizing deviant behavior in that labeling or implying a label for it stimulates the community to organize its response to the individual, to a degree segregating him by those special responses and encouraging him to accept the role of the blind man, the village idiot, or the cripple. In this sense, the "treatment" process may be said to create organized or stereotypical behavior. As Freidson says, "agencies for the physically handicapped have been observed to organize and stabilize deviant behavior into special roles, rather than eradicate it."

Freidson's analysis seems to suggest that institutional-environmental factors would contribute more than physical attributes to variance in social participation and citizenship behavior. An investigation of these institutional-environmental effects might be rewarding.

IMPLICATIONS FOR RESEARCH

For purposes of the present analysis, the following summary and concluding statements may be useful. Descriptive, demographic, and epidemiological research on such problems as social participation and citizenship have produced equivocal and minimally valuable results. What appears to be needed are ecological and intervention types of approaches. As Professor Copp points out and documents from the work of others, "Too often we fail to view the individual life history as a system." Further, it would seem evident that we fail in the same way to take research approaches which involve the whole ecological system of which the person who is visually handicapped is a part.

Professor Copp's objective and critical review suggests several considerations for those who would undertake behavioral research with reference to work with people who are visually handicapped.

1. The state of the art appears to motivate the view that to replicate with a blind population the types of studies that have been done with sighted individuals is unlikely to prove very fruitful.

2. If there is one finding that seems abundantly clear from research on blind populations, it is the fruitlessness of assuming that blindness as a physical disability produces a homogeneous group on any variable of crucial significance for research purposes.

3. Meyerson's canon[10] must be remembered. "Where a difference is found between disabled and non-disabled samples, the difference may not be interpreted as due to the disability if differences on other significant variables were not controlled."

4. It would seem that persons who are blind (in proportion to their incidence in the general population) should not be excluded from research studies on social participation and citizenship on the assumption that their blindness as a physical attribute is a critical or confounding factor. Persons who are blind should be included or excluded in terms of whether they meet the same criteria as normally seeing individuals, for example, age, sex, socio-economic factors, education, income, occupation, race, personality, and so on.

Professor Copp's review helps, in several ways, those who work with individuals who are visually handicapped. It suggests the limited value in pursuing the kinds of research which have been done in the past. Equally important, new approaches have been suggested, such as *The Triggering Phenomenon; The Benefit Contingency; "Plebiscitary Membership"* and *Career Stability*.

Perhaps the unfinished business is most important. Here he pleads for theoretical development, a plea frequently heard in connection with research on factors related to persons who are visually handicapped. The situation is similar with respect to the need for a taxonomy.

NOTES

1. S. C. Ashcroft, "Blind and Partially Seeing Children," in *Exceptional Children in the Schools* (New York: Holt, Rinehart and Winston, 1963), 413–462.
2. Mary K. Bauman, *Adjustment to Blindness: A Study as Reported by the Committee to Study Adjustment to Blindness* (Harrisburg: Pennsylvania State Council for the Blind, 1954).
3. ——— and Norman M. Yoder, *Placing the Blind and Visually Handicapped in Professional Occupations* (Washington: Office of Vocational Rehabilitation, Department of Health, Education, and Welfare, 1962).
4. ———, *Characteristics of Blind and Visually Handicapped People in Professional, Sales and Managerial Work* (Harrisburg: Pennsylvania Office for the Blind, 1963).
5. Thomas J. Carroll, *Blindness* (Boston: Little, Brown, 1961).
6. Hester Chevigny and S. Braverman, *The Adjustment of the Blind* (New Haven, Connecticut: Yale University Press, 1950).
7. James H. Copp, "An Interpretative Review of Research Dealing with Social Participation and Citizenship," (Paper given at the National Research Consultation on Problems Related to Blindness, The Pennsylvania State University, April 10, 1967).
8. T. D. Cutsforth, *The Blind in School and Society* (New York: American Foundation for the Blind, 1951).
9. Eliot Freidson, "Disability as Social Deviance," *Sociology and Rehabilitation*, Marvin B. Sussman, ed. (Washington: American Sociological Association, 1965), 71–99.
10. Lee Meyerson, "The Visually Handicapped," *Review of Educational Research*, Vol. 23, No. 5 (1953).

SESSION REPORT

Donald Granberg

In his response to Dr. Ashcroft, Professor Copp began by noting the importance of considering who is to be organized to support organizations for the blind: the blind or the non-blind. He also raised questions as to how homogeneous the blind people are as a social category. Dr. M. E. John, the moderator, indicated that the response of others to the handicap may be as important as the effects of the handicap itself. A comment from the floor suggested that gang behavior might constitute citizenship, to which Professor Copp emphatically replied, "no."

Dr. Copp seriously asked why a session on this topic was organized: That is, do blind people differ that much in social participation from the non-blind segment of the population? The indications, in fact, are that they do not. Mrs. Bauman found essential similarities, with about ten per cent of the blind people not participating. She used agency clients as the source of this data. Dr. Copp noted that blind males may be slightly better participators than their non-blind counterparts, but he added that Mrs. Bauman's study was limited in that an elite (middle class, professional) sample was taken.

The issue was raised as to whether it is better for blind people to attend schools for the blind or regular public schools, and also whether schools for the blind prepare their students to take an active, as normal as possible, role in society or whether they prepare the blind for permanent dependency or institutionalization.

Another issue centered on the basis and function of associations for the blind. The general feeling was that the blind should be citizens, not wards of society. It was suggested that the motives involved in organizing the blind be scrutinized. Dr. Ashcroft emphasized that institutionalization of the blind may not lead to independence, and he wondered whether schools for the blind actively seek to make blind people eventually independent.

The discussion then shifted to agencies for the blind because a question was raised regarding the number of blind people who have not been referred to such agencies. Interest was also expressed in learning how many people become independent once they have had contact with the agencies.

One discussant suggested the possibility that a blind person knows how best to treat another blind person. Another participant brought the discussion back to the effects of labeling, noting that organizations for the visually handicapped usually include the word "blind" in their titles, despite the fact that most members are not blind in the strictest sense. One person noted that recordings always state, at the beginning, that they have been prepared for the blind, and that this is resented by some blind people.

A research interest was expressed by one participant in analyzing the various organizations for the blind and, in particular, the relationships among these organizations. Another participant suggested that there was too much emphasis on legislation and too little concern with what the blind people, in fact, want. He also brought up the importance of examining the distinction between legislation and practice. It was noted that blind people do not seem to make concerted efforts for causes not directly related to helping blind people.

At this time, an underlying assumption of the discussion was pointed out by the moderator: interaction and participation are good; the more there is of it, the better. This remark turned the discussion toward the basic question: Is a high level of social participation necessarily good and desirable? Dr. Copp noted that people can live satisfactory lives with low levels of participation if neighborhood and family life are good. In fact, hyperactivity may be a symptom that something is wrong in these two areas.

Are the values of the agencies imposed upon blind people? This was referred to as "the problem of imposition." Should people be allowed to do what they want to do? Also discussed were the various gains and losses which blind people incur as a consequence of their blindness, and it was added that those helping the blind may be helping themselves in the process.

A few figures were presented: One half of all blind people receive, on the average, $81 per month. In Virginia, only 10 per cent of the blind receive public assistance.

The discussion shifted back to the question: Do agencies for the blind really seek to make blind people independent of them? Do blind people at times become entrapped within these organizations?

With regard to research, it was suggested (counter to Dr. Ashcroft) that comparisons need to be made between the "normal public" and blind individuals. It was felt that the attitudes of members of a society, and how they do or do not change, are of particular significance.

The difficulties blind people experience in carrying out civic responsibilities were also discussed. One blind participant noted that he was required to have one Democrat and one Republican in the polling booth with him when he votes. Also, the premise that it is wise and compassionate to pressure industries or civil service agencies into hiring the handicapped was challenged.

Problems of the blind with respect to voting were mentioned once again, one example cited was the problem of mobility: How does the blind person get to where he votes? This example related to the more general question of what makes the problems of the blind basically different from those of other handicapped people and from those of the population at large? How is he functionally different? Another research problem which emerged was: How are social participation and occupational success correlated for blind and non-blind people?

The occupation of teaching was then discussed with special reference to problems of blind teachers. The question was raised as to what the effects are, for example, of being able to achieve education so as to qualify oneself to teach and then being unable, legally, to teach in some areas. An interest in the parallels (or lack of them) which exist between blindness and other handicaps, was also expressed.

It was mentioned that blind people cannot enter the Foreign Service. This remark suggested to one discussant that a documentation of the legal barriers which exist for blind people, especially those which infringe on the exercise of basic civil rights and civic duties, would constitute an extremely useful project. The issue was also raised as to whether blind people can now marry everywhere without being sterilized.

Another potential research topic mentioned concerned the conditions under which the blind want to participate with other blind people and the conditions under which they would prefer interaction with non-blind people. The image that the public has with respect to these preferences of blind people might also be investigated. It was also brought out that there are times when a blind person may prefer to be alone and to do things by himself. However, it was noted that the nature of the handicap may place considerable restrictions on this kind of behavior.

In the concluding minutes, the discussion shifted back to questions of civil rights. Questions were raised such as: Does a blind person have the right to choose who will invade his privacy (for example, who will mark his ballot)? It was pointed out that attention should be given not only to existing laws but also to the logistics of initiating court actions and taking appeals.

MOTIVATION

MOTIVATION AND MOTIVATIONAL THEORY

Charles N. Cofer

MOTIVATION

Motivation, in the present century, has come to have a highly popular status as the postulated source of many of our individual and social problems, as an explanation for the failure of individuals to live up to their potentialities, and, on the other hand, as an explanation of why some people seem to exceed their potentialities or react constructively and successfully in the face of many difficulties and handicaps. It is not entirely clear to me why motivation has achieved this status, but there are perhaps several reasons. One is that in certain accounts of behavior, motivation, or something like it, is often accorded primary status. This has certainly been true in psychoanalysis, a viewpoint which has had wide currency, and it has figured centrally in those formulations which stress instinctive sources of energy as the mainsprings of action, as in William McDougall's account in his *Social Psychology* (1908). Likewise, in biologically oriented accounts of behavior, which use neither psychoanalytic nor instinct concepts, the notion of drive, as represented by such terms as hunger, sex, thirst, dependency, achievement, and power, is prominent. It is almost as if organisms, both men and animals, would do nothing at all were they not goaded into action by some drive.

There has, I think, been some change during the past decade or so in our conceptions of the nature of motivation and of its role as a factor in behavior. Some psychoanalysts, for example, have lessened the importance they attribute to motivation by postulating independent "ego structures" or processes as importantly involved in organismic functioning.[10] Instinct theories like those proposed by McDougall have fallen into disfavor, though the concept of innate behavior patterns has, if anything, received renewed emphasis in the work of the European ethologists and the Americans whom they have influenced. Recent advances in the neurophysiology of drive, together with experimental demonstrations that environmental contingencies are important to the appearance of drive-related behavior, have replaced simple, local-stimulus conceptions of drive, characteristic of an earlier day. Then, too, it seems now to be clear that organisms, from rat to man, can be activated by events external to them, such as novel or complex stimuli or by unusual situations or events. All of these trends have made our accounts of motivation more complex than they were a few years ago and perhaps lead to great concern for just what it is we have in mind when we use the term, motivation. (For a review of some of these developments and their implications, see Cofer and Appley,[7] especially chapters 3, 5, 6, 8, 12, and 16.)

For the purposes of the present discussion, however, it is not necessary to become involved in many of the questions to which I have just alluded. Rather, it is perfectly clear that people with handicaps, such as blindness and visual deficiencies, differ markedly in their reactions to their defects, to begin with, and in their adjustive means of coping with these defects over the long term. The differences between groups *A* and *C*, in Bauman's study,[1] are illustrative. The members of Group *C*, as you will recall, were and had been unemployed for some time and were not, generally speaking, well adjusted in their lives. Group *A*, on the other hand, consisted of employed persons selected because they were making satisfactory lives for themselves. Now it is true that Groups *A* and *C* differ in a number of respects from each other. But the distributions of their scores on many of the measures taken show great overlap, so that one would hesitate to say that any one factor, or perhaps any combination of factors, was the critical source for the over-all adjustment patterns of the group. I think Bauman means something of this sort when she says, ". . . no quality of vision, health, education, or family and social interaction has so much to do with adjustment as have the qualities measured by the Intelligence Quotient and personality inventory scores." [1] The aspect of her statement which concerns my topic, of course, is the emphasis on personality inventory scores. Traditionally, motivation is thought to have to do with these kinds of scores, whatever its relation to intelligence, or conversely. And in her other study, the one with professional and other successful people, Bauman[2] stresses the persistence, "in the face of unnumbered rebuffs," shown by the people in her sample and comments that many of them "decided what they wanted to do with their lives and went firmly ahead to do it." Surely these characteristics are motivational in nature.

Having made these opening and general remarks, let me say that I have not worked in the area of visual handicaps and have but a passing familiarity with the important problems. So what I choose to discuss will, of necessity, require further interpretation and application.

To begin with, it is evident that when one speaks of "the blind" or "the visually handicapped" he is not speaking of an homogeneous group of people. There are many differences, just as there are in any cross-sample of the general population. All, or many, of these differences may have much to do with the reactions to and the methods developed for coping with blindness. Motivation is only one of these factors and its importance may not always be great. I am certain, however, that its influence must be differentially important and that its import must take varied forms as we examine three broad classes of blind and visually handicapped people: (1) those blind from birth or from a very early age; (2) those for whom the onset of blindness was sudden; and (3) those in whom the visual handicap developed progressively and slowly over a period of years. It may be true of all three groups, but it seems especially evident in the case of the second group, that reactions will be vastly different for people of varying ages and of different statuses in life. Sudden onset in the elderly and in the retiree must have vastly different implications from those it has during the period of early adulthood, with its family responsibilities and its career aspirations. What I mean to convey is that workers with the blind must usually deal with the specific individual in the light of his specific capacities, capabilities, circumstances, and history.

I would like now to consider these three classes within the population of blind and visually handicapped people from the standpoint of notions from the area of motivation which occur to me as relevant to them. Let me start with the second class.

Sudden Onset

The sudden loss of vision must be, to those who have experienced it, a terrifying and traumatic event. It includes, so far as I can see, roughly three components:

(1) sensory deprivation, in the meaning that without sight the total influx of sensory input is reduced, perhaps markedly, unless and until the individual can come to attend to other sources of

stimulation, impinging on his ears, nose and skin, for example, which for the most part seeing people are unaware of.

(2) the loss of visually imparted direction and maintenance of elementary but vital activities, such as walking, dressing, cooking, and the like, and of visually important sources of information, entertainment, such as reading, looking at pictures and at scenery, attending movies or watching TV, and even girlwatching.

(3) the disruption of career and life plans, such as those involved in one's vocation, based as they are for many people on deep and abiding motives and aspirations, and of one's relations with other people, such as one's family and friends, important as they are in the lives of most, to one's comfort, security, and well-being.

I suppose that after sudden onset, these three components may occur in a temporal sequence but that at some point the awful and simultaneous reality of all three of them must ultimately become apparent to the individual. What I am proposing is that the sudden onset of blindness contains the features of *stress,* probably psychological stress[7] rather than systemic stress in the sense of Selye.[11]

SENSORY DEPRIVATION Although we are all more or less familiar with the effects of monotonous stimulation (we say we are "bored"), systematic and experimental studies of the reduction of stimulation were reported in 1954[3] and in subsequent years. The experimenters used college students as subjects and paid them twenty dollars a day to remain in a lighted, partially sound-deadened room, where they lay on a cot wearing translucent goggles, which permitted no pattern vision, and gloves and cardboard cuffs, which reduced tactile stimulation. The noise from the air-conditioner masked out other noises, and the subject rested his head in a U-shaped, foam rubber pillow. The subjects could not take this situation very long, seldom remaining in it for as long as two or three days. (They were free to withdraw from the experiment at any time.) Thus, they sacrificed the wage in order to be freed from the sensory deprivation. Later, the investigators themselves[8] each endured this situation for six days.

Among the phenomena which were observed in the isolated subjects were boredom, a wish to end the isolation, restlessness, irritability, and emotional lability. Likewise, the subjects experienced a desire for stimulation and listened with relish, during their isolated period, to an old stock-market report and a talk, prepared for children, on the dangers of alcohol. They were tested at intervals during the deprivation period and, while the tests were not easy and caused the subjects trouble, they looked forward to being tested. Another investigator[9] suspended himself in a tank of tepid water and wore a blackout breathing mask; he reported attempting to satisfy his hunger for stimulation by making such movements as touching his fingers together and twitching his muscles. Other investigators, studying animals, have found that the provision of external stimulation to isolated animals would serve as a reward or reinforcement to the animal to learn responses which would provide stimulation.

A number of sensory, perceptual, cognitive, emotional, and motor effects have been reported to accompany sensory deprivation of this kind, including visual hallucinatory experiences, although the various studies do not agree well in the specific effects they found. Berlyne[4] has suggested that sensory isolation may, over a period of time, produce emotional arousal.

Although the circumstances surrounding the people studied in these experiments are very different from those surrounding people who experience a sudden loss of sight, there may well be similarities in reactions. Reactions like these, combined with perhaps even more massive reactions to greater threats imposed by the second and third components mentioned earlier, are the bases for my suggestion that the sudden onset of blindness is a condition in which psychological stress may occur in many people.

Before going on to a further discussion of psychological stress, it is worth noting that a conception of motivation, which has emerged from consideration of the kind of work I have just summarized, is that deviations in amount or pattern of stimulation from what we ordinarily experience are motivating.[7] The idea is that we develop an adaptation—or expectancy—level, based on our past experiences. Small deviations from this level are thought to be the bases for our interest in novelty, exploration, curiosity, and the like, but large deviations are ordinarily seen as having negative or adversive emotional effects. Boredom, on the other hand, is thought to arise from sameness or constancy. These notions appear to be very different from at least some of the motivational ideas of early psychoanalysts, early instinct theorists, and early biological drive theorists.

PSYCHOLOGICAL STRESS Cofer and Appley[7] have defined psychological stress as an organismic state in which the organism or individual "perceives that his well-being (or integrity) is endangered and that he must devote all his energies to its protection." It is perhaps important to note that stress is an extreme state, one which not all people subject to similar traumatic or debilitating events would reach and, in any case, one which may be reached in stages. For example, if one is unable to satisfy his motives, thus being in a state of insufficiency, he will use his ordinary innate or acquired coping behavior in efforts to rectify the insufficiency. However, this coping behavior may fail, and the failure may then lead to further arousal which brings with it new or unusual efforts to cope with the situation. Failure of these further efforts to cope with the problem leads to the perception of *threat,* which gives rise to anxiety and an intensification of coping behavior (perhaps repetitive). The introduction here of threat presumably changes the attempts at coping from task-oriented, problem-solving behavior to ego-oriented, self- or integrity-sustaining behavior. Therefore, while insufficiency and frustration are bad enough, real threat to the self is worse and engages ego-defensive measures not necessarily involved in sheer frustration or insufficiency alone. Next, when both task-related and ego-oriented behaviors fail to change the situation effectively, a stress threshold is reached. At this point, the organism becomes exclusively preoccupied with protection of the ego, danger may be perceived, and desperation or panic may ensue. Finally, if no surcease comes or can be anticipated and if stress endures long enough, helplessness or hopelessness may arise, leading perhaps to apathy and an absence of caring or striving.

Appley, whose thinking is represented in what I have just said about psychological stress, would not of course expect these stages to have precise demarcations or to appear in pure or unmixed forms, and he adds, as a further *caveat,* the factor of individual differences in frustration tolerance and in stress tolerance, so that different individuals would go through these sequences at different rates, and some would, for a given kind of threat, go only part way.

I am not sure how far in this series of events terminating in psychological stress sudden blindness takes people, or whether many of them go all the way or a long way toward this condition. Interventions which occur on the part of physicians, nurses, relatives, and others may have ameliorative effects at any stage of the developmental sequence. But it seems that the potential for the appearance of psychological stress always exists in sudden onset of blindness.

It is perhaps worthwhile to consider two further points about stress, that is, the conditions giving rise to it and a more adequate characterization of the stress response. These aspects of the matter may suggest how to prevent its occurrence or how to cope with it when it does arise. Then we can comment further on the three components of the reaction to sudden onset of blindness.

Again, according to Appley,[7] the world, for most of us, develops through childhood into patterns of expectancy about ourselves and about the environment. The world, he suggests, divides itself into what is familiar, predictable, and certain, and into the opposites of these terms; self-integrity is bound up with this ordering of the world and the self-identity which accompanies it.

It is clear that blindness of sudden onset must disturb this stable set of expectations about the world and about the self. If one's self is organized in terms of interaction and coping with this world through the visual sense, further disruptions would presumably occur. The environment and the self, following sudden loss of sight, should be strange, unfamiliar and one to which past orientations are perhaps no longer relevant, or, worse, maladaptive. This is a condition for stress, or an approach to it: the effectiveness of one's normal coping responses is reduced, and the strangeness arising from the disruptions of expectations about self and environment in itself is emotionally disturbing and arousing.

One would guess that provision of stability would be a desirable step to take to counteract stress, but even stable expectations with respect to the familiar persons in one's environment may be altered, if one can no longer see their manner, facial expressions, and postures on which we all depend, to some extent at least, for our interpretation of what is said to us.

The response to stress, in many of the situations in which it has been studied, includes many systemic and physiological reactions, and I have little doubt that these often accompany the sudden onset of blindness. There will be expressed subjective feelings of distress; others may reveal the significant concerns of the patient over his condition. Such reactions of distress may offer a good way to assess the significance of the loss of sight to an individual. There will be defensive reactions, explanations and rationalizations, depressive and perhaps regressive reactions as means of coping with or controlling the situation. All such manifestations should be important in determining the kind of reactions the patient has to his defect and the personality and motivation factors which will be involved in his development.

I should remind you, once again, that I have sketched a general reaction pattern which, in the individual case, may vary markedly in terms of the significance of the factors contributing to it, the nature and the intensity of the stress response itself, the kinds of reactions to it that will occur, and the temporal development of these reactions. It would be very significant to know what interventions and by whom, or what hopes and expectations, realistic or unrealistic, delayed or prevented the perception of threat, where it does not develop.

GENERAL DISCUSSION You will recall that I mentioned three components possibly contributing to the stress reaction in relation to the sudden onset of blindness. They were sensory deprivation; the loss of visual guidance; and the disruption of career and life plans and of relations with other people.

When I think of the second component, I think at once of the *dependent* status of the individual who has experienced a sudden loss of sight. He cannot easily, without substantial training and practice, do the things he used to do for himself. I am sure that there are some who will welcome dependency and the surcease from enterprise, decision, and initiative which it promises. I do not know whether there is a dependency drive or motive; authorities[7] do not agree on this question. Dependent behavior can develop in the service of other motives and goals and become quite strong, without having the independent status of a drive or motive.

On the other hand, some authorities have proposed that an aroused state or motive can appear when the expectations based on the past experience of being cared for are frustrated. Such an arousal state would probably cause the individual to redouble his dependent activities. In any case, it would be difficult to differentiate such a state from other arousal states, such as anxiety, which dependency behavior can serve to allay. While the distinction I am drawing may be a rather fine one, it is useful to say that just because one is dependent does not necessarily mean that there is a need or motive to be dependent. Dependent behavior can serve many motives and goals, and the same can be said for many patterns of behavior, often thought to arise only because a motive or a need produces them; aggressive behavior is another good example.[5]

There will, of course, be other reactions to the loss of sight and the dependent role which it entails: Nonacceptance, attempts to do for and to entertain oneself, rage and aggression to the helpful efforts of others which are perceived as derogating, controlling, and insulting.

In this last comment, I have highlighted the interpersonal consequences of the dependent state into which the victim of sudden blindness falls. It is no less the case with those who welcome dependency that interpersonal ramifications will ensue. The overly dependent person can be annoying, especially if he is indirect and apologetic in his expression of his dependency and if his seeming gratitude exceeds what is appropriate. It is obvious that the management of this situation involves far more than intervention with the patient himself, although that will be necessary and desirable. Perhaps the most effective way to prevent the untoward acceptance of dependency, on the one hand, and the unrealistic rejection of it, on the other, is early contact and counseling or training of the significant caretaking persons.

In any case, it would certainly be desirable if there were assessment procedures adequate to uncover, at an early stage, the potential development of one or the other of these stages and to assess, at a later time, the progress toward or away from the kinds of development about which I have speculated. Bauman's comparisons of Groups *A* and *C* on the basis of personality measures came too late to determine whether the personality differences between the groups was an effect or a cause of the individuals being classifiable into either group. Unfortunately, it would seldom be likely that measures would be available ahead of the onset of sudden blindness, and I do not know of any entirely satisfactory way of making the assessments indicated. A detailed past history, with special attention to the extent to which the individual has taken responsibility in the past for those details of his life which are expressed in this second component and to how he has reacted to prior periods of dependency, might be useful. Some of the personality questionnaires, such as the MMPI, if administered in terms of former rather than present reactions might also aid in the assessment. I would be wary of projective procedures, because of their difficulties of interpretation. And most of them require that sight be present before they can be employed at all.

It is no easy task to ascertain how to allay the anxiety or other motives underlying dependency behavior without in some way rewarding the latter. But I suppose that a skilled and aware person can accomplish it. Perhaps those who reject dependency would be easier to cope with, once their rage reactions and interpersonal difficulties could be managed.

The third component, disruption of career and life plans and of relations with people, is the most difficult to discuss in the generality, because individuals perhaps differ most greatly in this component, whereas we could imagine that the first two components certainly must have elements in common. And to make matters worse, there are no available general and standard inventories of career goals and the motives that underlie them; no dimensional analyses of relationships with other people; and no prescriptions for a satisfactory life, aside from career and interpersonal relations. Furthermore, it is not at all clear to me that all people plan their lives, possess career goals, or have more than superficial relations with other people.

Where career goals and life plans are relevant, they are probably of several kinds and their relative importance will depend on the age of the suddenly blinded person and on the ages and composition of his family. I will comment on both of these aspects of this component separately though they are intimately interrelated.

Career goals are certainly important determiners of behavior, having both the functions of directing behavior in ways calculated to achieve them and of mobilizing the individual's energies and resources to their attainment. We can differentiate between general kinds of career goals and more specific goals, the latter involving a particular line of work or vocation. These specific goals I would judge to be more characteristic of the older person than of the younger, that is, of the person who has completed his schooling and has embarked on trade or profession. And it would be anticipated that his flexibility and mobility would tend, on the average, to decrease with age. The specific career goals, of course, represent a means of achieving the more general career goals.

The general career goals probably characterize the younger person before he has made a specific vocational choice, and they can be conceptualized in terms of the kinds of work he thinks he would like to do. The reason for this distinction is that the more general the goals the more varied are the ways of realizing them, the more specific the goals the fewer are the ways of accomplishing them. It follows, I think, that sudden blindness in the young is less of a threat to the achievement of career goals than it is in the older person.

How are these goals assessed? The motives on which some work has been done[7] are not numerous. This is to say that measurement and experimental analysis of motives in the literature of motivation have been largely limited to aggression, dependency, anxiety, achievement, and affiliation. These are general motives but, aside from achievement and possibly affiliation, they are not well attuned to career goals. Another kind of instrument, of course, is the interest inventory, some of which are designed to tap into general classes of interests, others of which get at more specific occupational kinds of interests. With these and a knowledge of interests, hobbies, and school work gleaned from an extensive history, the worker with the young blind person can probably help select a specific occupational goal which will be appropriately related to general goals and made consonant with visual handicap in terms of the training required, the work itself, and the circumstances under which the work is to be carried out.

For the older patient, whose goals have already become specific, it may be infinitely more difficult to find alternative ways, necessitated by the handicaps, to achieve them. For what jobs is it possible to reorganize skills so that they can be performed by the blind person as well as he performed them while sighted?

I have spoken also of life plans in conjunction with the third component. By life plans I mean the family plans, the retirement plans, the extra-career social life, the family savings and what goals they are intended to meet. They are intimately bound up with career goals but are aspects of life's responsibilities which are common to many, as specific career goals are not.

I have also spoken of interpersonal relations in the third component. Here the loss of a sensory avenue breaks off a source of communication and a way of evaluating communications from other people that come by way of voice and touch. How often do the seeing look at the speaker, watching his face, his gestures, and his posture, to determine not only what he says but also how to interpret what he says?

In spending so much time on the case of sudden onset of blindness, I have chosen an area which has, to me, the most obvious implications with respect to motivation. The components I have identified must lead to arousal, if they occur, and perhaps to threat and stress. Coping reactions will occur under conditions of arousal and threat, and their success or failure will have profound implications to the further adjustment to the new circumstances. Let me turn now to the other broad classes I identified early in this paper.

Congenital Blindness and Very Early Onset

The motivational problems which congenital blindness or onset at a very early age entail are very different from those that must accompany sudden onset at a later age. This is to say that there are no patterns of behavior or expectations to be disrupted. The individual has always been without sight; there is no abrupt point at which there was a change.

Given an infant healthy and normal in other respects but blind from birth or from an early age, I can see no necessary defect or difference in motivation as compared with the normal, seeing child. Of course, the sightless child will encounter less stimulation, unless he makes up for the absence of vision by emphasizing his other senses or by attempts at exploring the world through manipulation. In cases of this sort, it seems likely that the unique features of motivation would be those which develop because the child is special or exceptional, as compared to his siblings or his sighted peers. The world will react differently to him than it will to others.

At this point I am moved to ask, because I do not know the evidence, what is the competence of children born blind or blinded early so far as growth and development of behavior are concerned? I have read that they may talk more than other children and that they do not express their emotions in facial expressions as well as other children.[6] But if blind children are allowed a relatively unsupervised and unregulated environment, how do they behave? Do they suffer injury? How do they play? How do they relate socially with adults and other children, sighted and sightless? Perhaps the relevant evidence is not available or is impossible to obtain. But it is critical to the question of how different blind children are from sighted children and the question of what special consequences flow from the absence of sight. I would be fully prepared for the finding that there are *no* great differences from the sighted group on items that do not uniquely depend on sight. This guess leads me to stress the social environment in considering the motivational consequences of congenital and early blindness.

In needing special protection because he has always been protected and indulged, in being special or different because he has always been treated that way, in expecting to be taken advantage of because of often being exploited, in feeling left out socially because he often *is* left out—all these special motivational characteristics may be functions of the kind of child of whom I speak. How many of these developments result because of the importance of the visual handicap? And how many of them are imposed by the expectations of others as to the role of a blind person in society? The reactions and conceptions of seeing persons with respect to the capability and the competences of blind persons probably vary but, no doubt, include discomfort in their presence, uncertainty over what is expected of them, and confusion as to how much the special disability should be ignored.

To the extent that motivational differences characterize the congenital and early blind person as compared to the seeing person, one will have two major problems: The desire to be taken care of or the habit of manifesting dependent behavior; and the maintenance of self concept. If his evaluation of himself is largely negative, including features of inadequacy, self derogation, and self pity, steps will have to be undertaken to construct a more positive self concept consistent with whatever his real abilities and capabilities are. One would imagine that training should be programmed in small steps, the achievement of each of which should be accompanied by rewards, praise, or the satisfaction of accomplishment. In the case of the infant or young child, much work with the parents will be necessary to overcome attitudes they will have toward a blind child and to teach them the best ways to guide him in doing the things he can do. I would guess that many parents would fail to accept the permanent reality of their child's blindness, on the ground that his sight can be restored. This expectation must be dealt with as definitely and as firmly as the facts of the case permit.

My major point here is that if special motivational problems attend congenital and early blindness and if they stem from parents and others of the social environment, then an educational program may be the way to provide a social environment which will not be so conducive to the development of these motivational problems.

Progressive and Gradual Onset of Blindness

I would not perceive motivational problems of a unique character in those individuals in whom the onset of blindness occurred gradually. There would, of course, be a considerable reaction, bordering perhaps on stress, when the individual comes to realize that his failing sight will not improve and will end in total blindness. And there will, of course, be many of the problems occasioned by the social environment, as there were with the previous class of individuals. But the present group has some advantages over the other two. It can prepare itself for ultimate sightlessness over the period of time that it takes to develop. And it has had the advantage of having had some sight, so that thinking of things in visual terms should still be possible after sight is gone.

I would suppose the most difficult problem with members of this group would be for them to accept the progressive development toward loss of sight and to prepare for it. Perhaps the problem often is that people do not seek the aid of workers with the blind before the development of sightlessness has progressed very far. Or, possibly, a problem is to motivate the person to develop the skill of reading braille, for example, so long as he still has sight left. Events that will occur in the distant future frequently have little reality or motivating power in the present.

Can people of this kind be given sight examinations periodically and can the progressive decline of their visual effectiveness be demonstrated, simply and effectively to them? Can forecasts be made with reasonable accuracy of the course of the unfavorable development? Such information might have a motivating effect, at least for some people, whereas a vague, indefinite, poorly documented prognosis of future sightlessness may not.

As you can see from my discussion here, it is difficult for me to come up with ideas, from a motivational viewpoint, for these individuals. The opportunities are available to these people to learn to cope with blindness in effective ways before it occurs, thus avoiding at least some of the problems of the suddenly blinded and of the congenital and early blinded. But my only suggestions here are that any procrastination on the taking of the necessary steps must be offset by the effectiveness of a presentation of the facts and of the future in conjunction with what the individual wishes or hopes to do with his life.

MOTIVATIONAL THEORY

In discussing current trends in the area of motivation, I will take, to begin with, a rather historical orientation in order to indicate something of the background that there is in the area of motivation. I will emphasize some of the notions in the field that have come to the forefront in the last 15 or 20 years and will stress especially what seem to me to be the most provocative ideas to arise in this period.

I think it is fair to say that the history of concern with motivational problems is not really very old. The acceptance of the irrational, through the concept of motivation in its earliest forms, not as an exception but rather as a prevailing characteristic of the human organism, is primarily a 20th Century event. I would not wish to defend the proposition that, when we refer to the term "motivation," we are referring to the irrational! But I do think that the early workers in the late 19th and early 20th Centuries, who talked about motivational concepts, did so in order to admit the irrational into considerations of human nature.

As best as I can judge, an important development that led to acceptance of motivational ideas was Darwinian evolution. This theory was extremely influential on three movements which came to fruition in the early part of the 20th Century. One of these is well represented by a psychologist whom nobody reads any more named William McDougall. The second one is represented by a psychologist or a psychoanalyst whom everybody reads, or pretends to read, Sigmund Freud. And the third movement is not represented well by any individual but rather by a group of individuals who are responsible for the development of what I shall here call "drive theory." This formulation is seen especially in the writings of physiologists such as Walter Cannon, Herbert Spencer Jennings, and Curt Richter.

McDougall, in his book *Social Psychology* (1908), stated as his basic problem that man sometimes does behave rationally even though, according to McDougall's concept of the human condition or of human nature, it would be unlikely that man would ever behave rationally. He felt that man's behavior was the product of basic instincts. I will not list them, but these instincts were seen as powerful moving forces in the human psyche, and their control required the development of great and elaborate means in the individual under the impetus of society. I think that, in many ways, McDougall's discussion of the means by which the individual, in response to society, developed control over the powerful, irrational sources of conduct that he called instincts really anticipated many of the modern theorists who have had a great deal of influence. Among these is Harry Stack Sullivan, whose notions of the self and of control by the self of various motives are very similar to those McDougall enunciated 30 or 40 years before. I mention McDougall primarily to emphasize the fact that he realized that there are irrational forces which have to be controlled by very elaborate devices centering in the notion of the self, which he developed.

Very similar in many ways, although much more popular, were Freud's ideas. Freud developed what has been referred to as an hydraulic model of the instinct or drive basis of behavior: If an instinct or drive developed to a high degree of tension, it would seek inevitably some kind of discharge. Because of the nature of the instincts Freud postulated, that is, sex and aggression, this discharge would again have to be controlled in some way, and the instinct tension alleviated or modified by such mechanisms as displacement, substitution, and sublimation—to mention just three. These mechanisms were devices which the Ego, responding both to reality and to the demands of the Superego, developed in order to keep the organism from doing bad things. And so again we have, to some extent, the conflict, as we do in McDougall, between the rational and irrational with, in Freud, the instincts being the irrational sources and the ego acting as an adjudicating agent, serving to make some kinds of satisfactions possible for the irrational forces, while at the same time not offending society or, perhaps more importantly, not offending the

Superego so that the Superego would not arouse reactions of guilt or shame in the Ego.

The third of these formulations I identify with the names of Cannon, Jennings, and Richter. It was probably Cannon who was the most definite exponent of the particular point of view I want to discuss. Cannon studied hunger. He had an assistant named Washburn, whom he got to swallow a balloon. The balloon then was inflated and the pressure in the balloon was, of course, modified by any movements of the stomach. A recording system was arranged so that the contractions of the stomach, which modified the pressure within the balloon, could be recorded. It was discovered by Cannon, watching the recording, that the contractions of the stomach coincided with reports from Washburn that he had hunger pangs. Washburn tapped on a key to report his sensations of hunger and his taps correlated very nicely with the contractions of his stomach.

Cannon therefore was able to postulate that hunger arises out of the local stimulation from the stomach, caused by the contractions of the stomach. He could then describe "drives" (a term that was later introduced by Woodworth) as goading, urging kinds of stimuli. I think Cannon's ideas are responsible for the phrase, "We are scourged through life by goading internal stimuli," the stimuli representing drive or need states. Therefore, we (and other animals) are impelled to seek release from these goading stimuli. Cannon's formulation was that inner discomfort motivated goal-driven behavior in the organism's attempt to find satisfiers which would alleviate these internal tensions or "pains."

I mentioned Jennings and Richter with Cannon because, in their general orientation to the study of behavior, they were consistent with Cannon's ideas, although they were never so dramatic in their formulations as he was.

The 20th Century began or developed with conceptions of motivation which were essentially of the kind I have described: strong inner forces, irresolute in their purpose and demanding in their impulsive force, which then lead to behavior. And here is the Darwinian concept: Behavior is calculated to satisfy or to adapt the individual to the demands of these impulsive forces. I think that the real heritage from Darwinian evolutionary theory for the behavioral and social sciences was this notion that behavior is essentially a series of activities which are engaged in the service of the internal needs, drives, or instincts, that the individual's nature provides him.

It was difficult for theorists to discover, in the data for human subjects, the presence of hunger, thirst, sex, and aggression in quantities sufficiently great to account for their behavior with respect to careers, money, and things of that sort. And so the drive theory of Cannon (as opposed to Freudian theory, which explained these matters in terms of defensive maneuvers of the Ego) tended to be modified by the suggestion that there must be various kinds of learned or acquired drives which govern behavior in the adult human. In such individuals, who are relatively well fed and well watered and reasonably well satisfied in other areas of impulse, motivation cannot be very easily accounted for in terms of basic drives; so other sources of motivation were needed to explain continual striving in such areas as career, financial success, and creation of art and writing. The usual idea was that these kinds of behaviors could be accounted for by secondary or acquired drives which have their origins early in life in association with biological or primary drives. However, they were thought eventually to achieve a status independent of their primary origins and were able to maintain and support the goal directed behavior characteristic, at least, of the American middle class.

This was the theoretical solution to the problem of motivation which seemed satisfactory for a while. Recently we have seen, if nothing else, a substantial alteration in the ways in which we think about motivation. Changes have taken place in psychoanalysis which are, I think, in considerable contrast to the basic ideas that are implicit—if not explicit—in classical Freudian thinking. Perhaps the most important concept that emerged was the idea that there are conflict-free areas in the Ego. What this means is that the Ego, rather than arising solely from the Id as an agent charged mainly with gaining satisfaction for the Id, is to be seen as an independent, innate part of the organism—a considerable shift from the old doctrine which is well represented in Otto Fenichel's famous summary of psychoanalysis, *The Psychoanalytic Theory of Neurosis,* published about 30 years ago. Fenichel said, in effect, that without conflict, without difficulty and the necessity for adjustment, the concept of reality would never emerge in the individual. However, for these Ego-theorists, the idea is that there are processes or factors in the structure of the organism which would be able to cope with reality and would be able in various ways to handle reality with the cognitive processes that I have alluded to even if there were no sources of conflict to generate them.

So in this version of psychoanalysis we see a retreat from an exclusive emphasis on the role of motivational forces in the development of behavior and in the development of the Ego, and a replacement of it by the notion that there are intrinsic cognitive or Ego functions which would be there whether or not the Id and its vicissitudes made trouble for the organism in conjunction with its adaptation to reality.

Drive theory, aside from psychoanalysis, was, with its modifications in the direction of acquired drive, the dominant point of view in American psychology, sociology, and perhaps even social work in the middle part of the century. But a number of things were discovered around 1950 that seemed to throw doubt on drive theory. One of the implications of this theory—and probably of classical Freudian theory as well—is that organisms tend to seek a state of relative quiescence in which there are no great imbalances. Needs or drives produce imbalances which are a source of behavior; that is, to correct imbalances the organism must get up and do work. Under this approach, the ideal situation is that of the child in the womb. He is in a constant temperature and does not have to work for food or respiratory interchange or drink. This is obviously a relatively tension-free, work-free situation. The notion here is that in the classical version of psychoanalytic theory and in drive theory, the goal of the organism seems to be a state of quiescence. When we are goaded into behavior by an impelling hunger drive, our goal seems to be to ingest some kind of food so that the motivations arising from the hunger will be quieted and we can go back to inactivity. Such conceptions of motivation have been called homeostatic in character.

The discoveries that appeared in the 1950's seemed to throw into question the notion that organisms seek quiescence. These discoveries are reviewed by Cofer and Appley,[7] but let me list some of the phenomena that seem to question regulation of behavior entirely on the basis of homeostatic drives and learned drives derived from homeostatic biological drives.

One set of observations was that first made systematically in Canada at McGill University. Students there were asked to lie on a cot and do nothing for as long as they wished for $20 a day. They were shielded from sensory stimulation by wearing translucent goggles. (They could see some light but no patterned vision.) The subjects' ears were subjected to a constant masking noise so that there wasn't any real variation in the auditory signal that they received, and finally their hands and upper arms were encased in gauntlets so that the stimulation they could receive through these areas of the body was considerably limited.

The finding was that these students, as well as the staff members who tried the experiment, could not stand the sensory isolation very long. They became disturbed, some became hallucinated, and the general impression was that they could not tolerate sensory restriction for more than a day or two or, at most, three or four days, despite all of the secondary gains from the money and the scientific contribution.

The results have led to the suggestion that a certain amount of stimulation may be necessary to adequate functioning and for an adequate base of happiness or contentment. On the surface, these results appear to be incompatible with the notion that the goal of life is a Nirvana-like state where everything is in complete balance.

Other experiments have been conducted with animals. For example, Harry Harlow found that monkeys left with simple puzzles would manipulate them and disassemble them, rather than leaving them alone—even though the monkeys were neither hungry, thirsty, nor presumably otherwise motivated, and even though the act of manipulating these puzzles was not associated with a material reward of any sort. So Harlow postulated that there is in monkeys a manipulation motive.

In other species, a variety of experiments were carried out that seemed to show that in animals as well as in humans (even in fact in babies and very young children) there is a motivation to explore. In the process of exploration, the organism encounters stimuli that have some property such as novelty, complexity, incongruity, or surprisingness. Given the opportunity and given an environment in which certain kinds of changes are incident or coincident to exploration, organisms that are not particularly motivated in any way engage in exploration.

A good deal of work in the same period suggested that there may be such a thing as curiosity, a phenomenon which many of us have simply assumed to exist without evidence. Now there seems to be a lot of good evidence that there is such a thing as curiosity, as represented especially in the behavior of adults or children who will work to expose themselves to pictures that have properties and attributes that are unusual or novel. The period of the 1950's was associated with developments of these kinds.

From the results of the experiments on sensory isolation, manipulation, exploration, and curiosity, it seems that there is more to motivation and more to the determination of behavior in the motivational sense than the concepts that had been formalized earlier that we have attributed to classical Freudian theory and to drive theory supplemented by the notion of acquired drives.

I will try to summarize where theory and research regarding the topic of motivation seem to have gone since the years of the 1950's. It is worth noting that, correlated with the developments I have just described, there are pertinent discoveries in neurophysiology. The classic paper is one authored by Moruzzi and Magoun in 1949 which led ultimately to the notion that there is a structure in the brain called the reticular formation whose activity has a great deal to do with activity in the cerebral cortex and, further, that the arousal of the cortex by the activity of the reticular formation is integral to adequate intellectual functioning. That is, the unaroused cortex, not being activated by the reticular formation, is more or less asleep and can do nothing much with the sensory stimulation that comes in from the receptors and up the appropriate classical pathways to the brain. But if the cortex is to some degree in an aroused state, it can function and cope with these sensory stimulations that enter into the system.

These ideas seem to fit very nicely with the other kinds of observations I have mentioned. Perhaps we cannot endure sensory isolation because the brain is not functioning the way it would if we were getting adequate arousing stimuli, as we do in an ordinary rich environment, which perhaps stimulates the reticular system to activate the brain. Perhaps the manipulation of objects, or exploration, or dealing with novel, complex, unusual, or surprising stimuli all have the function, as far as the organism is concerned, of providing for some arousal of the reticular formation of the brain. When arousal occurs, one is able to avoid boredom and intellectual inefficiency.

I do not mean to imply that excessive arousal is desirable. The notion seems to be that there is some optimal level of arousal, and as long as the organism's arousal is at that level he will be relatively happy. Further, he will be reasonably happy if changes in expectation and changes in stimulation occur because they keep him aroused to some extent. He cannot stand boredom, and he cannot stand arousal to a level which far exceeds this optimum which I have mentioned.

In the field of motivation, we are now at a stage in which we think that optimal levels of arousal and optimal levels of stimulation are important in motivation, and that events in the environment such as the experiencing of complex or unusual or curiosity arousing stimuli are the kinds of things, in part at least, that will contribute to arousal. The monotonous dull environment that you might expect to be preferred from the earlier theories is not preferred, but rather bores the organism to a state of apathy.

With the impact of these ideas, motivation theory has undergone considerable change. We do not look, for example, entirely to internal sources for the bases of motivation. We can look at external things, such as the kinds of stimuli and the kinds of environment that the individual functions in, as perhaps giving him a source of motivation. Perhaps that is the most important idea that has emerged in the last few years.

Other evidence has come along that leads one to question the idea that internal states or drives alone have the capacity to evoke behavior. The basic observations were originally made on rats in activity wheels. The animals were fed once every 24 hours, and their activity was measured throughout the intervals over an extended period of time. The finding was that activity is cyclic, and that the cycle corresponds to some extent with time of deprivation. Specifically, immediately after feeding there is a quiet period; but as time elapses activity begins to increase, reaching a peak as the time for the next feeding approaches. This cycle was taken as evidence that drive, in this case, hunger, evokes activity and that the stronger the drive, that is, the longer the period of deprivation, the more behavior there would be.

These observations may be given an alternative interpretation on the basis of experiments which appeared in the 1950's. In one such experiment animals fed only once a day were fed at random intervals; the time of feeding was, in other words, unpredictable. Under these conditions there was no relationship of activity to time of deprivation. The inference, then, is that where cyclic activity appears, it arises because of the predictability of the time of feeding; some cues associated with feeding time evidently arouse or activate the animal so that he manifests activity. The drive alone does not evoke the behavior, but it is also true that the cues alone are usually not sufficient to arouse the behavior either. It takes both a period of deprivation and the cues in interaction to activate the animal. In the present example, the cues, of course, come through learning to signal the imminence of feeding time.

In other cases, learning may not be essential. The normal male rat, for example, shows sexual arousal and excitement when he encounters a receptive female. Without the female, he does not show arousal, and if he has been castrated for a period of time, a receptive female will not arouse or excite him. Here, too, we seem to have two factors: the presence of sex hormones (which are eliminated by castration) and the instigating or arousing stimulus. Both are necessary for arousal to take place. In this instance, however, it may be unnecessary, at least in the rat, for the arousing value of the receptive female to be developed through learning. It seems to be plausible, on the available evidence, to suppose that a male with an adequate hormone level is somehow sensitized, innately, to respond to receptive females, and that the arousal follows automatically when these two conditions, the hormone level and the female, are present simultaneously.

Motivational theory today, then, tends to stress stimuli, usually called incentives, in interaction with bodily states as requisite to the appearance of arousal or activation, which we refer to as motivated. This account has, I think, its greatest pertinence to the interpretation of what we have long called the primary "drives"—hunger, thirst, and sex. The analyses of fear, made in the past, have always stressed the evocation of fear, or of anxiety, by cues, external or internal, which have been associated with painful circumstances. The primary drives can no longer be thought of as automatic instigators of activity. Rather, incentives, innate or brought about through learning, in conjunction with bodily states are required for activity to be aroused.

How does what I have said about the role of incentives in the cases of hunger, thirst, sex, and fear relate to what I said earlier, in discussing optimal levels of arousal as playing an important role in motivation? The answer to this question is, I think, that both kinds of processes work and function in the same organism. We need the theory that organisms are motivated to seek and maintain optimal levels of stimulation because in that way we can account for curiosity, exploration, the aversion to sensory isolation and boredom. In other words, the argument is that these phenomena are essentially independent of hunger, thirst, sex, and fear. But we also require an account of the role of these latter conditions and that is how the theory of the interaction of incentives with bodily states enters in.

I have spoken primarily of work with animals but I think that the ideas I have outlined have applicability to humans. So far as we have much knowledge in detail about human motivation, the situation is complex. The need for achievement has received the greatest attention of all human motives, other than anxiety, in nonclinical investigations, and the work is mainly that of David McClelland and John Atkinson and their students and associates. Perhaps it will serve as a model or as an exemplar of the kind of analysis of human motivation which should be extended to other human motives.

Basic to McClelland's analysis of motivated behavior is that situational cues come, through learning, to evoke arousal. In his analysis the source of the arousal is an anticipation, for example, that an approach to the situation marked by the cues will produce pleasantness, or, alternatively, that withdrawal from a situation will avoid unpleasantness. So cues are important in this formulation, too. However, it is necessary to know a good deal more than this for the analysis of motivated behavior, or to predict that it will occur. The factors identified so far are:

(1) The state of the person's motive.

(2) The perception of the situation as relevant to the motive.

(3) The incentive value of achieving the goals the situation promises.

(4) The subjective probability of achieving the goals the behavior can obtain.

Let me say something about each of these factors.

THE STATE OF THE MOTIVE In the case of need for achievement (nAch), McClelland and his associates have developed a method of measuring the motive to achieve. In doing so, they obtain stories in response to pictures, the stories themselves being organized around several questions which are asked about each picture. The stories are scored, to begin with, as to whether they contain achievement imagery, which I will define loosely here as components that indicate that a goal is being striven for. If the story does concern achievement imagery, then it is scored further for other elements related to achievement.

Over a group of people, the scores for nAch vary, some people achieving high and others low scores, with still others in between these extremes. So individual differences appear here, in motivation, as they do in human characteristics generally. Further, it is now known that achievement scores have two components—hope of success and fear of failure. These components must be distinguished in evaluating an individual's achievement motivation.

PERCEPTION OF THE SITUATION AS RELEVANT TO nAch I can illustrate this point by saying simply that pictures will vary in their capacities to evoke achievement imagery. So we have this situation: some pictures clearly are achievement-relevant to everyone. Others are achievement-relevant to no one. If we can generalize from pictures to other situations, we would expect the same thing to hold —there will be some situations which have no relevance with respect to a given motive to anyone. And for the motive to be "engaged" differentially, the situation must have some but not too many aspects relevant to the motive in question.

INCENTIVE VALUE For adults in middle life, it is unlikely that to obtain a penny, a nickel, or a dime has much significance. A three-year-old, however, may be delighted with a dime, and an astute parent can even activate or direct the young child's behavior by means of such incentives. Incentive value then can vary, and we can expect behavior when incentive value is present but not otherwise, no matter what the motivating cue-value the situation may have or what strength of motive the person himself possesses. Many motivational programs engineered by middle class people may fail for just this reason. The incentives that have value for them have none for, say, people from a low socio-economic class.

SUBJECTIVE PROBABILITY OF OBTAINING THE INCENTIVE But even when a person is motivated, when the incentive has value, and when the situation is motive relevant, there may be little motivated behavior. If the possibility of obtaining the incentive is too remote, as the person sees it, then there is a low subjective probability of success with respect to obtaining the incentive. Perhaps an incentive with less value but greater likelihood of being achieved will be preferred. On the other hand, in the case of achievement, high probability of obtaining an incentive may at the same time decrease motivation to work for it. People with high nAch (and low fear of failure) desire a challenge: they will not work for something that is very easy to obtain, and they will not work for something which is virtually unobtainable. Rather, they are motivated to seek incentives which they perceive as having intermediate probabilities of being obtained.

This summary of factors identified in relation to behavior in the achievement case can, no doubt, be extended to other motives. It indicates, clearly, I think, that motivated behavior is complexly determined. Simple slogans about the importance of motivation will not be helpful in the absence of detailed knowledge about the person, the situation, the values of the incentive that the situation affords, and how likely the person thinks it is that he can obtain the incentives or reach the goals the circumstances provide.

Motivation is not everything. It still takes abilities, capacities, and training, regardless of the degree of motivation, to perform many of the tasks or to obtain many of the goals which people in the helping professions would like to see their clients perform or obtain.

NOTES

1. Mary K. Bauman, *Adjustment to Blindness* (Harrisburg: Pennsylvania State Council for the Blind, 1954).
2. ———, *Characteristics of Blind and Visually Handicapped People in Professional, Sales, and Managerial Work* (Harrisburg: Pennsylvania Office for the Blind, 1963).
3. W. H. Bexton, W. Heron, and T. H. Scott, "Effects of Decreased Variation in the Sensory Environment," *Canadian Journal of Psychology,* 8 (1954), 70–75.
4. D. E. Berlyne, *Conflict, Arousal and Curiosity* (New York: McGraw-Hill, 1960).
5. A. H. Buss, *The Psychology of Aggression* (New York: John Wiley, 1961).
6. L. Carmichael, ed., *Manual of Child Psychology* (New York: John Wiley, 1946).
7. Charles N. Cofer and Mortimer H. Appley, *Motivation: Theory and Research* (New York: John Wiley, 1964).
8. W. Heron, B. K. Doane, and T. H. Scott, "Visual Disturbances after Prolonged Perceptual Isolation," *Canadian Journal of Psychology,* 10 (1956), 13–18.
9. J. C. Lilly, "Mental Effects of Reduction of Ordinary Levels of Physical Stimuli on Intact Healthy Persons," *Psychiatric Research Reports,* 5 (1956), 1–9.
10. D. Rapaport, "The Theory of Ego Autonomy: A Generalization," *Bulletin of the Menninger Clinic,* 22 (1958), 13–35.
11. H. Selye, *The Story of the Adaptation Syndrome* (Montreal: Acta, Inc., 1952).

THE ROLE OF MOTIVATION IN THE REHABILITATION OF THE BLIND

Herbert Rusalem

Until recently the ideal of the well motivated blind person dominated rehabilitation practice in the United States. In this motivation model, the well equipped rehabilitation worker waited in splendid isolation in his office until psychic and environmental forces upset the psychosocial homeostasis of the blind individual and brought him to the agency threshold. In all cases, a variety of forces activating both positive and negative responses to rehabilitation contended with each other until an internal balance was achieved which placed the blind person at some point along a continuum of rehabilitation motivation.

Those positively motivated for rehabilitation tended to reach out for, and use, services. They were characterized as cooperative, feasible, and desirable clients. The others made few observable overtures to rehabilitation agencies. Perhaps they even avoided these resources and, as a consequence, established a long-term dependency status in their families and communities. When these so-called unmotivated blind persons came to the attention of the rehabilitation worker, their subsequent experiences tended to be unsatisfactory for all concerned.

The reasons for this dissatisfaction are evident. For most disability groups, the traditional rehabilitation process is built upon some initial level of client initiative and readiness for self-activity. In this context, the blind person must hold up his end of the bargain by engaging in certain well defined behaviors: for example, providing information about himself, agreeing to undergo various evaluations and examinations, taking responsibility for being in the right place at the right time, following directions, and sharing the rehabilitation worker's value system.

Individuals who do not conform to orthodox rehabilitation expectations perplex workers and agencies and fail in inordinate numbers to benefit adequately from rehabilitation services. In the process of failing, they usually feel defeated and become even less motivated to achieve independence. Essentially, the well motivated blind person in rehabilitation is cherished, respected, and valued. He fulfills the success needs of counselors and justifies the existence of rehabilitation services as they currently function. He conserves the professional worker's time and energy and contributes to readable and meritorious case records.

On the other hand, the resistant or reluctant individual often serves as a stimulus for low expectations. Years of experience have taught rehabilitation workers to recognize both the obvious and subtle evidence of defective motivation among blind users of their services. Perhaps, without being aware of it, rehabilitation workers react to such evidence with apprehension and avoidance. Thus, the avoidance or, at best, ambivalent attitudes of the poorly motivated blind person interacts with the avoidance or, at best, ambivalent attitudes of the rehabilitation worker to produce a transaction that increases for both the probability of failure.

The consequences of this situation are evident. In 1966 Cohen[4] estimated that there were 410,000 legally blind persons in the United States with an additional 31,800 individuals becoming blind for the first time each year. As he reported, the 1963–65 National Health Survey found that there were nearly 1.3 million Americans with visual impairments severe enough to cause limitations in at least one major life activity, such as work, school, or homemaking. The members of this group were unable to read ordinary newsprint with glasses.

In 1965 The Biometrics Branch of the National Institute of Neurological Diseases and Blindness, reporting on statistics relating to the Model Reporting Area for Blindness,[12] revealed that 42 per cent of the individuals in their register were in the age range 20–64 years. This 44-years span is usually considered the most suitable life period for the provision of rehabilitation services. If the Model Reporting Area generally reflects the nation as a whole, 42 per cent of 410,000 blind persons or 172,200 individuals currently are in the most favorable age range for rehabilitation. Obviously, not all of these 172,200 persons need or are accessible to organized rehabilitation services, for these reasons:

1. Some are functioning satisfactorily and have no need for additional assistance.

2. Some have already received services in the schools and from community agencies.

3. Some are so disabled by multiple handicaps that rehabilitation will not be effective.

4. Some are motivated for rehabilitation but do not have access to rehabilitation resources.

In 1965, 5,450 blind persons were given training and other forms of assistance by the Federal-State Vocational Rehabilitation Program. This total constitutes 3 per cent of the blind population estimated to be in the age range 20–64 years. Current data do not permit even the grossest of estimates concerning the percentage of blind persons who fail to enter or who enter and subsequently drop out of rehabilitation. However, it must be assumed that some proportion of blind persons is excluded from rehabilitation by reason of motivational factors. Although the size of the "unmotivated" group is still unknown, some clues may be found in data presented by McGuire and Sillen.[11]

During a 26-month period ending in September, 1965, a total of 612 blind individuals were reported to the New York State Commission for the Blind by ophthalmologists in New York City. Normally, the Commission refers such persons to one of four voluntary agencies in the city unless a specific request is made by the blind person or someone close to him that no referral be made. In the McGuire-Sillen study, 97 individuals (16 per cent) requested the Commission to make no referral to a local agency. The authors studied some of the blind persons who had received no help and found that major reasons reported for avoiding service were:

1. Specialized agencies for the blind are for the totally blind, not for those with residual vision.

2. Family members are available to assist them.

3. They are satisfied with their accommodation to visual loss.

As part of the same study, a list of possible deterrents to acceptance of rehabilitation by blind persons was submitted to 15 social workers and 10 rehabilitation workers employed by the Jewish Guild for the Blind in New York and to seven directors of hospital social work departments. The respondents were asked to select from this list those factors which seem to be most inhibiting to the acceptance of service by blind persons. An analysis of the data produced three major inhibitory clusters:

1. Factors relating to self-concept, including unwillingness or inability to accept visual loss, false hope that vision will improve, and gradual progression in the loss of sight.

2. Factors relating to attitudes, such as feelings about the stigma and shame of blindness, feelings about the client role *vis-à-vis* a voluntary agency, and feelings about being segregated as a blind person.

3. Factors relating to personality variables, such as apathy, resistance to change, and a need to retain the dependency role.

Despite the limited data available that relate to this problem, two assumptions seem justified:

1. A sizable group of blind persons who could benefit from rehabilitation services is prevented from doing so by motivational factors resulting in extensive personal and community loss.

2. Current rehabilitation procedures which depend upon some minimal degree of client motivation and initiative are not well adapted to the members of this group.

On the basis of the assumptions, the major theme of this paper is that research should be designed to develop new and innovative rehabilitation service patterns which can appeal to different and lower levels of client motivation than those currently demanded in rehabilitation and which, despite motivational insufficiency, can result in the achievement by blind persons of greater independence and community participation. In exploring this theme, we need to address ourselves to the following questions:

1. What do we know about the motivation of blind persons?

2. What types of research are needed to extend our knowledge about the rehabilitation motivation of blind individuals?

AN ANALYSIS OF THE REHABILITATION MOTIVATION OF BLIND PERSONS

Cofer,[3] in the previous paper on motivation, suggested these major points:

1. Visually handicapped persons differ from each other in many respects. One of these areas of individual difference is motivation.

2. One vantage point from which motivation can be studied is the age at onset of blindness. Within this framework, there are three major groups of blind persons with relevant motivational prob-

lems: the blind from birth or at an early age, those with a sudden onset, and those in whom blindness developed progressively and slowly over a period of years.

Cofer offers some general insights into motivation which can be applied to these groups, including:

SENSORY DEPRIVATION A deprivation experience can result in hunger for stimulation, restlessness, irritability, boredom, and emotional lability. Small deviations from customary stimulation levels provide novelty and interest but large deviations may be negative or aversive in effect. Sameness and constancy in stimulation tend to result in boredom. Sensory deprivation aspects of motivation apply with greatest relevance to those experiencing a sudden onset of blindness.

PSYCHOLOGICAL STRESS Psychological stress is a condition in which the organism perceives itself in danger and devotes its energies to self protection. It develops through a progressive process. As motives arise, one attempts to achieve the goal with one's customary coping mechanisms. If these fail, further arousal occurs followed by new, unusual, and, perhaps, repetitive coping efforts. If these fail, anxiety grows, further attempts are made to cope, and awareness sharpens of the existence of a threat. Finally, a stress threshold is reached.

In time, if the stress remains unrelieved, the resultants may include preoccupation with the protection of the ego, perception of danger, desperation or panic, helplessness or hopelessness, and, finally, apathy and cessation of striving.

The psychological stress concept seems most closely related to sudden blindness since in this condition well ordered visual coping patterns are disrupted and are no longer relevant or may even be maladaptive for the blind individual. Thus, guidance and reference points may be lost by the blind person in such areas as self-care activities, keeping informed about the environment, evolving and sustaining career and life plans, enjoying entertainments and amusements, and conducting interpersonal relationships.

One consequence is dependency which can serve many motives and goals. Some individuals welcome dependency as an extension of an already established pattern. Others rudely resist dependency, perceiving help as derogating, controlling, and insulting.

SOCIAL PERCEPTIONS OF DIFFERENCE Individuals who are different or special are treated in a differentiated fashion in the social environment. This differential treatment may be in the form of protection, a common response so far as the blind are concerned. This attitude is an outgrowth of shame, guilt, hostility, or succorance on the part of the sighted segment of society. Living through repeated exposures to this attitude, the blind individual may emerge with intensified needs to be indulged and protected. As time goes by, these motives tend to be perpetuated by the recurrent reactions and conceptions of seeing persons. The consequence is self-devaluation, feelings of inadequacy, self-derogation, and self-pity. This formulation is most relevant for those to whom blindness is congenital or by whom it was acquired early in life.

SPECIAL CONCERNS RELATING TO THE MOTIVATION OF BLIND INDIVIDUALS UNDERGOING REHABILITATION

It can be suggested that the so-called "unmotivated" individual in rehabilitation is an artifact of the rehabilitation contract and that the conditions set by professional rehabilitation agencies and workers fail to appeal to the motivational systems of some blind persons. In an attempt to endow this idea with theoretical significance, Dawis, England, and Lofquist [6] assumed a universal need to respond. As an individual develops, he experiences differential reinforcement from a variety of potential reinforcers in the environment. In time, he develops predispositions to some reinforcers and aversive reactions to others, depending upon his reinforcement history. Those toward which he is predisposed motivate him, but those toward which he feels antipathy evoke avoidant reactions.

Many behavioral scientists perceive such a reinforcement formulation of motivation as more relevant for simple organisms than for incredibly complex men and women. However, the supporting evidence derived from animal experiments is being confirmed increasingly by data generated by experimental studies with human subjects. In the absence of a single universally accepted theory of motivation, let us arbitrarily, but tentatively, explore the implications of a behavioral formulation for the rehabilitation motivation of blind persons. Turning to three of the foci of interest suggested by Cofer, let us examine each in turn starting with the assumption that an individual's motivational pattern is a function of his reinforcement history.

Sensory Deprivation

The deprivation of sight during one's developmental years creates a reinforcement history of a special character. Cutsforth [5] summarized this deprivation experience as follows: "No single mental activity of the congenitally blind child is not disturbed by the absence of sight . . . even in the cases of blindness occurring later . . . [in which] sensory stimulation is prevented. The organization does not continue as it has started but immediately is altered in the process of progressive reorganization."

Cutsforth proceeded to examine the relationship between sensory deprivation and such psychosocial phenomena as egocentrism, excessive verbalism, regressive fantasies, emotional disturbance, and social maladjustment. Lowenfeld [9] discussed the role of touch as a substitute for sight in the developmental process. Although definitive studies in this area are lacking, it is probable that a reinforcement history dominated by touch and hearing differs in some respects from such a history built primarily upon vision. If this is so, we should expect this reinforcement history to manifest itself in differentiated motivational patterns. Yet, congenitally blind persons reveal all levels of rehabilitation motivation. Some interact freely with rehabilitation agencies and move toward marked gains in achieving independent lives. Others do not. This observation is valid for all disability groups. Apparently, although it does influence one's reinforcement history, sensory deprivation is not *the* critical variable in determining rehabilitation motivation among those who were blind at birth or lost their sight early in life.

In the case of blindness acquired in adolescence or during the adult years, the individual enters the blindness experience with a rich reinforcement history in which selective reinforcing and aversive features of the environment are already well crystallized.

In virtually all societies, vision and the capacity to see are highly reinforcing and darkness and the inability to see are aversive. Consequently, the experience of blindness and everything related to it is usually aversive and, consequently, affects motivation. Cholden[2] described this aversive quality in a discussion of the "shock" and "depression" stages which seem to occur subsequent to the sudden loss of vision. Although interpretation of these stages varies from orthodox behavioristic formulations to orthodox psychoanalytic constructs, it has been observed by advocates of all approaches that rehabilitation motivation is at a low ebb during both shock and depression.

Consequently, for the adventitiously blinded, sensory deprivation functions as an aversive stimulus, negatively influencing rehabilitation motivation. Under these circumstances, rehabilitation achievements tend to be modest until a positive reorganization of the individual's motivational pattern occurs. In psychoanalytic terms, Cholden viewed this reorganization as follows: "The patient must die as a sighted person in order to be reborn as a blind man."

In reinforcement terms, the same phenomenon may be described in a comparable fashion: the potency of blindness as a negative reinforcer must be reduced before positive motivation for rehabilitation becomes firmly established.

Psychological Stress

Blindness and other disabilities are not necessarily productive of stress. Indeed, disability may bring a welcome fulfillment of lifelong goals to some individuals. Griffis[8] found that 39 per cent of 200 consecutive applicants for disability benefits under Social Security had caused their own disabilities by harmful health habits or retention of harmful or hazardous jobs. He concluded that a major reorientation of motivational patterns would be required in this group prior to successful rehabilitation.

Since disability and dependency can be reinforcing for some individuals, psychological stress is not universally experienced subsequent to disability and motivation, for rehabilitation is not universally activated. Under these circumstances, even though ambivalence may be operative a homeostatic balance is attained within the parameters of the nonrehabilitated state. Consequently, movement toward rehabilitation is not reinforcing.

On the other hand, an adventitious disability can elevate the stress level of an individual for whom independence and self sufficiency are positive reinforcers. Fenichel[7] described the effect of a trauma as a concentration of all mental energy on one task, that of mastering an overwhelming excitation with which the individual cannot cope successfully. In reinforcement terms, no available response suffices. Despite a mobilization of resources and frantic engagement in mental and/or physical activity, the stimulus continues to excite the individual without abatement, producing mounting stress. Blindness can be such an unfulfilled excitant for some individuals. In its early stages, blindness is a unique experience and no available response to it may be ever fully reinforcing. Consequently, the excitant of blindness motivates the individual to try one response after another in an effort to cope with his new psychosocial situation. If the failure to achieve reinforcement continues, stress may mount to an almost unbearable pitch. In time the individual may either withdraw into depression or fantasy, a process that dilutes rehabilitation motivation, or will make more frantic efforts to seek positive reinforcement. If the latter process can be controlled and directed, it can serve ultimately as a wellspring of rehabilitation motivation. Otherwise, the effort becomes an aimless uncoordinated activity without rehabilitation focus.

Social Perceptions of Difference

Barker *et al.*[1] reviewed the pertinent literature and concluded: ". . . blind persons are commonly perceived to be helpless and dependent and are frequently placed in underprivileged social situations."

In a comprehensive study on the subject Lukoff and Whiteman[10] confirmed the belief that the attitudes of family members and other sighted persons influence the blind individual's attitudes toward independence. It is as though the self-reactions of blind persons are a mirror of the sighted environment. When we look into this mirror, what really appears?

Lukoff and Whiteman analyzed blind persons' perceptions of sighted persons toward the blind. A majority of their blind respondents felt that sighted individuals are surprised if a blind person can do anything. In reinforcement terms, then, comforming to society's expectations of helplessness can be reinforcing to many blind persons. Although some proportion of blind people rebel against the role which society thrusts upon them, they do so at a price. In most cases, it is more reinforcing to play the assigned role. Indeed, even enlightened rehabilitation workers consider the tractable conforming client to be a more hopeful rehabilitation candidate.

The sense of social difference and the acceptance of society's expectations favors the continued use of specialized agencies for the blind in rehabilitation. In most cases, blind rehabilitation clients do need some differentiated types of assistance. However, separate agencies with separate workers and separate facilities may reinforce well established social perceptions of difference. Despite this, segregated services are kept alive because they reinforce many blind persons and many workers for the blind. Whatever the pros and cons of specialized agencies may be, the resultant probably is weakened client motivation to achieve integration into the mainstream of sighted society.

RESEARCH PROBLEMS

Rich research possibilities seem to emerge from the following assumptions made in this paper:

1. Rehabilitation success is related to positive motivation for rehabilitation.

2. Three major deterrents exert a negative influence on the rehabilitation motivation of many blind persons: sensory deprivation, psychological stress, and social perceptions of difference.

3. Each of these factors serves as a negative reinforcer of independence and self-direction among adventitiously blinded persons.

4. Rehabilitation programs have a responsibility for intervening in a positive and dynamic fashion to counteract and, perhaps, eliminate these negative reinforcers. Effective service to most blind persons cannot be achieved through the orthodox means of working primarily with blind persons whose rehabilitation motivation has already reached satisfactory levels.

5. If unsheltered living in regular society is a desirable goal for most blind persons, motivation for it may be achieved through participation from the start in a minimally segregated rehabilitation process.

Research tests of all these assumptions are a critical need in our field, but especially so in relation to such questions as:

1. Is an initially satisfactory level of rehabilitation motivation essential for rehabilitation success?

2. What kinds of results could be achieved through offering re-motivation services to "unmotivated" individuals undergoing rehabilitation?

3. What characteristics really differentiate successful and unsuccessful rehabilitation individuals?

In relation to the last question, emphasis has fallen traditionally upon demographic variables such as age, level of education, and sex. Data on reinforcement history and preblindness life style, self-attitudes, and autonomy may be even more significant in expanding our understanding of motivational factors.

Research is also needed on the temporal variable in rehabilitation motivation. Earlier in this paper, it was hypothesized that initial attempts to cope with adventitious blindness are usually unsuccessful because response patterns developed earlier in life are inadequate in the blindness situation. Motivated by a negative reinforcement history in relation to darkness and blindness, the sightless person often does seem to experience failure in his first coping efforts, strengthening even further the potency of blindness as a negative reinforcer. If this process really does occur, do we wait too long before intervening with rehabilitation services? Are initial shock and depression a necessary prelude to rehabilitation, serving as a period during which motivational patterns are reorganized enabling the blind individual to move forward in rehabilitation? Or are shock and depression products of dilatory rehabilitation tactics which could be prevented if rehabilitation were initiated almost immediately after visual loss?

Research is needed to demonstrate the values and limitations of 24–hour emergency service which swings into action as soon as visual loss is discovered by a physician, a hospital, a clinic, or a family. Such an experimental service could be conducted by indigenous, adequate adventitiously blinded persons who would attempt to reinforce positive fragments in the self-perceptions of the newly blinded person. This approach would be coupled with the provision of immediate successful experiences in some life activities; for example, retention of time orientation through the use of a braille watch and cooperative programs with previous employers so that certain aspects of the job are performed for pay by the newly blinded person as soon as medically approved.

Would such high-speed reinforcement function as a helpful first aid for the newly blinded, or would it inflict unnecessary stress upon the individual? Can rehabilitation motivation be built this early or will it be found that rehabilitation can begin too soon? Is a preliminary period of shock and depression necessary in human adjustment to sudden sensory loss?

Research is also needed in the desensitization of blindness as an aversive stimulus. The onset of blindness is superimposed upon a lifetime of reinforcement history in which blindness has served as a negative reinforcer. When blindness comes, this reinforcement history restricts rehabilitation motivation. Until now, intellectual approaches designed to reduce the potency of blindness as a negative reinforcer have had indifferent success. Pamphlets, car cards, lectures, and publications about successful blind persons have failed to desensitize large groups in the community. A research project could be structured in a public school setting in which students would gradually be accustomed to a reduced input of visual stimuli while in a favorable pleasant situation with a warm and trusted person present. Using this procedure followed, in time, by experimental total exclusion of visual stimuli with positive reinforcement given for independent behavior, would workers obtain a reduction in the potency of blindness as a negative reinforcer? If successful desensitization can be demonstrated experimentally in this situation, it may have important implications for attitude modification, in general.

Research is also needed to test various means of reducing feelings of social difference between sighted and blind persons. For example, under what circumstances will interpersonal contact between members of these two groups result in reorganized perceptions? What means can be used to create cognitive dissonance among sighted individuals through which changed perceptions of blind persons may be achieved? If blind persons did not have specialized agencies available to them, and had to use regular community agencies, what effect would this have on the sense of social difference and, consequently, on rehabilitation motivation?

NOTES

1. R. Barker, B. Wright, L. Meyerson, and M. Gonick, *Adjustment to Physical Handicap and Illness* (New York: Social Science Research Council, 1953).
2. L. Cholden, *A Psychiatrist Works with Blindness* (New York: American Foundation for the Blind, 1958).
3. Charles N. Cofer, "Motivation and Motivational Theory" (Paper presented at the National Research Consultation on Problems Related to Blindness, The Pennsylvania State University, April 10, 1967).
4. W. Cohen, "New Vistas for the Blind," *Health, Education and Welfare Indicators* (October, 1966), 20–25.
5. T. Cutsforth, *The Blind in School and Society* (New York: American Foundation for the Blind, 1951).
6. R. Dawis, G. England, and L. Lofquist, "A Theory of Vocational Adjustment," *Minnesota Studies in Vocational Rehabilitation Bulletin 38* (Minneapolis: University of Minnesota Press, 1964).
7. O. Fenichel, *The Psychoanalytic Theory of Neurosis* (New York: Norton, 1945).
8. B. Griffis, "Disability—How Often Self-caused?" (Paper presented at the Southeastern Psychological Association Meeting, Gatlinburg, Tennessee, April, 1964).
9. B. Lowenfeld, "Psychological Problems of Children with Impaired Vision," in *Psychology of Exceptional Children,* ed. W. Cruickshank (Englewood Cliffs, New Jersey: Prentice-Hall, 1963).

10. I. Lukoff and M. Whiteman, "Attitudes toward Blindness—Some Preliminary Findings," *New Outlook for the Blind,* 53 (1961), 39–44.
11. M. McGuire and J. Sillen, *Early Rehabilitation Services for the Blind* (New York: Jewish Guild for the Blind, 1966).
12. U.S. Public Health Service, *Statistical Report 1964 Model Reporting Area for Blindness Statistics* (Washington: Government Printing Office, 1965).

SESSION REPORT

Donald Granberg

Discussion after the session on motivation was limited to a few brief remarks.

Dr. Herbert Rusalem re-emphasized that the age at which blindness appears may have great importance, and that those who are born blind, those who experience a sudden onset of blindness, and those who have undergone progressive blindness should be kept conceptually distinct for research purposes.

From the floor Dr. Marvin Sussman noted the problems associated with the fact that agencies typically deal with the good "cooperative" individuals and eschew the "unmotivated" individuals. It might, he suggested, be especially fruitful to look at the reasons behind this fact. What is the relationship between the agency and the sponsor of the agency? Is there an emphasis on demonstrating success in dealing with individuals and may this, in fact, be the reason that agencies tend to deal with "good" rehabilitees? Has the financial perpetuation of the agency gained ascendancy over the basic reason for the agency's existence?

EDUCATION

A SELECTIVELY DRAWN PICTURE OF RESEARCH IN EDUCATION AND SPECIAL EDUCATION

Geraldine T. Scholl

This paper represents a subjective "selectively drawn picture of research" in education and special education. A review of research activity and research needs should be considered against a background of current trends in order to attain some perspective on the origin, purposes, and impact of research findings on the field. This paper is divided into three sections: a review of trends in education and special education, the status of research in education, and needed lines of research.

TRENDS

Education

Schools as social institutions are subject to certain cultural factors and influences that determine the direction of their operation. At least four such influences may be identified: a redefinition of the role and function of education; a movement toward providing equal educational opportunities for all; an emphasis on academic excellence; and the rise of the educator as a professional.

REDEFINITION OF ROLE AND FUNCTION Each society determines what it expects of the school in the education of its young; society's expectations are never static but change to meet the demands of new conditions. Two concurrent and interrelated trends may be identified in reviewing the history of education in the United States: the trend toward secularization and the trend toward assigning increasing responsibility for education to the state.

In colonial times, the purposes of education were chiefly religious, with emphasis on preparation for the next world. The support of education was a family affair. The wealthy hired tutors while the poor remained uninstructed, except for charity schools established in a few communities.

The birth of a new nation and the necessity for molding the nation into a national unit shifted emphasis to preparation for citizenship, both social and political; the newly formed states were delegated responsibility for the education of their citizens. Schools became the homogenizing agent for welding into a single nation the peoples of diverse cultural backgrounds. Education became separate from the church and the responsibility of the state; those citizens with strong religious convictions established their own schools. Concurrently with the emphasis on education for citizenship came an emphasis on preparation for economic efficiency since the new nation needed producers. Vocational and industrial training became a part of the school curriculum. As more adequate provisions were made for education, attention was directed toward the disadvantaged of that time—namely, the mentally ill, the mentally retarded, the deaf, and the blind. Institutions were provided for these handicapped citizens, since families could not care for them. While the first such institutions were established through private philanthropic sources, the responsibility of the state was quickly recognized and implemented.

As the United States assumed a leadership position in the world, education entered a new era. Schools came to be recognized as social institutions and were increasingly viewed as agents of social change exerting a positive force for human betterment.[56] In effecting this role and function as a social institution with broader responsibilities for changing society, education was called upon to expand both program and clientele, and to provide services that required the involvement of other disciplines such as social work and psychology. Its program was extended downward to include kindergarten and nursery school and upward to include those youth who in past years would have dropped out but who now remained in school because of compulsory school attendance laws. Enrollment of five-year-olds in school increased from 57.7 per cent in 1954 to 68.5 per cent in 1964; the per cent of the 16–17 year-olds in school increased from 78.0 per cent in 1954 to 87.7 per cent in 1964.[66]

Together with the emphasis on keeping youth in school until age 16 or longer and completing a high school curriculum, there is a trend toward providing post-high school education as a responsibility of the local community. Community colleges and junior colleges are becoming an accepted part of the public school system. In addition, schools now accept children previously thought to be outside the responsibility of public schools, such as the trainable mentally retarded and the severely physically handicapped. The trend toward secularism continues, with major modifications currently under way in many of the educational institutions formerly conducted by religious groups. The growing recognition that a segregated and parochial education does not prepare for leadership in the world of change is undoubtedly contributing to this movement.

The new role and function currently being assumed by education is closely related to another force: equalizing educational opportunities for all.

EQUAL EDUCATIONAL OPPORTUNITIES The Constitution assigns to the several states, responsibility for making suitable provisions for the education of its citizens. Consequently, education is administered and financed to a large extent on the local level. In general, there is minimal supervision and/or control from state departments of education. This de-centralized system has not proved to be an ideal or efficient arrangement. Great disparity exists among the several states in their willingness and ability to provide adequate financial support for quality education. In addition, local school districts vary in willingness and ability to provide financial support so that the quality of education varies even within each state.

At least two forces directed toward reducing these inequalities may be identified. First, there is a growing recognition that school districts must be a certain size in order to provide an adequate educational program. Reorganization of school districts provides a broader base, both for financing and program planning. While some loss of local control is inherent in this trend, the greater gains of a more efficient system and higher quality of instruction counterbalance this disadvantage. The second force is the increasing federal government support of education. Feared in the past because of "federal control," government aid is now recognized as the most feasible way of equalizing educational opportunities and providing quality education for all citizens regardless of where they live. The method of disbursement of federal monies to local districts through state education agencies represents an attempt to strengthen state departments, which in turn strengthen local programs.

Equalizing educational opportunities is further reflected in the emphasis on drawing all children, regardless of race, creed, or handicap, into the school program and planning appropriately to provide for the individual differences found in children.

ACADEMIC EXCELLENCE While, on the one hand, schools are called upon to provide an expanded curriculum for an ever growing and more heterogeneous population, improvement in the quality of education is also demanded. The launching of Sputnik exerted a great impact on our educational system. Schools were sorely criticized for not meeting the needs of a technological society. There is emphasis now on academic excellence, and pressures are placed on children both individually and in groups to achieve. These pressures have both positive and negative influences on schools, on those attending school, and on parents.

In an attempt to meet the demands for academic excellence, the schools are examining curriculum content and evaluating methods of teaching. More content is included at an earlier age than was truc ten years ago. While in the past there was concern with what was taught, or the input aspects of education, there is now increasing concern with what is being learned or the output aspects.

As pressures to achieve academic excellence increase, emotional and behavior problems increase in those children who are disadvantaged culturally, physically, or mentally. Frustrated, they present problems to a school which must keep them because of compulsory school attendance laws.

THE RISE OF PROFESSIONALISM The increasing importance and the improved status of education have given courage to educators to become a more powerful force in determining their destiny. Whereas, in the past school boards have exerted influence on such activities as curriculum development, teachers, through their professional organizations, are now demanding such rights. They are working toward increased recognition not only for their professional competence, but also for more mundane improvements, such as salary and working conditions including adequate time to plan, to work with individual children, to attend conferences, to improve themselves. Teachers are moving away from their previous subordinate role to a leadership role.[24,40]

Higher quality pre-professional preparation programs, as well as in-service education programs, are exerting their influence on the improvement of teaching. The special needs of the beginning teacher are receiving attention since no pre-professional preparation program can possibly equip a young teacher adequately.[62] With the financial encouragement of the federal government, industry, and philanthropic organizations, special study institutes to up-date knowledge in subject matter fields and in teaching methodology are sponsored by local school districts, state departments of education, and colleges and universities. The emphasis on quality preparation and constant attention to improvement of knowledge and skill is leading toward the concept of a career teacher, recognized as a professional on an equal status position with members of other professions, such as law and medicine.[63]

Special Education

Special education has moved from a family responsibility where the handicapped child remained at home usually hidden away and uneducated, to a state responsibility wherein custodial care was provided for the handicapped still hidden away, to the present stage. This is that of a community responsibility wherein habilitation and/or education are provided for the young handicapped person and sheltered work and living arrangements are provided for the adult. Both state and, to an increasing degree, federal financial support for community programs are being provided.

In addition, handicapped children are being integrated into the main stream of the school. They learn to evaluate their abilities against the norm, and the non-handicapped learn first hand that the handicapped have capacities and abilities. As regular school programs become more sensitive to providing for individual differences, there will be a decreasing need for special classes, but an increasing need for qualified personnel who will assist the regular teacher. The restrictions of the disability in the area of school learning will usually determine the kind and degree of assistance required to enable the handicapped person to compete with the normal individual.

The need for quality education is likewise felt in special education. Partly because of the stimulation provided by federal support of teacher education programs under the provisions of Public Law 85-926 as amended, more teachers are being prepared to work with handicapped children. The status of the special education teacher is rising, perhaps at a faster rate than that of teachers as a whole. The level of the curriculum in special schools for the handicapped is also rising.

There is at least one unique trend affecting special education: a movement away from medical and paramedical diagnoses to determine educational placement.[93] In its early days, special education provided special school or class placement for such children as epileptics, "delicates," polio-stricken individuals, and amputees. As time passed and special educators gained experience, it became evident that many of these children were not educational problems since their disability did not affect their ability to learn. Rather, they presented management problems: medical management, as in the case of epileptics, or physical management, as in the case of children confined to wheelchairs or wearing braces. To a degree, visually handicapped children may be viewed not so much as having "educational methodology" problems but rather "educational materials" problems. Provided with braille, large type, and recording aids, increasing numbers of these children are attending regular classes full time.

There is another factor influencing the movement away from the use of medically defined categories for special education placement: the number of children with multiple disabilities. A movement toward broader classifications and groupings that will embrace the particular educational needs of the child should enable schools to make better provisions for the disabilities of the multiple-handicapped.

STATUS OF RESEARCH

Education

Until recent times, research has been a neglected aspect of education. Most school districts, as well as state departments of education, allocated insignificant sums for this purpose. In addition, educational research was often conducted by university personnel who were not concerned with grass roots problems of the school; direct involvement of school personnel in research was rare.

Federal funding, first through the cooperative research program, provided much needed stimulation to educational research. Recent reductions in some programs and a hold-the-line policy in others have been attributed to the lack of information given Congress about the effects of educational research.[3] In addition to funds directly earmarked for educational research, Federal monies may be used for research and/or demonstration under provisions of such acts as the Elementary and Secondary Education Act.

Private industry is supporting educational research particularly in the area of technology.

Bloom estimates that the level of support for educational research was increased by about 2,000 per cent from 1960 to 1966.[19] However, support does not necessarily indicate quality or productive projects. He further states that in his opinion only 70 out of the 70,000 studies reported in the *Review of Educational Research* during the past 25 years are crucial and significant. Part of this opinion is attributable to the lack of qualified researchers. To help alleviate this situation federal funds are being allocated to the training of educational researchers.[3]

Lags in two directions are contributing to the somewhat discouraging status of educational research. There is often a lag of approximately a year from the time a manuscript is submitted to a book publisher and the time it appears in print; an even longer lag exists for research journal articles. To compensate, researchers often resort to duplicating their papers and circulating them in that temporary form or presenting research findings at national conferences. About 500 research reports for 222 sessions were listed in the Advance Program of the American Educational Research Association for the February 16–18, 1967 Annual Meeting.[2] It would be difficult to evaluate the quality of this quantity of research.

Perhaps more disturbing is the lapse of time between the publication of significant research findings and their implementation in the classroom.[19] This lag is variously estimated at between 30 and 50 years. To illustrate: if we assume that research efforts are directed at solving problems of concern to educators, then from a cursory review, we might say that a major problem lies in the area of individual differences, since much research is concentrated in this area. Apparently instruction in the classroom has not been planned in accord with the principle of individual differences long known and recognized.[45,67,68,101]

This paper discusses current research activity under three subheadings: individualizing instruction through organizational or administrative modifications; through changes in the teaching-learning process; and through maximizing the capabilities of individual children. Emphasis will be placed on what is happening in the education of the young from earliest years through high school.

ORGANIZATIONAL MODIFICATION In the public schools traditionally, teaching has been conducted on the one teacher with one class pattern; children in the class are considered as a homogeneous group and are said to be in a grade. Some early educational research efforts were directed toward grouping and the problems of grouping. Homogeneous grouping on the basis of intelligence and achievement has been tried, but the problem of individual differences remains: there does not seem to be one single criterion for successful grouping.[11,81,101] In fact, the country school concept with multigrade range has even been considered.

Having failed to find a solution to meeting individual differences through homogeneous grouping, educators are seeking other administrative or organizational solutions. Much of what is written in this area currently may not be classified as "research," since control groups are rare and reports remain descriptive and subjective. This situation is to be expected at the present stage of research in education. In an all-out effort to improve quality of instruction, many ideas are tried without benefit of evaluation through sound research.

Particularly in readiness for formal learning at the early elementary level, the wide range of individual differences has led some school systems to adopt the ungraded school plan.[11,39] In this plan, children are not "graded" according to the old grading concept but rather, during their first two or three years of schooling are allowed to proceed through "units" of instruction. Sometimes they remain with a single teacher for more than one year. A recent survey conducted by the National Education Association indicates that one large school system in three is using a nongraded scheme in at least one of its elementary schools.[65] The advantages as well as disadvantages have been enumerated in educational literature.[11,39,65] Little true research exists, however, partly because of difficulties in selecting control groups and the presence of uncontrolled variables. On a theoretical basis the plan might be defended as one means of providing for late developers.

There is little research evidence to indicate that any one class size is more efficient or more conducive to learning than any other. Teachers have known that a class can be too small or too large for certain activities but what is "too small" and what is "too large" is difficult to define.[11,101] School systems seem to adopt class size primarily on the basis of availability of funds and teachers. Since the experience of educators indicates that certain activities are better suited for small groups, while others are better for large groups, some schools are experimenting with variable groupings, particularly at the secondary school level [97] and more recently on the elementary level.[11] Modular scheduling, with emphasis on student determination of how long he will spend on any activity, is used by some schools. These plans require flexible scheduling and team work among teachers. Team teaching is usually used to implement the multi-group and large group pattern.[11,14,96]

A plan that seems somewhat contradictory to the nongraded school concept is the movement toward departmentalization.[64] Secondary school programs have traditionally been organized on a departmental basis, with subject matter experts teaching in their own fields. The push for academic excellence has undoubtedly influenced some school systems to carry the departmental plan to the junior high and even to the later elementary levels. During 1964–65, there were 97 large school systems identified by the National Education Association as using the departmental system in grades four, five, and six.[64]

The teacher shortage has led some schools to utilize the services of the nonprofessional, sometimes called the "teacher aide" or "teacher assistant." [11,96] The utilization of an unqualified person in the classroom has been criticized as taking away opportunities from qualified professionals for guiding learning through informal activities. It is hoped that the teaching profession will not assign to the subprofessional valuable learning opportunities to the detriment of the learner, but will utilize such personnel for the numerous routine jobs not directly related to the learning experience.

School building design is also receiving some attention.[20] Buildings are being planned with movable partitions that facilitate team arrangements and cooperative teaching as well as to accommodate variable groupings through creative architectural design.

Opportunities to view and to study new administrative plans should do much toward publicizing their merits as well as their disadvantages. The National Commission on Teacher Education and Professional Standards some time ago selected 60 centers in 26 states and the District of Columbia as models of new administrative plans.[61] These centers were selected as of December, 1966, and more will be added as they are investigated and approved. The identification of such demonstration centers should help to disseminate information and stimulate the replication of plans in other parts of the country. How much can or will be researched about organizational structure remains unknown.

THE TEACHING-LEARNING PROCESS The observer in a classroom may easily identify four variables: the learner, the teacher, the curriculum content and materials, and the method of instruction. All have been researched to varying degrees but what has apparently been lacking is a consideration of the interaction among the variables. A brief summary of current activity in the four areas follows.

Summaries of research in child growth and development are numerous. There is probably a greater body of knowledge from many disciplines in this area than in any other aspect of education. Some of the principles based on research most relevant to education include: sequence in the developmental process; individual differences in rate and pattern of growth; the unitary characteristics of the growth and development process; and the dependence on both nature and nurture to achieve maximum potential.[45] The role of culture in the growth and development process, particularly during the adolescent period, has received attention recently.[52,77,86,91] Current research activity seems to be directed toward investigating two areas of intellectual development, namely, language and cognition.[12,47] The language development of culturally disadvantaged children is being studied.[74] Studies of cognition by Bruner[21,22] and Piaget[31] are of particular relevance to educators.

While research in child and adolescent development has been productive in findings, and while most teacher education programs require courses in this area, actual application to the school program seems restricted. In general, children are treated as a group rather than as individuals; instruction is often pitched toward the hypothetical "average," with limited individualization of instruction; school programs, particularly at the secondary level, do not take into account the special needs of the age group. The lag in implementing research findings in this area seems critical.

The teacher variable has received considerable attention from research workers but questions of evaluating effectiveness remain.[59] The multifaceted nature of teaching competence, in addition to the lack of definition of who is an effective teacher, complicates the research picture.[16,37]

Educators have long been involved with the "what" of teaching. Subject matter to be taught and the relative allocation of time to each subject vary greatly from school to school. Each subject matter specialist attempts to crowd as much of his subject into the school curriculum as possible without regard to the contribution of other subjects to the education of the individual.[50] Most states minimally define what should be included in the curriculum, and frequently what is mandated reflects particular interests of legislators at that time. Curriculum content so legislated is often not followed by local school districts. To a degree, local school boards composed primarily of nonprofessionals have in the past determined curriculum content. In addition, textbooks written by middle class educators who often lack depth of knowledge in a subject matter field have determined curriculum. In general, curriculum content seems particularly sensitive to pressure groups.[85] The trend toward professionalism on the part of educators and the push for academic excellence are making inroads toward effecting change. Subject matter experts are becoming involved in developing curriculum content, and the new content is leading to new teaching methods and the development of new materials.[25,42,57,58,70,72,87,95,100] In general, the new content is characterized as being more sequential in presentation, with planned progression of content from early elementary through high school and on into college.

Until recently, few psychologists were interested in classroom learning and their research contributed little of practical value to the teacher. Learning theory developed from a study of animal learning or human adult learning in the laboratory or structured settings.[43] Application derived from such research to the classroom setting has not been productive in improving school learning, and the gap between the psychology laboratory and the school has not been bridged.[29] Principles of learning have been enunciated, but their incorporation and integration into a meaningful teaching theory or method are absent.[82,99] Bruner[22] would seem to be working toward this objective.

The current emphasis in research on improving classroom instruction seems to lie in technological directions, namely, programmed learning, television, and computer based instruction.

In the beginning, programmed instruction seemed wedded to the machine, and indeed much time and money were spent on experimenting with machine programs. However, research has not demonstrated the superiority of machine teaching over programmed texts,[28] which do have an additional advantage of being less expensive and more portable. In September, 1963, there were 352 commercially developed programs in 10 subject matter areas available to teachers; 56.6 per cent were in text form only; 19.6 per cent were in machine form only; and 23.7 per cent were available in both forms.[41] There were 190 reports of research in programmed instruction published from 1954 to February of 1963; 165 of which were reported since 1959.[84] Schramm[84] states that a disproportionate number of studies report "no significant differences." While many reasons may exist for this situation, one wonders if the value of programmed instructional techniques may not lie in an area not adequately studied; that is, how much time such aids save for the teacher to devote to other teaching-learning activities. Increasingly, educators seem to be viewing programmed materials for their special strengths; that is, to teach facts and to enable the child to teach and drill himself on content materials, leaving the teacher free to devote time to problem learners and to guide in the integration and application of content learned from programmed texts.[96] While much is written on programming and programmed materials, research evidence is lacking to demonstrate its superiority over any other type of instructional procedures. The language laboratory, a variation of the auto-instructional procedure, has demonstrated its value.[96] This may be due to the emphasis on aural-oral techniques in the development of skill in spoken language which lend themselves to such procedures.

Several years ago, educational television was widely heralded as a boon to educators and rapidly adopted. Again, research has not indicated any superiority of this medium of instruction over any other.[96] Recently, there seems to be a decline in its popularity. Instruction via television lacks one important element found in programmed instruction: individualization of instruction.

Since the computer now permeates a large segment of our lives, it is natural that it would also enter the field of education.[94] Computer based instruction represents a step beyond programmed instruction. With the computer, the learner gets immediate reinforcement in his learning and furthermore if he makes an error, he can be guided back to the correct response by a carefully programmed computer. The most serious disadvantage at this time seems to be cost: an estimated 8 per cent increase in cost of instruction per student would be needed to provide computer based instruction for a school system.[94] Thus far, educators have not apparently been as involved in research on computer based instruction as have engineers and psychologists.[38]

While much research is under way on the four variables of learner, teacher, curriculum content and materials, and methods of instruction, results seem fragmented and not too productive of change in the traditional classroom. What occurs in a classroom seems to be greater than the sum of the individual parts, and a research methodology with a more gestalt-oriented approach needs to be developed to explore the interrelationship of the variables. The interaction analysis technique developed by Flanders[30] may lead to more productive research findings and to improving the teaching-learning process in the classroom.

MAXIMIZING EACH CHILD'S CAPABILITIES While educators seek a solution to individualizing instruction through organizational modifications and through improving the teaching-learning process, individual children, for a variety of reasons, are not able to take full advantage of the education that is offered them. Some are deprived of the experiences of early childhood that prepare them for school; some receive inferior schooling or inappropriate and meaningless schooling because of their racial, cultural, or socio-economic backgrounds; and some have become so frustrated with the system that they have developed emotional problems that interfere with learning or else have left the system entirely. Educators attempt to meet the needs of such children primarily through trial and error.

To compensate for the deprivation of experience sustained by many children during pre-school years, pre-school programs, including Project Head Start, have been initiated. The contribution of nursery school and/or kindergarten experience to the future academic achievement of the so-called normal child remains in doubt.[34] Programs for the culturally disadvantaged at the pre-school level have not demonstrated long range effects.[102] Since such programs seem to be based on sound theory, one wonders why research evidence is lacking to support their value. There are a number of explanations. Highly individualized instructional procedures are found in pre-school programs; creativity is nurtured; and freedom to seek out learning on the basis of interest is encouraged. These conditions do not exist in the typical public school program which, particularly from the third grade onward, tends to force children to fit a mold. A stereotyped curriculum does not meet the needs of children who are different. Another reason may be that pre-school training is primarily a program of prevention, and the result of any program of prevention cannot be measured easily. A third explanation might possibly lie in our crude research methods and measurements.

Much attention is currently directed toward providing better educational opportunities for minority group children. Almost every school district in the country is faced, to a greater or lesser degree, with problems of integration. While, in the past, separate schools have been provided for racial groups in the South, the North has also had its segregated schools because of the neighborhood school concept and segregated housing. Various plans are being tried to change this situation and to provide quality education for all. Some school systems are pouring into schools in disadvantaged areas all possible auxiliary services, such as remedial reading, school social work, recreational programs, parent education, in addition to reducing the class size so that much individual attention can be given. Research under such conditions is difficult to conduct since few school superintendents would be willing to assign certain children to a control group and incur the wrath of parents and pressure groups. Consequently, the results of such programs are and will probably continue to be reported in descriptive terms with minimal objective evidence of their efficacy.

Another procedure for affecting integration is the practice of bussing children within communities so that racial balance can be achieved in the schools. This practice is too new to determine its long range effects, but it does lend itself to more rigid research methodology since, over a period of time, intelligence and achievement test scores may be compared.

Mental health of Americans has received considerable attention in recent years.[76] The problem may be resolved if approached on a preventive level. The incidence of mental illness has led to federal and some state legislation to provide for community mental health programs.[92] New approaches to treatment are being sought since traditional psychotherapy has not been demonstrated as a successful therapeutic technique.[71,76,80,92,104]

The school provides a logical setting for a program of mental illness prevention.[71] Some school districts have initiated school social work programs.[48,53,54] While therapy was at first handled on an individual case work basis, in most of these programs there seems to be a trend toward utilizing group techniques since schools are group oriented.[71] Mental health consultants are also provided in certain school systems. Since many of the early behavior problems in school are the result of temporary frustration or reaction to a situation, some schools are providing assistance to the temporarily disturbed child through life space interviewing and work with teachers on preventing the development of more serious problems.[60] No one technique will work in every school, and a variety of techniques should be available. Again, because of the preventive nature of these programs, research will be difficult to conduct and currently the literature is primarily descriptive in nature.

Some writers are viewing prevention of behavior and emotional problems from a broader perspective, namely, that of society's contribution to producing problem behavior. Behavior problems, particularly in the adolescent, are attributed to the ambivalence of the culture.[32,52]

One of the most crucial problems facing educators is the dropout.[46,66] The necessity for completing at least a high school education in order to obtain employment makes it imperative that students stay in school, and yet the school curriculum at the secondary level continues to be directed toward meeting the needs of the college bound student. Those who cannot compete tend to drop out or be pushed out.[83,98] In spite of this, modifications in school programming are not instituted at a very rapid pace.[46]

Special Education

If the status of research in the field of education in general is rather discouraging, it is even more so in special education. Many educational practices in special education are derived or adapted from work with the so-called normal child; some are based on what seems good, reasonable, or logical; others are adopted directly from regular education. In the past, little money has been allocated to research in special education. The initiation of the cooperative research program stimulated some research activity in the area of mental retardation.

The passage of Public Law 88-164 in 1963 marked a milestone in special education research. During the first year of operation $2 million were allocated for research related to handicapped children. Increasing sums of money are authorized each year under this program. For fiscal year 1966, $6 million were appropriated although a portion of that sum was designated for a research and demonstration center in the education of handicapped children.

The titles of papers listed in the recent program of the American Educational Research Association may shed light on the status of research in special education within the discipline of education.[2]

THE REVIEW OF EDUCATIONAL RESEARCH The appearance of a section devoted to "learning disorders" in recent issues of *The Review of Educational Research* probably reflects the rise of a new concern of educators and perhaps the beginning of considering educational diagnosis and remediation rather than the older more widely accepted categorical approach based on medical or paramedical diagnosis.

Much of what is reported is descriptive in nature, however, and tends to be subjective and applicable to only a small segment of the population with few valid generalizations that may be applied to the total population. Research in all areas might be characterized as fragmented and nonprogrammatic.

There are several reasons for this state of affairs. There are usually small numbers of subjects available for study by any researcher, and frequently the variability between subjects is too great to permit any generalizations regarding the findings. Control groups are difficult to identify since the total sample is often too small to divide for experimental treatment, or else one particular setting or group does not lend itself to comparison with another setting or group. Hence, control and experimental groups often must be selected from different settings. Special educators in all areas are plagued with the problem of definition. Who is hard of hearing? Who is mentally retarded? Who is emotionally disturbed? Because there seems to be no commonly accepted definition in most categories, comparison of research findings from similar studies is difficult if not almost impossible. As a result conflicting findings are often reported.

ORGANIZATIONAL MODIFICATIONS In the past, the education and/or habilitation of certain groups of exceptional children have been conducted in settings away from the child's family and community. This is particularly true of the visually impaired, the deaf, and the mentally retarded. Increasing numbers among these groups are being educated in regular public schools.[23] While this trend may be attributed in part to the increasing responsibility of public schools for the education of all children, there is some research evidence indicating that retardation in certain aspects of mental, social, and emotional growth and development may be attributed to the somewhat sterile atmosphere of an institution.[73,89,90] Many physically handicapped children are required to spend varying periods of time in a hospital for medical remediation. The deleterious effect of such hospitalization has been recognized, but programs of remediation seem difficult to implement.[15]

Early public school programs for the handicapped were primarily on the segregated special class pattern. Gradually the advantages of integration were recognized so that the trend is toward more integration.[23] Research has not demonstrated that the practice of placing handicapped children in special classes has a beneficial effect on academic achievement although social benefits have been reported.[17,38,49]

THE TEACHING-LEARNING PROCESS Except in the area of the gifted, longitudinal studies of the growth and development of handicapped children are conspicuous by their absence. The area of mental retardation has been active in attempting to describe variations from the norm in intellectual characteristics, but conclusions appear contradictory and studies are short-term and fragmented.[17,55] A fresh approach to studying problems of cognitive development in retardates may evolve in the future from the three theoretical models (factor analytic study, Piaget, and Bruner) presented at a recent research conference.[36]

The acquisition of language is, of course, a central problem in the education of the deaf and has received attention from researchers.[35,78,79] Research findings have not filtered down to the classroom to improve instructional procedures, however; and the education of the deaf has been criticized as being ineffective.[1] Language development of retardates and the socially disadvantaged has also been studied.[17,55,74]

The increased interest in the area of learning disabilities[13,69] and the development of remedial techniques for such disabilities may prove in the future to be the unifying characteristic for classifying and planning appropriate programs for all types of handicapped children.

Research related to the special education teacher may be characterized as descriptive.[18] The recent Council for Exceptional Children study[27] on the competencies of teachers of various types of exceptional children represents a step toward describing the special teacher on a theoretical basis. Whether these competencies are necessary in actual practice remains to be determined. Personality characteristics of prospective special education and elementary teachers have received some attention and may point the way toward more effective recruitment procedures in colleges and universities.[103]

NEEDED LINES OF RESEARCH

Educational research must develop an identity of its own. Currently, there is dependence on the exact sciences for methodology, treatment of statistical data, and so on. Such techniques tend to lead to an analysis of parts rather than of the whole and in the educational process, the whole is greater than the sum of its parts. Educational research may need to be satisfied with less rigorous controls than the exact sciences, and develop, more thoroughly, techniques of descriptive research.

Too often the researcher seeks a problem that lends itself to his particular research design interest rather than identifying a problem and seeking a research design to solve it.[19] Future educational research must find ways of studying the classroom as a totality with teachers, learners, methodology, and subject matter interacting. If education is to meet the challenge society is assigning to it—namely, to be an agent for social change—the school must be studied as a social institution by interdisciplinary teams.

Future educational research should emphasize longitudinal and long-term studies of growth and development, learning, cognitive development, acquisition of language, effects of special programs, and so on. The complexity of researching educational problems would seem to demand a team approach with more cooperative ventures. Such teams need to include educators from various sub-specialties as well as professionals from other disciplines.

In special education we need to identify what is really unique about the learner and his needs, the classroom setting, and the procedures. We must find the best ways for conducting an educational program. We also need to take a close look at our products and how they have adjusted to adult life. Continuing educational practices that are not contributing to future adult adjustment should be discouraged.

If educational researchers face the current status of research realistically, and if public schools recognize the ability of research to improve classroom procedures and practices, we may enter a new era in education wherein the application of research findings to the school program will enable each individual child to achieve his maximum potential.

NOTES

1. Advisory Committee on the Education of the Deaf, *Education of the Deaf* (Washington: U.S. Department of Health, Education and Welfare, 1965).
2. American Educational Research Association, *Advance Program for the 1967 Annual Meeting* (Washington: AERA, 1967).
3. ———, *Educational Researcher,* 17 (December, 1966), 1–3.
4. ———, "Education of Exceptional Children and Minority Groups," *Review of Educational Research,* 11 (June, 1941), 253–329.
5. ———, "Education of Exceptional Children and Minority Groups," *Review of Educational Research,* 14 (June, 1944), 201–263.
6. ———, "Education of Exceptional Children," *Review of Education Research,* 23 (December, 1953), 391–507.
7. ———, "Education of Exceptional Children," *Review of Educational Research,* 29 (December, 1959), 395–570.
8. ———, "Education of Exceptional Children," *Review of Educational Research,* 33 (February, 1963), 5–136.
9. ———, "Education of Exceptional Children," *Review of Educational Research* 36 (February, 1966), 5–198.

10. ———, "Methodology of Educational Research," *Review of Educational Research* 36 (December, 1966), 487–617.
11. R. H. Anderson, *Teaching in a World of Change* (New York: Harcourt, Brace and World, Inc., 1966).
12. D. P. Ausubel and Pearl Ausubel, "Cognitive Development in Adolescence," *Review of Educational Research* 36 (October, 1966), 403–415.
13. R. Batemen, "Learning Disorders," *Review of Educational Research* 36 (February, 1966), 93–119.
14. D. W. Beggs III, ed., *Team Teaching: Bold New Venture* (Bloomington: Indiana University Press, 1964).
15. Thesis Bergmann, *Children in the Hospital* (New York: International Universities Press, Inc., 1965).
16. B. J. Biddle and W. J. Ellena, eds., *Contemporary Research on Teacher Effectiveness* (New York: Holt, Rinehart and Winston, 1964).
17. L. S. Blackman and P. Heintz, "The Mentally Retarded," *Review of Educational Research,* 36 (February, 1966), 5–36.
18. B. Blatt, "The Preparation of Special Education Personnel," *Review of Educational Research,* 36 (February, 1966), 151–161.
19. B. S. Bloom, "Twenty-five Years of Educational Research," *American Educational Research Journal,* 3 (May, 1966), 211–221.
20. C. W. Brubaker, "What's New In Urban School Buildings," *NEA Journal,* 55 (December, 1966), 26–29.
21. J. S. Bruner, *The Process of Education* (Cambridge, Massachusetts: Harvard University Press, 1961).
22. ———, *Toward a Theory of Instruction* (Cambridge, Massachusetts: The Belknap Press, 1966).
23. L. F. Cain, "Special Education," *Encyclopedia of Educational Research* (3d ed.; New York: Macmillan, 1960), 1324–1330.
24. R. F. Campbell, "Tomorrow's Teacher," *Saturday Review* (January 14, 1967), 60–64, 73.
25. J. B. Carroll, "Research on Teaching Foreign Language," in *Handbook of Research on Teaching* (Chicago, 1963), 1060–1100.
26. H. D. Carter, "Gifted Children," *Encyclopedia of Educational Research* (3d ed.; New York, 1960), 583–593.
27. Council for Exceptional Children, *Professional Standards for Personnel in the Education of Exceptional Children* (Washington: Council for Exceptional Children, NEA, 1966).
28. W. Dick, "The Development and Current Status of Computer-Based Instruction," *American Educational Research Journal,* 2 (January, 1965), 41–54.
29. W. K. Estes, "Learning," in *Encyclopedia of Educational Research* (3d ed.; New York: Macmillan, 1960), 752–770.
30. N. A. Flanders, *Teacher Influence, Pupil Attitudes, and Achievement,* U.S. Department of Health, Education and Welfare, Office of Education, Cooperative Research Monograph No. 12 (Washington: Government Printing Office, 1965).
31. J. H. Flavell, *The Developmental Psychology of Jean Piaget* (Princeton, New Jersey: D. Van Nostrand Co., Inc., 1963).
32. E. Z. Friedenberg, *Coming of Age in America* (New York: Random House, 1963).
33. ———, *The Vanishing Adolescent* (Boston: Beacon Press, 1959).
34. E. M. Fuller, "Early Childhood Education," *Encyclopedia of Educational Research* (3d ed.; New York, 1960), 385–398.
35. H. G. Furth, *Thinking Without Language: Psychological Implications of Deafness* (New York: The Free Press, 1966).
36. M. Garrison, Jr., ed., *Cognitive Models and Development in Mental Re-*

tardation, Monograph Supplement to *American Journal of Mental Deficiency,* 70 (January, 1966), 3–149.
37. J. W. Getzels and P. W. Jackson, "The Teacher's Personality and Characteristics," *Handbook of Research on Teaching* (Chicago: Rand McNally, 1963), 506–582.
38. H. Goldstein, J. W. Moss, and L. J. Jordan, *The Efficacy of Special Class Training on the Development of Mentally Retarded Children* (Urbana: Institute for Research on Exceptional Children, University of Illinois, 1965).
39. J. I. Goodlad and R. H. Anderson, *The Nongraded Elementary School* (New York: Harcourt, Brace and World, 1963).
40. C. J. Hannan, "Professional Negotiation for Improving Education," *NEA Journal,* 55 (December, 1966), 56–57.
41. L. F. Hansom, ed., *Programs, 1963: A Guide to Programmed Instructional Materials Available to Educators by September 1963,* Bulletin 1964, No. 3 (Washington: Government Printing Office, 1963).
42. K. B. Henderson, "Research on Teaching Secondary School Mathematics," *Handbook of Research on Teaching* (Chicago: Rand McNally, 1963), 1007–1030.
43. E. R. Hilgard, *Theories of Learning* (2d ed.; New York: Appleton-Century-Crofts, 1956).
44. N. Hobbs, "Helping Disturbed Children: Psychological and Ecological Strategies," *American Psychologist,* 21 (December, 1966), 1105–1115.
45. M. L. Hoffman and L. W. Hoffman, eds., *Review of Child Development Research* (New York: Russell Sage Foundation, 1964).
46. D. E. Hunt, "Adolescence: Cultural Deprivation, Poverty, and the Dropout," *Review of Educational Research,* 36 (October, 1966), 463–475.
47. J. Huttenlocher, "Children's Intellectual Development," *Review of Educational Research,* 35 (April, 1965), 114–121.
48. A. Johnson, *School Social Work: Its Contribution to Professional Education* (New York: National Association of Social Workers, 1963).
49. G. O. Johnson, "Special Education for the Mentally Handicapped—A Paradox," *Exceptional Children,* 1 (February, 1963), 21–27.
50. N. C. Kearney and W. W. Cook, "Curriculum," *Encyclopedia of Educational Research* (3d ed.; New York: Macmillan, 1960), 358–365.
51. S. A. Kirk, *Educating Exceptional Children* (Boston: Houghton-Mifflin, 1962).
52. W. C. Kvaraceus, *Anxious Youth: Dynamics of Delinquency* (Columbus, Ohio: Charles E. Merrill Books, Inc., 1966).
53. G. Lee, *Helping the Troubled School Child* (New York: National Association of Social Workers, 1959).
54. H. W. Lundberg, ed., *School Social Work: A Service of Schools,* Bulletin 1964, No. 15 (Washington: Government Printing Office, 1964).
55. J. J. McCarthy and R. C. Scheerenberger, "A Decade of Research on the Education of the Mentally Retarded," *Mental Retardation Abstracts,* 3 (October-December, 1966), 481–501.
56. S. M. McMurrin, "What Tasks for the Schools," *Saturday Review* (January 14, 1967), 40–43.
57. H. C. Meckel, "Research on Teaching Composition and Literature," *Handbook of Research on Teaching* (Chicago: Rand McNally, 1963), 966–1006.
58. L. E. Metcalf, "Research on Teaching the Social Studies," *Handbook of Research on Teaching* (Chicago: Rand McNally, 1963), 929–965.
59. H. E. Mitzel, "Teacher Effectiveness," *Handbook of Research on Teaching* (Chicago: Rand McNally, 1963), 1481–1486.
60. W. C. Morse, *The Crisis or Helping Teacher in the Public School: Theory*

and Practice (Ann Arbor: School of Education, The University of Michigan, 1966).
61. National Commission on Teacher Education and Professional Standards, *Annotated Listing of Selected Demonstration Centers* (Washington: Council for Exceptional Children, NEA, 1966).
62. ———, *The Real World of the Beginning Teacher* (Washington: Council for Exceptional Children, NEA, 1966).
63. ———, *Remaking the World of the Career Teacher* (Washington: Council for Exceptional Children, NEA, 1966).
64. National Education Association, "Departmentalization in Elementary Schools," *NEA Research Bulletin,* 44 (February, 1966), 27–28.
65. ———, "Nongraded School Organization," *ibid.,* 43 (October, 1966), 93–95.
66. ———, "Who's In School?" *ibid.,* 44 (October, 1966), 93–95.
67. W. C. Olson, *Child Development* (Boston: D. C. Heath and Company, 1959).
68. ———, "Developmental Theory in Education," *Concept of Development* (Minneapolis: The University of Minnesota Press, 1957), 259–274.
69. W. Otto and R. A. McMenemy, *Corrective and Remedial Reading: Principles and Practices* (Boston: Houghton-Mifflin Company, 1966).
70. M. B. Parke, "Teaching Materials and Their Implementation," *Review of Educational Research,* 36 (June, 1966), 380–387.
71. M. Peters and W. W. Wattenberg, "Adolescence: Behavior Disorders and Guidance," *Review of Educational Research,* 36 (October, 1966), 474–484.
72. M. G. Phillips, "Learning Materials and Their Implementation," *Review of Educational Research,* 36 (June, 1966), 375–379.
73. S. Provence and R. C. Lipton, *Infants in Institutions* (New York: International University Press, Inc., 1962).
74. J. B. Raph, "Language Development in Socially Disadvantaged Children," *Review of Educational Research,* 35 (December, 1965), 389–400.
75. N. Ridemour, *Mental Health in the United States* (Cambridge, Massachusetts: Harvard University Press, 1961).
76. F. Riegsman, J. Cohen, and A. K. Pearl, *Mental Health of the Poor* (New York: The Free Press, 1964).
77. M. Rosenberg, *Society and the Adolescent Self-Image* (Princeton, New Jersey: Princeton University Press, 1965).
78. J. Rosenstein, "The Deaf and Hard of Hearing," *Review of Educational Research,* 36 (February, 1966), 176–198.
79. ——— and W. H. MacGinitie, *Research Studies on the Psycholinguistic Behavior of Deaf Children* (Washington: Council for Exceptional Children, NEA, 1965).
80. E. A. Rubenstein and M. B. Parloff, *Research in Psychotherapy* (Washington: The American Psychological Association, Inc., 1959).
81. D. H. Russell and H. R. Fea, "Research on Teaching Reading," *Handbook of Research on Teaching* (Chicago: Rand McNally, 1965), 865–928.
82. J. M. Scandura, "Teaching-Technology or Theory," *American Educational Research Journal,* 3 (March, 1966), 139–146.
83. W. E. Schafer, *Deviance in the Public Schools: An International View* (Ann Arbor: The University of Michigan, School of Social Work, 1966). (Mimeograph.)
84. W. L. Schramm, *The Research on Programmed Instruction: An Annotated Bibliography* (Palo Alto, California: Stanford University Institute for Communication Research, 1962).

85. F. Shaw, "The Changing Curriculum," *Review of Educational Research,* 36 (June, 1966), 343–352.
86. Carolyn W. Sherif, "Adolescence: Motivational, Attitudinal Personality Factors," *Review of Educational Research,* 36 (October, 1966), 437–449.
87. L. S. Shulman and E. R. Keislar, eds. *Learning by Discovery: A Critical Appraisal* (Chicago: Rand McNally, 1966).
88. B. F. Skinner, "Teaching Machines," *Science,* 128 (1958), 969–977.
89. L. M. Smith and P. F. Kleine, "The Adolescent and His Society," *Review of Educational Research,* 36 (October, 1966), 424–436.
90. M. B. Smith and N. Hobbs, "The Community and Community Mental Health Center," *American Psychologist,* 21 (June, 1966), 499–509.
91. R. A. Spitz, "Hospitalism: A Follow-up Report," *The Psychoanalytic Study of the Child* (New York: International Universities Press, 2, 1946), 113–117.
92. ———, "Hospitalism; An Inquiry into the Genesis of Psychiatric Conditions of Early Childhood," *The Psychoanalytic Study of the Child* (New York: International Universities Press, 1, 1945), 53–74.
93. G. D. Stevens, *Taxonomy in Special Education for Children with Body Disorders* (Pittsburgh: University of Pittsburgh Press, 1962).
94. P Suppes, "The Computer and Excellency," *Saturday Review* (January 14, 1967), 46–50.
95. D. Tanner, "Curriculum Theory: Knowledge and Content," *Review of Educational Research,* 36 (June, 1966), 362–371.
96. W. C. Trow, *Teacher and Technology* (New York: Appleton-Century-Crofts, 1963).
97. J. L. Trump and D. Baynham, *Guide to Better Schools* (Chicago: Rand McNally, 1961).
98. R. D. Vinter and R. C. Vinter, "Malperformance in the Public Schools: A Group Work Approach," *Social Work,* 10 (January, 1965), 3–13.
99. N. E. Wallen and R. M. W. Travers, "Analysis and Investigation of Teaching Methods," *Handbook of Research on Teaching* (Chicago: Rand McNally, 1963), 448–505.
100. F. G. Watson, "Research on Teaching Science," *Handbook of Research on Teaching* (Chicago: Rand McNally, 1963), 1031–1059.
101. G. Watson, *What Psychology Can We Trust?* (New York: Teachers College, Columbia University, 1961).
102. D. A. Wilkenson, "Programs and Practices in Compensatory Education for Disadvantaged Children," *Review of Educational Research,* 35 (December, 1965), 425–440.
103. E. William, *A Comparison of Prospective Special Education and Elementary Teachers on Selected Personality Characteristics* (Unpublished doctoral dissertation, Ann Arbor, Michigan: The University of Michigan, 1966).
104. J. Wolpe, A. Salter, and L. J. Reyna, eds., *The Conditioning Therapies: The Challenge in Psychotherapy* (New York: Holt, Rinehart and Winston, Inc., 1964).

RESEARCH IN EDUCATION OF THE BLIND

Carson Y. Nolan

Broad conceptualizations of research in education of the blind must be concerned with problems which are foreign to educational research as generally conceived. These problems arise from two principal sources: the small population of blind students available for study; and, consequently, the small number of researchers who become attracted to this field.

In 1966, approximately 19,000 legally blind children were registered with the American Printing House for the Blind. About 8,000 of these students were enrolled in 47 residential schools for the blind whose enrollments ranged from 372 individuals down to 16. About 11,000 students were placed in public school programs where enrollments varied from about 400 students down to one. However, even in large public school programs, the number of students to be found at a single site is small.

There are probably no more than 15 year-round college training programs for teachers of the blind. Fewer than half of these offer training to the doctoral level; and there is, probably, less than one doctorate degree awarded in this field each year. At the doctoral level, the total number of faculty people primarily concerned with teacher training in these college and university programs probably does not exceed ten. In addition, probably no more than five additional persons possessing the doctorate have a full-time concern with research on education of the blind.

GUIDELINES FOR RESEARCH

The consequence of the small number of subjects and the small number of potential researchers is that research in this field is severely limited. For this reason, it is critical that what research is undertaken be planned to provide maximum returns for the efforts expended. The following guidelines are suggested to help achieve this end.

1. Research should be programmatic in that problems should be pursued to their solution. Wherever applicable, this solution should include a product and the necessary instructions for its use by students, teachers, or other workers.

2. Emphasis should be on applied instead of basic research. More return can be expected from those projects that study the application of what is already known about behavior and education to problems of educating blind children. Important exceptions to this rule, of course, exist. For example, basic research is required in the area of tactual perception.

3. Research on educational fads should be left to those agencies which enjoy a surplus of subjects and researchers. If such research yields worthwhile results, studies can then be made of applicability to the education of the blind.

4. Every effort should be made to offset the effects of the small numbers of subjects available for study through use of precise experimental designs. Emphasis on multivariate designs, statistical control of critical variables through analysis of covariance, and use of sequential analytic techniques can do much to offset the problems induced by small numbers of subjects.

5. On the other hand, concern for the precision of experimental designs should not preclude seizing unique opportunities for study. In many instances, case studies carried out over a long period of time present the only opportunity for systematic study.

AN OVERALL VIEW

The overall view of the field of education of the blind is that education of blind children is essentially identical to the education of all children. Certainly the goals are the same. Why, then, is there a need for a special research effort? The reason lies in the fact that the perceptual development of blind children and their subsequent perceptual behavior often are different from those of sighted children. In areas where this is so, the means of intervention between the individual blind child and the common educational goals must differ from those customarily employed. Such means include educational media, educational techniques, and educational measures.

When broadly conceived, educational research for the blind should concern itself with three general areas. The first of these is the area of perceptual development, where research should have as its purpose the delineation of the effects of visual handicaps on the perceptual development of the child, and the detailed analysis and description of his characteristic modes of perceptual behavior. The second area is that of educational technology, where the concern should be the development of educational media and techniques best suited to enable the visually handicapped child to reach the common educational goals in light of his characteristic perceptual development and behavior. The third area, research and development in educational measurement, should have as its purpose the development of predictors of academic success and criteria to assess the degree to which the outcomes of research in educational technology enable the child to meet curricular goals.

Ideally, the ultimate goal of research in this area should be the development of educational systems for the visually handicapped. Briefly stated, this approach requires description in detail of the learning tasks imposed by the school goals or curriculum, description in detail of the capabilities of visually handicapped students for attempting these tasks, and development of the necessary interventions to maximize the probability that handicapped students master these tasks through the fullest use of the capabilities they possess. As mentioned above, these necessary interventions include educational media, educational techniques for learning and teaching, and the means of assessing task mastery.

SPECIFIC AREAS FOR RESEARCH

With this background in mind, one can consider specific areas of needed research. The list of research areas and problems that follows represents the range of most important problems.

Cognition

Cognition refers to the process by which the individual gains knowledge of or becomes aware of an object. It is within this realm that critical differences exist between the blind and sighted which have such significant implications for education. The following problems seem significant.

THE DIMENSIONS OF TEXTURE Although some work has been done in textural dimensions,[12,26] we still have no clear idea of the dimensions by which textures are tactually discriminated. Such information is critical, of course, for the design of maps and other tactual graphics. At the same time we have no formal information of development of ability to discriminate textures.

FORM PERCEPTION Some work has been done on form perception by Schiff and Isikow.[28] No information exists concerning what factors determine figure–ground relationships in tactual stimulus fields. Are differences in surface texture sufficient; or, in order to be a figure, must a tactual form be higher than its surroundings? Can a tactual figure be depressed below the surface of the stimulus field? How is a total form synthesized out of piecemeal tactual inspection of its parts? How valid and complete is the perception? How do these factors vary with size and complexity of the stimulus field? These questions have yet to be explored.

STRUCTURE IN PERCEPTION No information is available describing the degree to which patterning occurs in the perceptual organization of tactual stimulus fields. That such phenomena are common in visual perception is well known. Results of inspections of many tactual maps and charts in braille books and other sources appear to indicate that designers of these assume such patterning takes place. No empirical evidence exists to support this notion, and pilot work by the author indicates that it may not occur.

PERCEPTUAL CONSTANCIES What about perceptual constancies in the tactual realm? Are there relationships between the perceived size of an object and its weight or shape or surface texture or combinations of these?

PERCEPTION OF SPACE How do the blind develop their concepts of space? How accurately is space perceived? What are the roles and limitations of the various sensory channels in space perception? Answers to these questions have implications for mobility instruction as well as instruction in mathematics and the sciences.

VISUAL PERCEPTION Most individuals who qualify as legally blind have some residual vision. However, very little information describing the effects of types and degrees of visual handicaps on visual perceptual processes is available. An exception is the recent study of strabismus and amblyopia by McLaughlin.[19] Study is also needed of ways in which the visually handicapped can make use of residual vision. Development of training techniques to maximize use of residual vision is of great importance.[2]

CONCEPT DEVELOPMENT Visual deprivation results in a great reduction in the possible amounts of direct and vicarious contact with the environment. As a consequence, the proportion of experiences that must be classified as abstract is greatly increased for the blind. The significance of this factor for concept development has long been of interest.[11,5] However, its implications for education have never been fully explored.

Communications in Education

Educational communications is an area that is affected greatly by the perceptual differences between visually handicapped and normal children. Rates of communication are much slower when either braille or large type media are used. In the education of the blind, greater emphasis is placed on aural communication. Many problems for research exist in this area.

The inability of the visually handicapped child to contact many aspects of his environment directly or vicariously can result in retarded cognitive development in the preschool years. The possibility of retardation is increased through the ignorance of parents, and the effects of ignorance are facilitated by emotional problems resulting from the entry of a visually handicapped child into the family. Research and development can bear on the readiness problem in several ways:

1. Development and evaluation of programs to work with parents and/or children in the homes prior to school entry.

2. Development and evaluation of materials and techniques for use within preschool training sequences. While many toys and materials commonly available should be suitable for use, special adaptations and routines for their use may be necessary.

3. Development and evaluation of measures of readiness for school are required. Measures for reading readiness should include especially designed tests of cognitive development as well as measures of tactual readiness.[17,27]

BRAILLE READING For many years educators have drawn close parallels between visual and tactual reading. Recent research[1,16,23] indicates that the perception of braille material departs considerably from the patterns of perception necessary for efficient reading of ink print material. Further exploration of these differences is required.

In the past the techniques and materials used in teaching braille reading have been taken directly from those used with normally sighted materials. Enough information on perceptual factors specific to braille reading is now available to allow us to design and evaluate specific techniques and materials.[13]

Further efforts to develop training methods for maximizing braille reading speeds are needed. While results of efforts to use mechanical devices for this purpose are inconclusive, results of manipulation of motivational factors appear to hold promise.[7,16]

Development of measures to evaluate progress in braille reading skills as well as methods of diagnosing the causes of braille reading deficiencies are still in their infancy.[1,30] Work in this area is very much needed.

LARGE TYPE READING Many of the reading techniques and materials suitable for use with normally sighted children are printed large enough for use with children who have residual vision. For these children, however, it would appear that training in basic types of visual discrimination might be a profitable antecedent to common reading readiness programs.[2,10]

Optical aids have been shown to be a means of increasing ability to read print.[29,14] However, little is reported in the literature about comprehensive programs for training students in the use of such aids.

The question of appropriate type sizes for large type publications is still of interest in spite of recent studies.[3,6,20] However, the wide range of visual conditions, coupled with the difficulties of obtaining sufficient varieties of large type books, may make this question more academic than practical. Other typographical factors needing study include line length and leading.

Legibility is also a problem with pictures and other non-verbal graphics.[21] Development and evaluation of techniques for reproducing legible graphics of these types is critical.

The data on large type reading behavior presently available are secondary findings of research designed for other purposes.[24] It would be useful to produce a variety of measures of reading in large type and use these to explore systematically this behavior and evaluate its efficiency.

LISTENING AS A SUBSTITUTE FOR READING The very slow rates at which both braille and large type are read by most visually handicapped students impose a severe handicap in gaining access to educational information. Use of recorded texts is one means to increase the rates at which these children can gain exposure to knowledge. Lack of availability of books (particularly college texts) makes study by listening important in its own right.

Prior studies have shown that learning by listening at regular speech rates compares favorably with learning attained through reading braille or large type.[18,22] Precise identification of the grade levels and curricular areas where this learning occurs—as well as a determination of relationships with such factors as intelligence—is necessary.

Several means exist for increasing the word rates of aural messages. Research indicates that for some materials the comprehension of blind children is equal whether they read or listen at word rates three to four times as rapid as their reading rates.[8] Precise identification of the grade levels and curricular areas where this phenomenon occurs is necessary. In addition, it is desirable to determine if children can be trained to listen to rapidly presented materials. The implications of factors such as levels of grade, age, and intelligence for listening to accelerated word rates need exploration.

Recent research has identified serious problems arising from incompatibilities which exist among the materials and devices used.[4,24] Research is needed to develop a complete system for study using recorded tests. Coordinated within the system should be designs for playback equipment, recorded textbook formats, response equipment, and user techniques.

Research is needed to define and outline the most efficient study techniques. For example, research has shown that the better students who use recorded texts engage in heavy note taking.[4,24]

TACTUAL NONVERBAL GRAPHICS In spite of the experience gained from producing tactual maps, graphs, and charts for over a century, we still do an inadequate job. Both techniques and media need research. Such research should be tied firmly to what is now known about perception generally and tactual perception specifically. It should be closely coordinated with the research in tactual perception suggested earlier.

Mathematics Instruction

For decades, mathematics has been a source of major frustration for blind children and their teachers. Research is needed in several areas.

READINESS Concrete materials should be developed to teach number concepts to blind children. Techniques for the use of these should be developed and integrated with the reading readiness program suggested earlier.[9]

Retardation of 20 per cent in mathematical skills has been consistently found among the blind. Rapid development of modern mathematics curricula and their injection in the mainstream of education present at least a short-term threat of a decrease in the relative standing of the blind. Research to adapt modern mathematics curricula for the blind is imperative.[25]

Over the years early stress on mental arithmetic and its accompanying high level of abstraction have complicated, for the blind, learning in this subject.[9]

Research on design of tactual drawings, graphs, and charts, as indicated earlier, is also necessary. Development of materials should be paralleled by development and evaluation of techniques to teach children to use such materials.

Natural Sciences

Teaching science to the visually handicapped child, particularly through use of laboratory methods, has long posed a problem. In regular science classes, many of the phenomena of the physical and biological sciences are encountered visually. Visual interactions may range from direct unaided observation of phenomena to observation of the results of indirect effects. Consequently, the blind child has been denied instruction in many areas of science or has been cast into the role of a passive bystander, while a sighted partner or instructor orally describes what is occurring.

Consequently, a great need exists for research designed to encourage the development of science experiments and demonstrations which blind students can perform independently. This development should be closely related to modern science curricula, and should help convey science concepts by presenting natural phenomena within the limits of the sensory capabilities available to the blind. Indirect observations should be minimized, particularly at the lower grade levels.

NOTES

1. S. C. Ashcroft, "Identification of Braille Reading Errors," (Doctoral dissertation, University of Illinois, 1960).
2. Natalie C. Barraga, "Increased Visual Behavior in Low Vision Children," *American Foundation for the Blind Research Series,* No. 13 (1964).
3. J. W. Birch, W. J. Tisdall, R. Peabody and R. Sterrett, *School Achievement and Effect of Type Size on Reading in Visually Handicapped Children,* U.S. Department of Health, Education and Welfare and Office of Education Cooperative Research Project No. 1766 (Pittsburgh: University of Pittsburgh, School of Education, 1966).
4. B. Carter, "How to Use Educational Recordings Effectively—A Survey of Blind College Students," *New Outlook for the Blind,* 32 (1962), 332–334.
5. P. R. Dokecki, "Verbalism and the Blind: A Critical Review of the Concept and the Literature," *Exceptional Children,* 32 (1966), 525–530.
6. W. M. Eakin, R. J. A. Pratt and T. L. MacFarland, *Type Size Research for the Partially Seeing Child* (Pittsburgh: Stanwix House, 1961).
7. P. J. Flanigan, "Automated Training and Braille Reading," *New Outlook for the Blind,* 60 (1966), 141–146.
8. E. Foulke, C. H. Amster, C. Y. Nolan and R. H. Bixler, "The Comprehension of Rapid Speech by the Blind," *Exceptional Children,* 29 (1962), 134–141.
9. V. E. Haas, "The Development of a Tangible Mathematics Laboratory for Teaching Modern Arithmetic Concepts to Blind Children," (Master's thesis, University of Washington, 1963).
10. Carol Halliday, "Findings and Implications of Experimental Teaching in Visual Stimulation," *Proceedings of the 48th Biennial Conference of the American Association of Instructors of the Blind,* Washington, June 26–30, 1966.
11. R. K. Harley, Jr., "Verbalism Among Blind Children," *American Foundation for the Blind Research Series,* No. 10 (1963).
12. W. R. Heath, "Maps and Graphics for the Blind: Some Aspects of the Discriminability of Textural Surfaces for Use in Areal Differentiation," (Doctoral dissertation, University of Washington, 1958).
13. Freda Henderson, "The Rate of Braille Character Recognition as a Function of the Reading Process," *Proceedings of the 48th Biennial Conference of the American Association of Instructors of the Blind,* Washington, June 26–30, 1966.
14. International Home for the Blind, *Optical Aids Service: Survey—First 50 Cases* March, 1953 to December, 1955 (Brooklyn, New York: International Home for the Blind, 1957).
15. C. J. Kederis, "The Legibility of Braille Characters," (Master's thesis, University of Louisville, 1963).
16. ———, C. Y. Nolan and June E. Morris, "The Use of Controlled Exposure Devices to Increase Braille Reading Rates," *International Journal for the Education of the Blind* (in press).
17. I. Kurzhals, "The Factor of Touch in the Reading Readiness Program for Blind Children," (Master's thesis, Utah State University, 1959).
18. B. Lowenfeld, *Braille and Talking Book Reading: A Comparative Study* (New York: American Foundation for the Blind, 1945).
19. S. C. McLaughlin, "Visual Perception in Strabismus and Amblyopia," *Psychological Monographs,* Vol. 78, No. 12, Whole No. 589 (1964).

20. C. Y. Nolan, "Readability of Large Types: A Study of Type Sizes and Type Styles," *International Journal for the Education of the Blind,* 9 (1959), 41–44.
21. ———, "A Study of Pictures for Large Type Books," *International Journal for the Education of the Blind,* 9 (1960), 67–70.
22. ———, "Reading and Listening in Learning by the Blind," *Exceptional Children,* 29 (1963), 313–316.
23. ———, "Perceptual Factors in Braille Word Recognition," *Proceedings of the 48th Biennial Conference of the American Association of Instructors of the Blind,* Washington, June 26–30, 1966.
24. ———, *Reading and Listening in Learning by the Blind,* Progress Report: 1 September 1963–31 August 1966. U.S. Public Health Service Grant No. NB-04870–04 (Louisville, Kentucky: American Printing House for the Blind, 1966).
25. ——— and R. E. Bruce, "An Experimental Program in Elementary Mathematics for the Blind," *International Journal for the Education of the Blind,* 11 (1962), 71–74.
26. ——— and June E. Morris, *Tactual Symbols for the Blind,* Final Report: OVR-RD-587 (Louisville, Kentucky: American Printing House for the Blind, 1963).
27. ——— and June E. Morris, "Development and Validation of the Roughness Discrimination Test," *International Journal for the Education of the Blind,* 15 (1965), 1–6.
28. W. Schiff and H. Isikow, "Stimulus Redundancy in the Tactile Perception of Histograms," *International Journal for the Education of the Blind,* 16 (1966), 1–11.
29. Louise L. Sloan and Maria D. Jablonski, "Reading Aids for the Partially Blind—Classification and Measurement of More Than Two Hundred Devices," *Archives of Ophthalmology,* 62 (1959), 465–484.
30. R. W. Woodcock and S. G. Bourgeault, *Construction and Standardization of a Battery of Braille Skill Tests,* U.S. Department of Health, Education and Welfare and Office of Education Cooperative Research Project No. 1650 (Greeley, Colorado: Colorado State College, 1964).

SESSION REPORT

Adrienne V. Little

The problem of defining the multi-handicapped child was often noted during the session. Should a diabetes-blind child, for instance, be included in this category, as well as blind children who are retarded or emotionally disturbed?

The possibility of doing behavioral research on teachers was suggested. For example, how do teachers resist change? Are they being overwhelmed by the increase in research? Are they hindered by state programs and administrative control? Perhaps schools should have a special staff member to interpret research and suggest applications to the administration. The effectiveness of such an approach might then be studied. These were the suggestions of Dr. Douglas C. MacFarland and R. Paul Thompson.

Dr. Carson Nolan expressed a need for research on persons with multiple handicaps, especially for descriptive research on the behavior of people with such problems and research on how to train teachers. Strict categories of teachers (for the blind, for the retarded) were seen as unfortunate. Greater communication between these teachers is needed, as well as special training for teachers of children in several categories. Team-teaching was also suggested by Dr. Geraldine Scholl as a possible solution to this problem.

The sources of the increase in multiple handicaps (for example, rubella babies) are not well documented, and it was thought that research in this area might be fruitful. There may also be a need for basic research on a new way for the blind to read. Braille and large type books were thought by Dr. Scholl to be inadequate.

The lack of coordination between various research projects was seen as a serious problem. Both Mr. Thompson and Dr. Nolan suggested that an institute (for example, in a university) be established to handle this problem. Such an organization could plan and structure research on a large scale.

Communication between investigators and sponsoring agencies was seen as seriously lacking. Delegates from agencies rarely visit research sites; nor do they evaluate the projects and progress reports. Yet where such evaluation does exist, it is generally effective. The use of contracts was thought to be a possible improvement over outright grants. These were the views of Dr. Robert J. Teare, with Dr. MacFarland concurring.

The major portion of this session was devoted to discussing the lag between completion of research and its implementation in the classroom. This problem was attributed to a lack of interest in applied aspects on the part of researchers and in their isolation from the practitioners. It may also be due to teachers' inability to interpret research journals. It was suggested that more publication in teachers' journals be emphasized. Lack of prestige in publishing in such journals was noted by Dr. Scholl. Having investigators become involved in classroom work and teaching practitioners to interpret research journals were two other suggestions.

Dr. Scholl went on to speculate that many teachers want to be involved in research in their schools and want feedback from the researchers. Dr. Norman M. Yoder agreed, saying that steps should be taken to include the practitioners in research and to see what new ideas they provided. Small research projects could be conducted in the class by the teachers themselves.

Dr. Teare also thought that more applied aspects should be mandatory in journal articles; or, a series of monographs could be written to discuss the application of research.

STRESS: REACTION TO LOSS

ADJUSTMENT TO MISFORTUNE—A PROBLEM OF SOCIAL-PSYCHOLOGICAL REHABILITATION

Tamara Dembo, Gloria Ladieu Leviton, and Beatrice A. Wright

At particular times in the history of science, particular problems become ripe for investigation. It is therefore understandable that during World War II the need was felt to investigate the problems of social-psychological rehabilitation of the physically handicapped and that someone should look for a place and the means to set up a research project that would try to solve some of these problems. In pursuit of such a goal a research group was established at Stanford University on February 1, 1945. Conducted partially under a contract between Stanford University and the wartime Office of Scientific Research and Development (recommended by the Committee on Medical Research), partially under a contract between the University and the Army Medical Research and Development Board of the Office of the Surgeon General, War Department, the work continued until April 1, 1948.

To investigate the personal and social problems of the physically handicapped, two groups of subjects were needed—people who were considered handicapped and people around them. Therefore, both visibly injured and noninjured people were used as subjects of the research. Interviews were employed as the primary method of investigation. The great majority of the 177 injured persons were servicemen or veterans of World War II. More than half the subjects had suffered amputations and almost one fourth facial disfigurements. The injured man was asked questions designed to elicit his expectations, experiences, and feelings in his dealings with people around him. Sixty-five noninjured people also were interviewed in regard to their feelings toward the injured man.

A first task in the research project was to determine the meaning of the relationship between the injured and the noninjured. Was it primarily that of the helper and the helped, of the curious onlooker and the one who is looked upon, of the independent and dependent person, the one who rejects and the one who is rejected, the person who pities and the one who is pitied? Some of these relationships were described during the first period of the research program.[1,5,8] As the research proceeded, it was seen that one particular relationship between the injured and the noninjured was more "basic" than others—in the sense that it underlies and determines the character of other relationships. This underlying relationship is the one which exists when a person who regards himself as fortunate regards another as unfortunate. We learned that to understand this one has to see "being unfortunate" as a value loss and, furthermore, that the adjustment of this relationship involves the problem of acceptance of loss—a case of value change.

In current psychology, the problem of acceptance of loss is hardly investigated. Loss is usually seen as an end-point of unsuccessful, goal-directed behavior (failure) or else it is investigated in terms of the effect of failure on further goal-directed behavior (such as on setting the next "level of aspiration"). But it is important to know what loss means to the person himself, how it affects the opinions and behavior of others toward him, and what acceptance of loss implies. Too often life is seen as a series of goal-directed acts, whereas the *consumption of gains* and the *acceptance* (or nonacceptance) of losses which result from those acts are disregarded.

Almost all people are at some time faced with the necessity of adjusting to loss. In investigating the problems of injured people, therefore, we are dealing not only with special problems of a special group but with problems important to all. If we state that the injured need psychological rehabilitation or adjustment, this in no way implies that they are not "normal." The impact of loss which they experience produces suffering and difficulties. The overcoming of psychological suffering, whether or not it threatens mental illness, is a problem of adjustment.

Three years in a new and relatively unexplored field had to be considered a pilot period. After exploration the field was seen to be fruitful, both for the growth of ideas on the specific topics and also for the development of more general theoretical problems in psychology. But only a beginning was made, and the material here presented is therefore properly viewed only in the light of its pioneer character.

Many of our findings may from the theoretical standpoint be seen as more precise statements of problems awaiting further investigation.

From the practical standpoint, the study may be useful to those who critically examine the findings, not with the orientation of translating them into rules of behavior but so that their understanding of the problems involved in loss may be broadened.

METHODOLOGICAL AND THEORETICAL CONSIDERATIONS CONCERNING SOCIAL-EMOTIONAL RELATIONSHIPS

Some Characteristics of Social-Emotional Relationships

We shall present a list of pairs of words designating social-emotional relationships. We ask you, the reader, to think about the feelings connoted. Specific points to consider may be seen in the first example, the idea of "abandonment." How does the abandoner feel? How does the abandoned feel? How do they feel toward each other? How do you, as a person not involved in the interaction, evaluate abandonment? As you proceed down the list, you should ask yourself these and any other questions you think of which bring out the emotional meanings of the interaction concerned. We ask you to work hard because in so doing we think that you will see the problems of the psychology of emotions in a very different way from the orientation given them traditionally. You will see this field not only as unexplored but also as full of psychological resources available to those who are ready to dig. Here is the list:

To abandon—to be abandoned.
To abhor—to be abhorred.
To feel that someone is able—to feel that another considers you able.
To consider someone abnormal—to be considered abnormal.
To be abrupt—to be exposed to abruptness.
To consider someone absurd—to be considered absurd.
To abuse—to be abused.
To accept another person—to be accepted.
To feel in accord with someone—to feel that another person is in accord with you.
To accuse—to be accused.
To become accustomed to someone—to have someone become accustomed to you.

To consider someone as an acquaintance—to be considered an acquaintance.
To acquit someone—to be acquitted.
To act in a given way, without actually feeling that way—to feel that someone is just acting.
To adapt yourself to someone—to feel that another person is adapting himself to you.
To help someone become adjusted—to have someone try to adjust to you.
To admire—to be admired.
To admit to someone—to get an admission.
To adopt—to be adopted.
To adore—to be adored.
To advise—to be advised.
To feel affable—to feel that another person is affable.
To give affection—to get affection.
To affront—to be affronted.
To be against someone—to feel that another person is against you.
To aggravate someone—to be aggravated by someone.
To be aggressive toward someone—to feel that another person is aggressive toward you.
To agree with someone—to feel that another person agrees with you.
To aid someone—to be aided.
To alarm someone—to be alarmed by someone.
To give an alibi—to get an alibi.
To consider someone an alien—to be considered an alien.
To allow someone to do something—to be allowed.

Only a few of the diverse emotions or feelings are mentioned above. They were selected from the first 20 pages of *The Pocket Oxford Dictionary* (New York, 1927), which has 1010 pages. The list might have impressed you with the tremendous number of unexplored problems in the area of emotions. The psychological structure and the functions of the majority of emotional relationships are unknown. Yet these problems practically do not exist as topics of systematic investigation.

We do not wish to imply that emotional problems are completely disregarded by psychologists. The psychology of personality, social psychology, and abnormal psychology *do* take them into account, but within these divisions other problems, particularly problems of needs and goal-directed behavior, have been in the center of attention.

Evaluation by the Outsider

We are concerned with emotional relationships which are considered by people at large, with or without the permission of the scientist, as desirable or undesirable, good or bad. It is simply an undeniable psychological phenomenon that evaluations are made, and as phenomena they cannot be disregarded. In fact, these evaluations, as shall be seen, are important for the understanding of the dynamics of emotional interpersonal relationships and the problem of adjustment of these relationships.

If one considers the relationships in the list, it is noticed that, even though no specification is given of the conditions under which they exist, some of them connote undesirable feelings and states, others more desirable ones. Examples which fall into the negatively evaluated group are "to abuse," "to abhor," "to accuse," "to affront." Examples which fall into the positively evaluated group are "to accommodate," "to admire," "to allow." There are others which seem less definitely to belong to the negative or positive group. For example, "to get accustomed," "to admit." Such abstract evaluations are not made specifically in terms of the meaning of the relationship to either of the partners. They are given by a person who psychologically takes the position of an outsider.

Evaluations of outsiders very often show a high level of agreement, as is easily demonstrated by a simple experiment. The list of words can be presented rapidly to a group of subjects who are asked to evaluate the relationship as positive or negative from the standpoint of an outsider to the relationship. In only a few instances will there be disagreement, and these disagreements will be due largely to what amounts to a violation of the instructions: for instance, the subject may "take sides" with one of the partners, or the subject may base his reply on the circumstances of particular situations.

Evaluations of outsiders might be considered standards of cultural judgment. It may be the high agreement in the evaluations of outsiders which make them appear to have the role of common cultural standards.

Evaluation by Donor and Recipient

In any relationship, the person who bestows the emotion may be called the "donor," and the person upon whom the emotion is bestowed may be called the "recipient." The difference in the meaning of the relationship for the donor and the recipient is frequently very great. To give an appreciation of this difference, the list was arranged in pairs. You were asked to feel the way the donor in the relationship might feel and the way the recipient might feel. "To abuse or to be abused, to accept or to be accepted" are emotionally far apart. Sometimes both donor and recipient will evaluate a given relationship in the same way. But since the meaning which the relationship has for one partner is not the same as that given to it by the other, their evaluations often differ, and this difference may produce difficulties in the relationship. Help, for example, is almost always seen as positive for the recipient as judged by the donor, but as judged by the recipient it often has both positive and negative aspects. It is important for adjustment of relationships to know the conditions under which the donor and the recipient give the same evaluations and, when they do not, to find ways of producing a change which will lead to agreement in evaluation.

The donor and recipient not infrequently attempt to overcome the difficulties resulting from their different evalutions by urging each other to "be objective." But objectivity, in the sense of assuming the position of an outsider and giving abstract evaluations, is not what is really desired. What each *really* wants is that the partner should "understand" him, that is, should understand the meanings the relationship has for him. He wants the other to take his position and from this standpoint to think, evaluate, and act.

Scope of Meanings and Structure of Relationship

It is seen from the list that a great variety of social-emotional relationships exist and that each is characterized not merely by pleasantness or unpleasantness but by a diversity of qualitative connotations. It might be agreed, for example, that one feels lost and hurt when abandoned or that one may feel free and at the same time guilty when abandoning someone. It may also be agreed that one will feel aversion for, and a desire to escape from, one abhorred and that one would feel rejected and resentful if a person abhorred him. Each connotation will be referred to as a "meaning" of an emotional relationship. The diverse, sometimes apparently contradictory meanings which an emotional relationship can have for different people under different circumstances build the "scope of meanings of a social-emotional relationship."

As an illustration, we present some of the meanings which "being helped" has for the injured: it means that a goal is made accessible; it means that another person is courteous and polite; it means that the injured person is in a position of lower status; it means dependence, burden, and so on.[5] We assume that these meanings are not merely a congeries of separate entities attached to the same word. Instead, we believe analysis will show that many of them hang together, that they may be integrated within one or more coherent structures.* When the structure of a relationship has been determined, it is sometimes found that some of the meanings which subjects give to the word do not belong to the relationship in question but to a different one. For instance, in the case of the sympathy relationship, some of the subjects gave meanings which belong to the relationship of "pity," a relationship which has a different structure.

The determination of the scope of meanings seems to us an essential problem because it is the first step toward determining structures of relationships. The structure is a better description of the social-emotional relationship than is the scope of meanings. Even before the development of the structure of a relationship, however, the determination of the scope of meanings has practical value. It permits realization of possibly disturbing connotations and encourages precautions and safeguards against them.

Qualitative Versus Quantitative Approaches in a New Field

The selection of problems which are scientifically promising is an extensive qualitative research job. Essential questions are those which promise to become an integral part of an interrelated group of problems and to lead to the development of corresponding systems of concepts. In a new field neither the problems nor the systems are known. They have to be discovered by giving a "qualifying examination" to the problems and preconcepts which occur to us, since these include both promising and unpromising ones.† The qualifying examination consists of a test which shows whether a particular problem and preconcept with other "candidates" promise to form an interdependent team. When they not only develop but also add to the development of the emerging system, they acquire the position of fruitful essential problems and preconcepts.

Consider an example of a problem which does not seem promising, in the sense that it is likely to remain an isolated problem. It is

* By "structure of a social-emotional relationship" we mean those characteristics which, when interrelated, are necessary and sufficient to describe the nature of the relationship.

† By "preconcept" we mean a term which lacks either a rigid conceptual definition or a precise operational definition.

noted that some of the items in the list connote what may more frequently be called feelings (for example, "to abhor," "admire," "adore"). Others have the character of emotional acts ("to accuse," "advise," "acquiesce," "admit"). Still others reflect social distance ("to consider someone an acquaintance or an alien"). These categorizations seem, however, not to lead to further understanding. In this example, categories rather than preconcepts are relied upon to "order" the facts. Only an orderly catalog instead of a system of interrelated dynamic concepts can be built up in such a way.

An example of a problem which we consider promising is the determination of value structures held by those people who are undergoing difficulties and by those who have overcome these difficulties. This, we believe, is one of the first steps in conceptualizing adjustive change.

Another example of what might be considered promising for future investigation relates to the "mutual" relationship. Partners may abuse each other, accept each other, or admire each other. Each may be in the position of donor and recipient at the same time.

It frequently happens that when a one-sided relationship is unpleasant for the recipient, he will try to change it to a mutual one. For example, if he is being abused he may begin to abuse the other. What effect does this change produce? The question will be sharpened if we consider the following hypothetical statement:

$$R_p^{rd} = R_p^r + R_p^d,$$

where R_p indicates the person p's relationships, and d and r indicate the donor and recipient positions, respectively. In this statement, p's mutual relationship is a simple summation of his relationships as donor and recipient. Can this actually be the case? Are the *meanings* for p in the mutual relationships (R_p^{rd}) equal to the sum of meanings which the one-sided relationship has for him when he is only a recipient (R_p^r) plus the meanings it has for him when he is a donor (R_p^d)? This question is important, for if the addition of the new meanings of the donor relationship does not change the old meanings of the recipient relationship, then the addition will not diminish the previously existing conflicts or difficulties.* Actually, the "adding" of new meanings may not be an addition at all but rather a restructurization of the first one-sided relationship (that is, a change in some of the meanings which the relationship originally had for the person). In the latter case we would have to study the type of change produced

* Though it may increase them.

by the restructurization and the circumstances under which the change is adjustive.

At different stages of research, the "candidate problems" must be subjected to further test. For a time they might drop out from the "team," and then later their participation may again become fruitful. Within this process they may change their character and gain a new role.

The Position of Measurement in Psychological Research

The attitude, "Investigate what you can measure," is not infrequently found in psychological research practice. But there is such a thing as primitive quantification. Quantification of data on systematically unimportant questions is primitive. And there is also such a thing as premature quantification. That quantification which is done before the laborious task of qualitative description of problems and concepts is sufficiently advanced is premature.

The determination of statistically significant differences between two sets of data does not ensure that these data are important either practically or for further theoretical advance. Instead of regarding the statistical fact as an observation which needs anchoring in an explanatory system before its import can be judged, all too frequently such observations, by sheer virtue of their statistical nature, are held up as contributions in themselves. We do not declare that measurement should not be done without a well-developed theoretical framework. But we do assert that such measurement often produces statistically significant differences on inessential details. And we further assert that where problems well grounded in theory have not as yet been formulated, data analyzed qualitatively may contribute far more to the understanding of important problems.

Where there is a well-defined theoretical system, however, measurement has a very important and different position. Measurement in this case, as we see it, means measurement of conceptually defined constructs and the determination of interrelationships among those constructs. Preliminary to such measurements, one has to determine whether the constructs used permit metrization or whether nonmetrical mathematical (topological) statements should be made. The particular problems involved in this type of mathematical determination in psychology were first realized by Kurt Lewin[6,7] in regard to problems of goal-directed behavior. Such mathematical determination will have to be made in the field of emotions as in any other field, though it may take years before it is possible. In the meantime, sound investigation, systematic in nature, will have to be primarily qualitative.

There also may be considerable practical value in qualitative investigation before quantification is possible. The knowledge of *what* affects a given social-emotional relationship, even if we are unable to indicate the strength of that factor, is of value.

Concerning Frequency Counts

At any stage in theoretical development, one may tally the number of times a given observation occurs in the sample studied. But the meaning of such frequencies needs to be examined. The sheer number of occurrences does not indicate the relative importance of the event.

One function of frequency counts is to permit a more accurate prediction of the number of occurrences of like events in like populations. This function, however, is often limited by failure to define the research population in terms of systematically important factors.

Some Problems of Sampling

To "select" a population for research in a new field which lacks systematization is harmless but also meaningless and therefore to be rejected as impractical. The traditional parameters of age, IQ, socioeconomic status, and geographic location should not be thought of as automatic principles of selection. Their usefulness for the particular research has to be determined in each case. It may be, for example, that in research on the injured it would be more appropriate to define the sample in terms of pre-injury attitudes toward the handicapped, relative evaluation of beauty and physical prowess as compared with other personality characteristics, and sensitivity to status position. A group which is homogeneous with regard to some arbitrarily selected factors will actually be heterogeneous with regard to those factors which prove to be of systematic importance.

Heterogeneity is, however, not a disadvantage. In an unstructured, new field, where the first task is to determine fruitful problems and the concepts to be used in their solution, the danger lies in overlooking diversities which should be taken into account. Heterogeneous groups which yield a wide range of differences in behavior are therefore welcomed. To narrow down the range of subjects is permissible only for a good reason. This reason has to be specified. In the beginning stages of our research on the social-emotional relationships between visibly injured and noninjured persons, it was legitimate to include a variety of subjects.

In later stages of research, the original sample might legitimately be narrowed down or enlarged, depending on the particular problem being pursued. For example, we have indications that a person's status values affect his attitudes toward such social-emotional interactions as sympathy, help, curiosity, and so on. This suggested systematic relationship could be tested by narrowing down the sample so that but two groups would be included, one strongly status-minded and the other not, according to certain criteria. Whether the expected differences are to be found could then be determined. As an example where an even more heterogeneous sample than the original one is indicated, we can present again an instance from our research. The understanding of problems of loss became clearer to us when the concept of misfortune was introduced. In light of this theoretical orientation, it undoubtedly would be fruitful for further research to enlarge the sample to include, in addition to the injured, other persons regarded as being in an unfortunate situation. In short, throughout research, the sample taken for study should be determined by the requirements of the problem being studied and not by applying sampling procedures which are either extraneous to the purpose of the research or else actually interfere with it.

The Interview as a Tool for Investigating Emotional Contents

The interview as an experimental tool is in disrepute with many present-day investigators. Some investigators will go as far as to withdraw the honorable title of "real scientific endeavor" from a study which uses "just interviews" because interviews do not deal with how the person "actually behaves." In this section we shall examine the validity of this argument.

Reflection Units and Interaction Units

Consider this example: A young girl gets an invitation to a ball. She is full of anticipation—perhaps she will be the belle. Perhaps a certain young man will dance often with her. She decides what gown she will wear and how to arrange her hair. She plans imaginary conversations with gallant partners. But she is anxious too. Maybe she will be a wallflower; maybe the young man will not even notice her. Finally, after a succession of alternating moods, the ball arrives. The social interaction which has occasioned so much thought and feeling actually takes place.

If, in the investigation of social-emotional relationships, only interaction units were studied, a large part of the course of events would be neglected. Periods of reflection which include planning, expectations, evaluations, struggle with one's feelings and moods, would be excluded from study. Similarly, if in the investigation of personal-emotional events only action units were studied, periods of reflection would be overlooked. The interactions or actions themselves might not be fully understood without the consideration of reflection units.

The high status position of interaction data as compared with the data of reflection units seems in part to be based upon a vague feeling that only interactions are "real facts." But the types of reflection units enumerated above are all *real in the sense that they exist as psychological phenomena.* Even if reflection units had a segregated existence and did not influence interaction units, they would still have to be studied as real psychological phenomena within the life of the person. The reflections themselves may produce pain and consequently require adjustment; for instance, a man with a scarred face believed that "no woman in her right mind could possibly accept me now."

Is it meaningful to ask whether interaction units are *scientifically more real* than reflection units? The frequently stated criterion of scientific reality, "What is real is what has effects," concerns not observable facts but the reality of descriptive, explanatory concepts. The reality of the effects is not under discussion in the criterion; nothing is implied about them but their virtue of being available for observation. Scientifically, reflection units and interaction units are both legitimate observable facts. It is true that in the case of reflection units the content must be communicated to the interviewer. But this mediation should be no more disturbing than that of other instruments. The criterion cited does not specify that the observable facts must be observed directly.*

What conclusions can be drawn as to the relative merits of the two types of units for study? Both interactions and reflections are real phenomena and legitimate observable facts; psychological difficulties requiring adjustment may exist in either case. They differ in that interactions can be observed directly, whereas the content of reflections must be communicated to the investigator by the subject.

* The validity of the interview as an instrument is a separate problem.

For an investigator, the difference between them is simply one of kind and not of value.

Interviews versus Behavior Observations

We submit that the richness of emotional life can be more fully realized through the use of the interview than through observation of behavior. It is true that we can infer something about underlying emotions from behavioral observations, but the understanding gained in this way is usually more limited. If we could have observed the girl smiling over the invitation, taking from her wardrobe first one gown and then another, being absentminded about her everyday tasks, and so on, we might have been able to infer something about her feelings. But the complexity of her feelings, the content of her hopes and fears, remains largely unappreciated. On the other hand, for particular problems observation of behavior would be required, for example, in order to study the effects of reflections on behavior, such as how fear of failure affects performance, or whether verbal attitudes correspond to behavior.* Only when a particular problem is specified may one method be judged better or worse than another.

Validity of Interviews versus Validity of Behavior Observations

It is frequently stated that the subject willfully or otherwise does not tell the interviewer what he actually feels.

The need to hide during an interview, it might be argued, may frequently be less strong than in interaction units. It might be considered whether hiding of feelings from a person with whom they are connected is not frequently more necessary than when discussing or reflecting about these feelings with a third person. It is likely that feelings of guilt or shame will be less strong in regard to statements than to acts. Especially if the third person takes a nonjudgmental position or the position of an ally will the true feelings as far as they are recognized by the subject be expressed more openly than in interaction units. Of course the need to hide particular emotions will exist during interviews, but the interaction units cannot be turned to as the better ones in this respect.

---

* One would wish that instead of imputing a lower quality to interview data, instead of stressing that "How a person thinks he will act does not always correspond to how he will act," attention would be given to the specific conditions under which intentions and attitudes, given an "action test," either are or are not carried out.

Knowledge of the Subject about His Own Emotions

Interviews are sometimes held in disrepute on grounds that people do not know their own feelings. Fortunately, people do not learn to cognize feelings in college only. Much of what one feels when someone nags him, for example, or helps him, or when he is jealous, can be perceived without special psychological training* If the objection is raised that the conscious meanings which feelings have for the subject are less important and more superficial than those of which he is not aware, we would say that such a statement is premature. Explicit criteria of importance have first to be given.

If important feelings are those which affect a person's behavior, we say that those consciously given share the same honors as the hidden. And if it is asserted that unconscious feelings are more important because they explain *more* of a person's behavior, one is called upon to compare counts. This has never been done, nor does it make sense to do so. For immediately the question arises as to what weights to assign to the individual behavior units. Are they more important because they are resisted? Then what is the rationale for considering the resisted more important? We suspect that all too often the hidden is identified with the important by sheer virtue of the fact of its covertness. Clearly missing is a link which must be supplied before such an evaluation can have scientific merit.

As far as we can see, it is scientifically meaningless to argue about the importance or superficiality of perceived meanings of feelings before the criteria of such judgments are made clear. One criterion does exist. If important problems are those which are essential (that is, problems which attempt to relate observable facts to systems of concepts) then there is nothing which leads us to exclude feelings as perceived by the subject as "candidates." Criticisms regarding essentiality of problems are applicable to overt and covert meanings alike.

Feeling Level versus Intellectual Level of Discussion

Emotional topics can be discussed with almost anyone who is willing to participate in an interview. The discussion, however, may take

* In no way do we believe that the subjects' conscious perceptions of their feelings are the only data worthy of study. Many other clues during an interview give us indications of hidden meanings which broaden the understanding of the person's feelings.

place on an intellectual level or on a feeling level. One can "just talk about" feelings, in an abstract, impersonal way (intellectual level), or one can analyze one's feelings in terms of the particular intimate meanings they have for the individual (feeling level). Psychotherapy, whether directive or nondirective, strives for such a feeling analysis by the patient. It has been commonly recognized that, in order for feeling analysis to take place, the person must have a need to examine his feelings, and he must expect the interviewer to be tactful, understanding, trustworthy, and so on. In the study of the meanings which social emotional relations have for the donor and for the recipient, however, a further important condition must be realized. To approach such meanings on the feeling level, the subject must *actually feel* the position of a partner in the relationship. He must feel something of the hurt involved in being stared at, for example; or in the case of the donor position, something of the curiosity. It is more advantageous to select subjects who in actual life are donors or recipients in the relationship investigated. Otherwise the subject tends to discuss on the intellectual level or evaluate as an outsider, and in neither case can he convey the emotional impact which the relationship has for a partner.

Analysis of Data in the Area of Emotions

The principles which guided us in choosing methods of collecting data apply no less to its handling after it has been gathered. The whole flavor of the emotional meanings which one was at such pains to obtain can be lost if the approach to the data is unwisely rigid. The investigator is forced to perceive and to feel emotional relationships from the point of view of the donor and recipient before he can understand the meanings and evaluations ascribed to them. Not being involved in the particular relationship, the investigator has to find equivalent relationships in his own experience. Frequently in our research we had to feel through relationships from our own personal histories in order to be able emotionally to understand the subject's comments. Though the occasion at which sympathy, for instance, was given to us differed from the occasion leading to sympathy relationships in our subjects, the tool of self-analysis was useful. There is an obvious danger of analyzing superficially similar relationships instead of equivalent ones. Self-analysis, therefore, should be used for the purpose of getting "hunches" which can be applied to the data obtained from the subjects. Such an approach leads to aspects of data which an investigator, viewing the data as an outsider, will overlook or misinterpret.

There is nothing unscientific about being a subject and an investigator at the same time. In perception psychology, for example, the investigator frequently takes his double role. He can perceive and then cognize what he is perceiving. In the area of emotional problems, the investigator should try to feel the emotional situations being studied and then to examine what he is feeling. Physical, physiological, and psychological laws which hold for the object of the investigation hold for the investigator also. In investigating emotional relationships, to feel is at least as essential as to think.

In attempting to find aspects under which the data may be fruitfully seen, complete freedom should be given to the investigator. He cannot be free enough and "wild" enough in looking for interpretations and possible implications of the raw data which might lead to hunches, hypotheses, and conceptual formulations. Hunches are freedom-loving birds which do not hatch in supervised, restricted areas. This does not mean that the data will be distorted or that the results will be "only speculation" and not "facts." The test is whether, when a category has been well defined, independent observers will agree that given items of the raw data fit the category. If they do agree, then this aspect is indeed "an observable fact." If we are too "wild" in our interpretations, then we shall be caught by another observer. But if we are unwisely rigid we shall not be able to make a step in the direction of theoretical progress.

STUDY ON THE VISIBLY INJURED: A GROUP CONSIDERED UNFORTUNATE

Research Procedures

Our approach to the problems of the social-emotional relationships of the visibly injured was based on the theoretical and methodological considerations discussed previously. Because the task was that of determining essential problems in the new field of social-emotional relationships, qualitative methods were chosen as the appropriate ones. Measurements at this time would have been premature. Frequencies of observations and statistical analysis are therefore not presented, since they would only be misleading.

SUBJECTS Heterogeneity of subjects, as has been seen, is an asset for such a study. The subjects (177 visibly injured and 65 noninjured persons) varied as to age, race, intelligence, socio-economic background, occupational interests, marital status, and so on. The injuries varied. The relationship of the noninjured to the injured persons varied. To have narrowed the groups for the sole reason that they should be homogeneous would have given us a more limited picture of the emotional meanings of the relationships existing between the injured and the noninjured.

If, at the beginning of our investigation rather than at the end of it, we had known that the relationship of misfortune was especially important to the understanding of the problems studied, we would

Table 1

DISTRIBUTION OF INJURED SUBJECTS WITH REGARD TO INJURY

Physical Defect	Hospitalized Servicemen	Veterans of World War II	Civilians
Amputations: leg			
below-knee	20	16	1
above-knee	18	13	1
bilateral	3	1	—
Amputations: arm			
below-elbow	10	2	2
above-elbow	6	1	3
bilateral	2	—	—
Amputations: one arm and one leg	1	—	—
Facial injuries:			
(plastic surgery)	38	2	—
Injuries:			
leg	4	1	1
arm	—	1	—
hand	14	—	1
Residua of:			
arthritis	—	1	—
poliomyelitis	—	—	3
spinal meningitis	—	—	1
tuberculosis of bones	—	—	1
Congenital deformity	—	—	3
Transverse myelitis (in wheelchair)	5	—	—
Multiple sclerosis (in wheelchair)	—	—	1
Total	121	38	18

have considered it profitable to have included persons who experienced misfortunes other than injuries. But our research was an outgrowth of interest in the problems of the injured, and thus misfortunes other than visible injuries were not studied. Orthopedic cases and cases involving plastic surgery were chosen because the visibility of the injury is important in relationships with noninjured who are not close to the injured. Blind and deaf persons were excluded as subjects since it was felt at the time that the specific additional problem of communication between them and the noninjured would have in the beginning of the research unnecessarily complicated the data.

The ages of the injured subjects ranged from 19 to 58 years, the duration of their disabilities from two months to 33 years. Of the 177 injured subjects, 121 were hospitalized servicemen of World War II and four were women. *Table 1* presents the distribution of the subjects according to type of disability; *Table 2* gives the distribution of the noninjured according to relationship with injured persons.

Table 2

DISTRIBUTION OF NONINJURED SUBJECTS ACCORDING TO RELATIONSHIP WITH INJURED PERSONS

Wives of injured men	18
Other close relatives	4
Professional personnel dealing with injured (surgeons, occupational therapists, manufacturers of artificial limbs)	12
Other noninjured (friends, acquaintances, distant relatives)	31
Total	65

INTERVIEW PROCEDURES After having tried out several techniques of investigation, we found that the scope of meanings of socio-emotional relationships could most adequately be determined by interviews. Prior to the interview much work was done on the selection and formulation of questions, the purpose being not to set up a questionnaire for the interviewer to follow rigidly but rather to prepare him for the interview. We wish first to point out why we think it unnecessary and often disadvantageous to follow a rigid order and formulation of questions; then we would like to explain what we mean by "preparing the interviewer for the interview."

It was observed that, for at least three reasons, the actual course of events in an interview might require deviations from a prearranged interview. In the first place, identity of questions and order does not ensure that the psychological situation will be the same for different subjects. In many instances, a question will have the same meaning for each subject only when it is put in a different form. Thus, in our study, as well as in many investigations where comparisons among the subjects are made, rigid interview procedure is contraindicated. That we deny the necessity of maintaining a rigid formulation and order of questions does not imply that we disregard the influence of preceding events upon a given question. Rather, we assert that this kind of influence can be validly determined only when the analysis of data is made. A rigid order gives an "appearance" of the same conditions and illegitimately relieves the experimenter from investigating the effects of the actual psychological conditions upon the responses of the subject.

Secondly, a rigid interview leads in many cases to a more superficial intellectual discussion than is the case when the interviewer follows the natural course of the discussion. If a subject is developing a topic in a given direction and the interviewer goes on to the next question on the list, the interruption might be emotionally disturbing. Such interruptions promote the feeling that the interviewer is not really interested in what the subject is saying but just has to complete the task of getting answers to "twenty questions."

Finally, in a nonrigid interview the subject may introduce new topics which, in the exploratory stage of research, are often worthy of consideration.

To "prepare" or train the interviewer, the design and redesign of questions that might be asked in the interview are of extreme value. First, the process of developing questions sharpens the sensitivity of the interviewer to the scope of meanings which may be implied in a question and in possible answers to it. It prepares him to listen for the shades of meanings which the subject may bring out. Second, the interviewer, when later analyzing the interviews, will also be more sensitive to the shades of meanings implied in the subjects' statements. Third, the attention given in the training to the problem of the logic of transitions from one question to another and to the possible negative effects implied in some transitions is also important. The interviewer is then better able, when the subject waits for him to take the lead, to introduce a new topic without disrupting the relationship. And finally, the training on design of questions makes the interviewer realize what questions may be seriously disturbing to the subjects, a matter especially important with the injured subjects and their sharers for whom the injury is a vital problem not limited to the interview situation.

The design of questions to be used as guides for interviews in a new area is a serious and laborious task. During the research, changes in the original questions were made; some were dropped, others added. In successive interviews, the improved interview form served to suggest the areas to be brought up for discussion, but when and how they were to be introduced was left to the judgment of the trained interviewer. We present below one of the prearranged lists of questions which was developed during the training period and used as a guide in some interviews with injured subjects:

1. How do people act?

    1*a*. How should they treat you?

2. How about their asking questions?

3. How about help?

4. Do you think that noninjured people are uncomfortable when they are with you—for instance are they at a loss for words?

    4*a*. Do you think they are afraid of hurting your feelings?

    4*b*. Do you try to put them at ease?

5. Do you think it wise for the uninjured to make light of the injury?

    5*a*. Do you think a person who is not injured should kid the man about the injury?

    5*b*. Is it good for them to tell an injured man about all the things that another injured man can do?

    5*c*. Is it good for them to tell a man that his injury is not noticeable?

6. Do you like to hear it said that the injured man is courageous?

7. What do you think comes into a person's mind when he sees someone with an amputation?

    7*a*. Do you think many people would feel sorry for him?

    7*b*. Would many people feel respect for him?

    7*c*. Is the opposite ever true? Would anybody look down on him?

8. Do other people react any differently from what you expected at first?

9. What percentage of people do you think act very well and really badly? How many in between?

10. How would you check whether a person has the right feeling toward injured people? Do you do anything like that?

11. Did you ever know anybody who was injured, before you were hurt?

11*a*. How did you feel about him?

11*b*. Do you feel differently about him now?

12. What would you be careful of now when you're with another injured person?

13. Do you ever feel sorry for anyone around here?

14. Is there a bad kind of sympathy and a good kind?

14*a*. Is there a kind you can't help?

15. Is pity different from feeling sorry?

16. Quite a number of things may be important for other people who are injured to know about—the stages one goes through. It would help them to know they are not the only ones who have these feelings in the beginning. How was it at the beginning? What are the stages one has to go through and the things you have to get used to?

17. Do you think a person should try not to think about his injury?

18. Is it better if he thinks and talks about his injury in a matter-of-fact way, whenever there is any reason to think or talk about it?

19. What would you do if you saw a fellow patient who was feeling sorry for himself?

20. What kind of person will let his injury lick him, or get him down?

21. Do you think you would have been able to take it if it had been worse?

22. Does it help to know that another person was injured worse than you?

22*a*. Is it because the other person is in a worse condition, or because even though he is in a worse condition he can still take it?

23. What things have you learned to do since you were wounded?

23*a*. What things do you still have to learn?

24. Which is more important, the looks, or the things you can't do?

24*a*. Does it matter much how it looks, either to other people, or to you? Do you have to get used to it?

25. Is an injury easier to take for a woman or a man?

25*a*. Would you object to marrying an injured woman?

26. Do the men feel that their injuries will make a difference in their getting married?

26*a*. Let's say that about 70 out of 100 men are married in the general population. What would you expect about wounded people, would there be more of them married, or less, or about the same?

27. Are you satisfied with your stump?

27*a*. Some people say that they get mad at the stump and try to hurt it. What do you think the reason might be?

27*b*. Have you ever felt that way?

28. Are there some words you object to?

28*a*. How about the word "stump"?

29. Do you think that after an injury a man gets more interested in new things that didn't interest him before—that he looks on life differently or that things that were important before don't seem important now while new things do?

29*a*. Do you have any new plans for a job?

29*b*. Do the same kind of people interest you?

30. There are a good many things we haven't talked about that might be very important, and we'd be glad to have your suggestions. Is there anything else that occurs to you that would be good for us to talk about?

30*a*. Anything you think the wounded man ought to know?

30*b*. Anything the public ought to know?

The interview usually lasted about an hour and a half. In a few instances, there were repeated interviews with the same subject. About half of the interviews were recorded by the interviewer himself as verbatim as possible, the others by a stenographer or a trained recorder.

The cooperation of the injured subjects was obtained by telling them that the purpose of the study was to determine difficulties existing in the relationships between injured and noninjured people and how these difficulties could be overcome. The subjects were asked to help in finding out "how people act" and "how they should act." The injured considered the endeavor a worthy one. Many of them challenged the usefulness of current magazine articles, and some felt that correct information might improve matters. The social-emotional relationships discussed had a high potency for them. Many of the subjects were recently injured, but all of them had had contacts with the noninjured—contacts in which they were the recipients of help, of curiosity, of sympathy, of being considered an unfortunate person. For them, such relationships were real and vital. Because they mattered to them they discussed problems not only intellectually but also on the feeling level.

In the interview the injured subjects were first asked "how the noninjured behave and how they should behave." This confirmed the feeling which we had attempted to convey when we first approached them—that we valued their opinions and knowledge as they "are the ones who really know." This open-ended question was also a precaution against feelings in the subject of intrusion into his privacy. Later in the interview, when the subjects became involved and felt secure and free with the experimenter, they frequently shifted to their own personal feelings and were even willing to discuss private matters brought up by the interviewer.

At the beginning of the interview it was a difficult task to achieve real emotional involvement on the part of those noninjured who were not close to injured persons. Noninjured persons who are in the position of sharers, wives and mothers of the injured for example, do feel that relationships between the injured and noninjured really concern them. But for other noninjured, the area of problems is not a vital one. Some time was therefore spent with subjects of this group at the beginning of the interview in discussion of injured persons they knew and how they felt about them in an attempt to bring the discussion to a more basic feeling level. In order to keep the subject on the feeling level, the interviewer also attempted to bring out the conflict in the noninjured between ethical demands and emotional feelings. Because it is considered "good" by the noninjured to believe that the injury does not matter to them, they may try to convince the interviewer and themselves that they do not have any "special feelings toward an injured person." When the interviewer responded to the underlying emotional feelings rather than to the overt ideological statements, the noninjured not infrequently became aware that the relationships involved important meanings for them and not merely intellectual or ideological ones. Discussion on the feeling level could then take place.

ANALYSIS OF DATA The analysis of data in a new field, where the aim is to discover essential problems, requires a great flexibility on the part of the investigator. Because the search is for "hunches" and connections among them and not for frequencies of occurrences, an attitude of a single subject in its ramifications requires much thought and understanding. For those who will work further in this field, we wish to mention some points which are well to keep in mind when analyzing interview material.

The understanding of the emotional meanings implied in the statements of the subject requires taking into account the context of the discussion. It is important to consider the interplay between the responses of the subject and those of the interviewer. Sometimes contradictory statements made by the subject in different portions of the interview lead to understanding of basic feelings. Always it is necessary to try to put oneself in the position of the subject and to feel with him. Often, in order to appreciate the subject's subtle feelings, it helps to examine one's own feelings in situations similar to those evaluated by the subject. Frequently the impact of the subject's own feelings is further enhanced if the investigator assumes the position of the other partner in the relationship he was talking about. In our work this was especially true in analyzing the noninjured records. The covert meanings appeared most clearly if we tried to see the implications which a superficially innocuous statement might have if an injured person were to read it.

A rigid scheme of analysis of interview material may lead to superficial conclusions; since in such a case one is obliged to cover the material in a technical, automatic way, the many-meaningfulness of the single answer of the subjects is apt to be overlooked. Thus, for our purpose, the interview material was more fruitfully analyzed by developing categories as the analysis proceeded rather than by following a predetermined scheme. This meant categorizing, recategorizing, and again recategorizing. When a new category was added it sometimes required a re-examination of parts of interviews in the light of the new insight gained. Not all of our theoretical statements, however, are based on category analysis of all the interviews. Sometimes the attitudes expressed in single cases gave us hunches which led to the development of hypotheses and theoretical understanding. In these ways we tried to determine the scopes of meanings and structures of social-emotional relationships.

Misfortune

Many kinds of social-emotional relationships exist between injured and noninjured people. Which should be investigated as more essential? We began with those which were frequently pointed out by the injured themselves, namely, "to help—to be helped," "to question—to be questioned," "to stare—to be stared at," "to sympathize—to be sympathized with," "to accept—to be accepted." [1,5,8] During the analysis of data, a different relationship emerged as more basic for understanding the social-psychological problems of the injured—the relationship "to consider someone unfortunate—to be considered unfortunate." This relationship enables us to tie together many of the phenomena observed and indicates the direction which further research should take. The finding and description of this essential relationship is a *result* rather than the historical beginning of our investigation.

MISFORTUNE AS AN EVENT A painful event which does not have farreaching consequences may be called "a mishap." If the event produces prolonged and more inclusive suffering, if it affects a large part of the life space of the person, it is called "a misfortune." Other people will tend to shift the position of the sufferer downward on the fortune scale. The circumstances surrounding the event may themselves be important. But this is a special problem, and fruitful investigation of it presupposes knowledge of the nature of the misfortune relationship. We shall, therefore, disregard such differences as whether an arm was lost in a car accident or because of shrapnel wounds.

For an investigation of the effect of the circumstances surrounding the event upon the feelings of the person himself, simple grouping into war and accident casualties, for example, would be too superficial. The groupings have rather to be made in terms of the intimate psychological meanings which the circumstances have for the person. Moreover, one would have to know whether after his injury the person believes that his loss was for a worthy cause, or whether he became disillusioned, and so on. We shall emphasize not the nature of the event which produced the change in position on the fortune scale but the consequences of the persisting difference in position between those who are considered fortunate and those who are considered unfortunate.

MISFORTUNE AND SUFFERING That an unfortunate person suffers is the fact which is outstanding from the point of view of common-sense observation. It is also the suffering aspect of misfortune to which people who are close to the sufferer and who share his difficulties predominantly react. We can then ask, "Is the judgment that a person is in an unfortunate position only a statement that he suffers and nothing more?" Are "unfortunate" and "suffering" equivalent? We shall see that there are instances in which the judgment of unfortunate is made in spite of the fact that the person does not suffer, at least not directly from the event itself, and that there are other instances in which suffering occurs and yet the judgment of unfortunate is withheld.

Let us first consider the fact that when suffering is not perceived the person may still be considered unfortunate. This is true, for instance, in the case of a person having a facial disfigurement. It may be objected that, even if the suffering is not perceived, people "realize" that he suffers, and this may have something to do with considering him unfortunate. But, we ask in a provoking way, may it not be this "realization," the opinion of others that he is unfortunate, which makes him suffer, rather than anything independent of these opinions?

It is also puzzling that not all people who experience suffering are considered unfortunate. Boxers, pioneers, members of an arctic expedition are not considered unfortunate. The argument that in such cases the suffering is of short duration does not always hold; the hardships of the pioneers lasted a lifetime. Nor does it help to point out that these sufferings are self-imposed and are therefore not misfortunes. It is not strictly true that they are self-imposed, especially when they are necessary to gain a livelihood. Moreover, someone who imposes an injury upon himself in attempting to commit suicide is still judged by many to be an unfortunate person.

It should be clear from the foregoing that the statement, "One considers somebody unfortunate when one perceives that he suffers," is unprecise. We shall see subsequently that a statement which is almost the reverse will, paradoxical as it seems, lead us further: "When one considers somebody unfortunate, one will not only expect him to suffer but may even feel that he *ought* to suffer!"

MISFORTUNE AS A VALUE LOSS In order to understand many of the social-emotional relationships arising between the fortunate and the unfortunate we must make explicit one important aspect of misfortune: a misfortune involves, in the eyes of the judge, a loss or absence of something valuable. But the word "misfortune" is sometimes used when the person has experienced no unfortunate event, for example when the injury is congenital. In this case, the absence of a value may be felt psychologically as a loss.

THE REQUIREMENT OF MOURNING Since a misfortune is, in the eyes of the judge, a loss of something valuable, the person who experiences a misfortune is generally expected to suffer and mourn his loss. Sometimes these expectations may even have the character of a judgment as to what is proper: it is *natural* and *normal* to mourn one's loss when struck by misfortune. It may therefore be disturbing and uncanny to the noninjured to find an injured person who is not distressed. The noninjured will tend to suspect that the injured person is putting on a good act, or they may conclude that he does not yet realize what has happened to him but "will in time."

We venture to say that these feelings of the donor do not arise solely from the possible intellectual consideration that emotional acceptance of a loss is inconceivable. It is likely that they stem also from the need on the part of the fortunate to keep high those personal and social values which he possesses or cherishes. He therefore objects to the apparent disrespect shown these values as implied in the nonacceptance of the unfortunate position by the person who is deprived of them. When the recipient does not show that he feels unfortunate, the implication is that the loss is not so great, and therefore the donor requires that the recipient mourn. We are now ready to state the following hypothesis: When the fortunate person has a need to safeguard his values, he will either (*a*) insist that the person he considers unfortunate is suffering (even when he seems not to be suffering) and that he ought to suffer, or will (*b*) devaluate the unfortunate person because he ought to suffer and does not.

We expect that the noninjured will resist the implications of this hypothesis. It implies that they *want* the unfortunate to suffer, which is in direct conflict with prevailing ethical codes. An analysis of several examples will, however, make the hypothesis more convincing.

Consider a woman to whom "position is everything in life." She must consider as unfortunate those who are omitted from the social register. If she does not it would mean that her position is not so valuable after all. If they do not accept the fact that they are unfortunate, she must consider them either too stupid to know better, or insensitive, or shamming; otherwise her own position is threatened.

To one who is proud of her beauty, whose sole stock in trade it is, the ugly duckling who flirts and seems happy would be disturbing. The beauty may laugh at the plain one and comment on her appearance so that she will "know her place." If she accepts this place, then she supports and does not challenge the values of the beauty.

For like reasons, it is considered scandalous if a widower remarries too soon. He should have observed a "decent" period of mourning. He is heartless and disrespectful. He threatens the value of strong interpersonal ties. He undermines the value of dependence upon each other in close relationships.

The feelings of the judge which are implicit in the requirement of mourning will tend to be expressed, however, only in covert ways because of the conflict between these feelings and ethical demands. Thus in the following example, though the demand for suffering is not overt, the noninjured subject makes it clear that an injury is devaluating and that the injured should be ashamed of and hide the injury:

> The last place I worked there was a girl there who had been born without an arm. It was about to here [indicates above-elbow]. And she had fingers on it. She didn't care. She used it to hold bobbie pins, etc. . . . I didn't think it was very nice. Right in front of the other girls she would uncover it. Would you think that was all right? [Interviewer: What did you feel about it?] It was repulsive. If it had been an amputation it would have seemed cleaner. I thought at the time that I would have gone into the dressing room and do that and not be where so many people could see it.

MISFORTUNE AND DEVALUATION It has been seen that if a person does not mourn his loss when the donor believes that he ought to he will be devaluated. Mourning his loss does not, however, insure the unfortunate against devaluation. He may be devaluated whether he mourns or not. There remains then the task of determining other conditions under which a person who experienced a misfortune is devaluated.

Devaluation of a person implies comparison. The comparison may be made between two persons in respect to particular characteristics, or between the current state and a previously existing or predicted future state of the same person, or a person may be compared with some abstract norm. The standard of comparison has a position which is evaluated positively and below which any position is negative. Thus, when there is devaluation, the comparisons are not made in neutral terms indicating likeness or difference. Instead, there is always a judgment of better or worse. The position of the person being judged and the standard against which he is compared may be represented on a value scale.

Summarizing, we may say that devaluation presupposes comparison on a value scale on which a person is judged to be in position *x*, the standard occupying position *y*, which is higher on the scale. Close consideration of this statement, which sounds so self-evident, will show the problems actually involved. Several terms used require further specification. These specifications will help in the task of determining the conditions which lead to devaluation. The terms are "value," "person," "position of the person," and "standard."

VALUE We raise the question: Does devaluation occur when a person has lost or lacks *any* value, or does it occur only when particular values are involved? It would seem that even when something is evaluated highly, the nonpossessor is not necessarily devaluated. Two kinds of values which preclude devaluation can be distinguished —possession values and asset values.

Possession Values. If a value is seen only as a possession of a person and not as a personal characteristic, devaluation of the person cannot take place. Thus beautiful pictures may be evaluated highly, yet those whose homes do not boast of even one old master are not devaluated. Though this seems clear, the terms "personal characteristic" and "possession" are in themselves problematic. Psychologists are uncomfortable when they have to draw a boundary between the person and the environment. Whether something is seen as a part or characteristic of a person or as a possession seems to depend upon the judge. Even a part of the body may be thought of simply as a possession rather than as a characteristic of the person, as the following statement of an injured man would seem to imply:

> In other words, I kind of think now that the hands and legs are just merely tools. Where if you haven't got the right tool there are some jobs you cannot do. It is not the handicap that holds a man down. It is his head. In the beginning one does not see it—that they are tools.

The general problem will have to be solved: What are the conditions under which a value will be seen as a personal characteristic or simply as a possession?

Asset Values. Even when a value is seen as a personal characteristic, the nonpossessor is not devaluated if the value is regarded as an asset value. When asset values are involved, the person does not base his evaluation upon comparison with any standard. He may, for example, simply enjoy the musical performance of his acquaintance without comparing it with the performance of anyone else. Should the judge not be talented in this regard, he is not disturbed because he is inferior to another. Musical ability in others and himself is seen as an asset value. More generally, the existing state of a person may be felt to be satisfying (or disturbing) without comparing it with a standard. A woman, for example, who is forced because of family and children to give up a vocation which until then had made up a large part of her life will not feel inferior if a vocation represents to her an asset value which is a "fine thing to have" if circumstances permit.

From the above, it is clear that it is not inherent in a value to be considered an asset value. Among other things, the needs of the judge will determine whether or not he is in a comparison frame of reference. Thus, though musical ability may be an asset value under certain circumstances, when the judge is in a comparison frame of reference because he has to select members of an orchestra it is not. In the latter case, we may speak of musical ability as a comparative value, a value used in making comparisons for the purpose of evaluating the person.

We wish to make a sharp distinction between comparative values and the possibility of making comparisons when asset values are in question. In the latter case, comparisons which might be made are intellectual ones which do not affect the evaluation of the person. In the former case, the comparison is the main aspect; whether or not the person is meeting the standard with all its consequences is most important.

PERSON We have to distinguish between what we call "total person" and "characteristics of a person." By "total person" we mean all the characteristics which are taken into account by the judge at a given time whether they are clearly or only vaguely perceived. Devaluation can exist in regard to single characteristics and not in regard to others. If the characteristics on which the person is devaluated are "decisive" for the judgment of the total person, total devaluation will take place. But if these characteristics are seen as unimportant, then the person is not devaluated as a total person though he is devaluated on single scales. Moreover, when the single characteristics on which the person is devaluated are the only ones that enter the evaluation of the judge, then "total person" is equivalent to these characteristics and total devaluation takes place.

Consider the example of the noninjured girl who said:

> He's correct in not proposing if he couldn't earn a living because of his handicap.

This subject evaluated the injured person as a husband in terms of a single characteristic or scale on which she feels he has an inferior position. Because other characteristics of a good husband are not taken into account, he is necessarily devaluated as a husband. If other characteristics which are felt to be the decisive ones are considered, such as affection and understanding, he may be judged equal to whatever is taken as the standard. He will be devaluated only if the girl feels that earning a living is of primary importance.

Examine similarly the self-devaluation of an amputee who says:

> You feel like a heel lots of times when kids are playing on the street with their sleds. Other fathers can play with their kids.

The subject devaluates himself because other characteristics which may be considered more important for a good father than those on which he falls short are not considered at the moment.

Devaluation of the injured is not limited to bodily values only. When the injured person is devaluated because of physical performance, appearance, or aptitude for particular roles, a jump is not infrequently made so that he is also devaluated in regard to assumed mental characteristics. Some people directly indicate that abnormality of the body means abnormality of the psychological make-up. Thus we have the following statements made by noninjured subjects:

> You'd be very conscious of your own deformity; it would hurt you psychologically.

> Some have a disposition to arrogance. "You are going to accept me whether you like it or not" like a midget, you know, inferiority complex. Some overdo the matter of being congenial. [Note that even positive traits are seen as negative.]

> After she [girl with short bowed legs] had been with us for a short while, we accepted her as normal, except for that handicap. [This implies that at first they didn't accept her as normal.]

We should like also to point out that devaluation of the total person does not always occur by way of single characteristics. Sometimes there seems to be a direct, all-inclusive judgment of devaluation of the total person. It seems that the broader the meaning of the word "person" the less clearly does the judge perceive how the single scales determine his evaluation of the person. He has a vague feeling, for example, that a "cripple" is somehow "an inferior person."

In speaking about devaluation of a person, then, we must ask two questions. Is his devaluation limited to particular characteristics or is he devaluated as a total person? Is he devaluated because only those scales on which he has a low position are taken into account or because these scales are given considerable weight when the scope of values is enlarged to include other characteristics of the person.

POSITION OF THE PERSON To a judge, the permanence of a person's position with respect to the standard is important in his evaluation of the person. We may expect that devaluation will be less severe if, when taking the "time perspective" [4] into account, the position of the person is seen to shift in the direction of the standard. The judge may expect the shift for different reasons. In some cases, he may feel that the loss can be replaced in whole or in part. Thus, even a person who considers "home-owner" as a characteristic of the person, and a minimum requirement for the role of a responsible community member, may not devaluate someone who suffers the misfortune of having his house destroyed. The judge may expect that he will again be able to establish a home and thereby regain his former position. The loss is only temporary.

In other cases, the person may be expected to adjust to his loss even though the lost value cannot be regained. The position of the person, then, is felt to shift so that he can meet the standards in regard to such values as, for example, adequate personality, social usefulness, and the like. For problems of injuries, the shift due to perception of adjustability is of particular importance. Even in those instances in which physical improvement can be limited only, the recognition that one can adjust to the injured state will minimize devaluative feelings. A noninjured woman says:

> When I thought of the courage it took to ignore those handicaps, I felt humble. I felt that anyone who overcomes a handicap like that wins an added amount of respect from everyone.

For this subject, the fact that the injured men were able to adjust to their handicaps led her to evaluate them not as inferior but, on the contrary, as persons meriting respect.

We believe further that the judgment of adjustability will depend upon the adjustment of the judge. A person who feels in essence "What a terrible misfortune to be injured, I could never stand it. I would rather die," we consider maladjusted with respect to injuries. The following comments were made by noninjured people:

> It wouldn't be worth while to live.
>
> I'd develop a complex and go off in my little hole.
>
> I'd go into hiding and not show my face for the rest of my life.

To such people it will seem impossible that one can adjust to injuries.

STANDARD In connection with the term "standard," we have previously noted that the standard may be another person, the same person at a different time, or some abstract norm. Frequently the abstract norm has the character of the minimum requirement for a certain role. If the person does not meet the minimum requirement, he will be judged as an unacceptable candidate for whatever role is in question or he will be devaluated as unfit to continue in the role.

In the extreme case of devaluation of the total person, the person will be thought of as an outcast. He does not meet the minimum requirements on a value scale which, in the opinion of the judge, everyone "ought to possess" in order to be a normal human being. Though such extreme devaluation is not often directly expressed, we do find, in the records of the noninjured, statements such as the following when severe handicaps are being discussed:

> If you have no limbs you are not a person really.
>
> With both arms and legs gone the person isn't of any use, a detriment to society.

When a person is above the level of minimum requirements or "ought-standard" (either for a particular role or for a "normal" human being), he may still be devaluated as inferior, for example in comparison with some other person, but the devaluation will not be as severe.

There are individual differences in regard to where the ought-standard is set. For some it is simply undeniable that a man ought to be able to support his family entirely by his own efforts. If he is disabled so that his wife must work, or if state assistance is required, he will be seen to fall short of this minimum requirement and will be judged unworthy to have a family. Some people may not see this as an ought-standard at all; others may apply it to themselves and yet not require anyone else to meet it.

We can now state that the most severe type of devaluation (devaluation as unworthy or unacceptable) will occur when the person, in the eyes of the judge, falls below the ought-standard on a value scale.

CONCLUSION It is obvious by now that the value structure of the judge is of utmost importance. Devaluation will depend upon whether the judge regards the values in question as possessions or as personal characteristics. It will depend upon whether the judge considers the values as comparative values or as asset values. It will depend upon whether the judge regards the person only in terms of single value scales on which he has a low position; whether the judge regards these values as decisive in the context of other characteristics of the person, that is, when the scope of values is enlarged; or whether in this context they are felt to be nonessential. It will depend upon whether or not the judge regards the state of the person as an unadjustable one. It is up to the judge how high the standards will be set, whether he considers a particular standard an ought-standard for *his* concept of the role of husband, father, and so on, or of a "normal" person, and whether the standards are flexible or rigid. It is not the objective loss but the values of the judge which determine devaluation. A remedy, therefore, is a change in the value system of the judge. The judge may be another person, or the person himself who experiences the loss. In the first case we speak of the devaluation of someone else, in the second case of self-devaluation.

CONFLICT IN THE NONINJURED Devaluation of the injured, like the requirement of mourning, conflicts with ethical prescripts as well as with spontaneous, positive feelings toward the injured. The noninjured person does not want to hurt the injured. He tries to be tactful. He will not address the injured with an emotionally loaded word like "cripple." He will be reluctant to say that the injured man is inferior, to be pitied. He will not point to the injured part of the body. He will hesitate to mention handicaps in the presence of the handicapped person. He might sometimes dare to mention handicapped people who "get along amazingly well" (almost as good as a noninjured person) or who, like Roosevelt, are as good as the best noninjured. He might dare to say that he "would never have noticed it" or that someone else has not noticed it. He might feel a strong positive tie with the injured person and feel genuinely sympathetic toward him.

Because negative, devaluating attitudes conflict with positive feelings toward the injured which are ethically prompted or which are spontaneous and genuine, we can expect that devaluation will seldom be manifested simply and directly but will tend, instead, to be covered up. For example, a noninjured subject who showed concern and warmth toward the injured could not admit his attitude that a handicapped person is less acceptable. But this status-discriminatory attitude is covertly expressed when he says:

> I can readily understand how they [people with less severe handicaps] might resent being classed with those who are totally handicapped.

Another subject is able to express his devaluative feelings when speaking about himself if he were injured:

> Without doubt I would be tremendously depressed [if I had an arm or a leg off] at the thought that your usefulness is over now and that you will be nothing but a burden from now on.

But he is unable to leave the discussion on this negative level. He hastens to right the situation, to pay deference to the other side of the conflict, and adds:

> But I presume that that would pass and with a little bit of expert help one could return to a normal life.

It is also often difficult to disentangle just when the favorable, verbalized attitudes correspond to the underlying feelings and when they do not. When our subjects speak of the courage of the injured, their cheerfulness, perseverance, they are expressing attitudes which overtly are favorable. Sometimes these attitudes seem to be prompted by ethical demands and sometimes they seem to reflect genuine feelings. One suspects that the positive feelings expressed by the following subject are glib and superficial:

> I have met one woman in particular with both legs gone and she had artificial limbs and she got along beautifully. She lost her legs about a year before I met her. And she was very happy. I have more sympathy, and I thought she was very brave.

On the other hand, in the following account a noninjured subject reveals a feeling of warmth and respect for the injured:

> I went to a dinner party the other night for the wounded Japanese soldiers at ——— Hospital. There were about a dozen of them —one completely blind, two with partial sight, another with a leg

> off, another without an arm. When I first arrived I thought, "I can't bear this. I have never been able to look at suffering." I wanted to go away. I stayed. I got acquainted with these boys. They not only had the physical handicap. They had the racial handicap which is a serious one in this country. I stayed until midnight. I felt each one could have been a friend of my son. They were so courageous, so gay, so sympathetic and generous with the blind boy. They helped him so unobtrusively. I felt I had learned a great deal. I felt there was nothing we could do for them. They were doing for us. . . . The way I felt about those boys—I felt inferior.

The conflict in the noninjured may be evaded or diminished in different ways. We should like to mention two phenomena which might be less obvious than simple avoidance of the injured as a means of escaping the conflict. These phenomena are aversion and spread—emotional reactions which make it easier for the noninjured to avoid the injured. Aversions have the useful quality of enabling the noninjured person to feel that he does not voluntarily avoid the injured but that he does so for reasons beyond his control.* Spread, or the exaggeration of negative effects of an injury, may provide the noninjured with an excellent reason for excluding the injured from participation in activities which might, for example, be somewhat strenuous. And if one exaggerates the injured person's sensitiveness and withdrawing tendencies, ethical demands will not be obviously violated, since one can assert that the injured person would feel uncomfortable in the group or decline the invitation anyway.

Sympathy

Sympathy is brought about in the donor by the suffering aspect of misfortune rather than by the value-loss aspect. Our approach to the study of the sympathy relationship was to consider the total scope of meanings assigned to the word and then to extract those which were tied together by a coherent underlying structure. Pity and other devaluative meanings which the subjects sometimes give to the word "sympathy" do not belong to the same structure.

---

* We do not imply that *the* reason for aversions is a need to escape the conflict. Nor is the reason something inherent in humans which makes it natural for them to be filled with aversion at the sight of deviations from the "normal" human form. The ideal of beauty, the Venus de Milo, is a bilateral amputee. The stunted feet of Chinese women were considered beautiful. The heavily padded shoulders of a few years ago exceeded the normal body form. Aversions are "visual allergies," symptoms of more general psychological maladjustment and not only of conflict between positive and negative feelings toward the injured.

PRIMACY OF NEEDS AND EMOTIONS In the older treatises, sympathy was considered an instinctive, or at least an immediate, response to the perception of emotion in another; the perception of pain would bring about discomfort in the observer, the perception of joy would give him satisfaction. We would have no great objection to such a "theory" as far as it goes, but there are difficulties in its incompleteness. For example, we would be reluctant to term "sympathetic" one who, because of his discomfort on perceiving the distress of another, tries to escape the situation.

It is essential for the sympathy relationship that the donor set aside his own needs and feelings in favor of those of the suffering member. The recipient will then feel that his needs and emotions are given primacy, and only then will he feel that the donor is sympathetic. The conditions leading to the existence of primacy of needs and emotions of the other are not known to us and require further study. Most frequently it arises in what we call "we-groups." The partners in a we-group feel bound together by strong ties of friendship, family, etc. They like each other, enjoy being together, need each other. But relative contributions are not measured; comparison of values possessed is not in order; what is important is "we" rather than "you as compared with me." The group is characterized by the sharing of the feelings of one member by the other. The partner is pleased with the joy of the recipient; he is made sorry by the recipient's sorrow. As an injured man says:

> Love for a certain person, that is why you feel sorry. I know my mother feels awfully sorry that I lost my arm. Every time something happened to me my father too felt awfully sorry for me. It was just that he loved me. You just can't get away from it I guess.

Primacy of needs and emotions, however, does not arise in we-groups only. It may exist between people who have no lasting relationship with each other, whose relationships are as tenuous as being fellow-Americans in a foreign country or even passers-by. What the forces are which keep the donor in the negative distress situation in these instances are not known.

What primacy of needs and emotions implies in the sympathy relationship may be described under the headings *Congruence, Understanding,* and *Readiness to Help.*

CONGRUENCE The injured sometimes state that no one can ever really know what it is like to be injured unless he is himself injured. Those who would urge this against the possibility of real sympathy would probably subscribe to the "identity theory" of sympathy. This as usually stated is "seeing and feeling the distress as the other person sees and feels it." An injured person who rejects sympathy gave this as a reason:

> It's very easy for a person to sympathize who hasn't had the experience himself. It would be a very shallow thing. It wouldn't mean anything to me. . . . How can you sympathize with me if you haven't lost your father and I have? You wouldn't know what it is like. How can a fellow sympathize with you if he hasn't lost the leg or the arm? I don't think he could do it.

It should be clear that primacy of needs and emotions does not imply identity of feeling. We doubt that the feelings of the donor and recipient can be identical. Nor would identity have advantages. The donor cannot *see* the situation as the recipient sees it. He cannot know all the emotional ramifications of being injured. He does not suffer the actual social deprivation nor the self-devaluative feelings of the recipient. The recipient is distressed over the loss itself, the donor because the recipient suffers. The *content* of their distress is therefore different. Even in the case of a sharer who may himself experience loss, the content is still different.

The donor need not approach the *mood* of the recipient in intensity, nor is it necessary that his mood be the same qualitatively, as long as it is not incongruous. Moreover, were the donor to feel precisely the same way as the recipient, it is questionable whether any *action* he could take would be effective in diminishing the distress. The anxiety and fearfulness of the recipient, for example, would prevent him from realistically evaluating his situation. A similar anxiety and fearfulness in the donor would also act as a barrier to adjustive effort.

Thus the donor and the recipient *perceive* differently, feel differently, and *act* differently. Congruence rather than identity is required in each of these instances. What makes for congruence is an important problem meriting special investigation.

UNDERSTANDING In a distress situation there are in the recipient two conflicting needs that must be taken into account by the donor. On the one hand the recipient wishes to remain in the area of preoccupation with his loss because of attachment to the object of loss, desire for clarification, and so on. On the other hand, he wishes to leave the area because of the negative character of the situation (the unpleasantness of the state of depression, a feeling of unproductiveness, or whatever). A clear example of both tendencies is found in a bereavement situation in which, in spite of the negative characteristics of grief, one wishes to continue to mourn as an expression of devotion to the person he loves.

The first thing the donor must understand, then, is this conflict in the recipient. He must not only be concerned about the emotional state of the recipient in the sense of wishing to help him leave the negative area; he must also give sufficient weight or respect to the reasons which produced the distress and which keep the recipient in the area of preoccupation with the loss. When either of these attitudes is felt to be lacking, the recipient feels that he is not understood.

The wish for respect to the cause of distress is seen in the following statements made by injured subjects:

> [People say] "Now before long you'll be as good as new." That's a bunch of posies all for naught. . . . They don't know what they're talking about. . . . Though people say, "Oh you'll forget it in a few years," they're always the people who aren't injured.

> People would come in and tell me how lucky I was. It was just that they were trying to put a whole new set of values on my misfortune. If there is anything you feel about it, it is that it was not lucky.

The sympathizer cannot take lightly any features of the situation which are of great moment to the injured even though, in his efforts to bring about emotional relief, he may try to emphasize certain positive aspects.

It is important to point out that the word "understanding" is misleading when it is taken to imply only a conscious intellectual appreciation of the diverse meanings which the loss has for the injured. When the injured speak of a person who understands, they sometimes speak in these terms:

> Probably that girl could not answer your questions but she just knew. Some people are like that. . . . There is a person that just has an instinctive good taste and quality in her.

It seems as though there is such a thing as emotional understanding—that is, grasping the emotions of the other person directly on the emotional level without the intermediate step of intellectual realization of these emotions. The distinction between intellectual and emotional understanding is clearly brought out in the following statement of a noninjured woman:

> Every mother thinks about the possibility of her son coming back wounded or disabled. . . . I don't know just how I would react. . . . You would have to feel your way along and learn every day. But if

> you really love and understand them, you would learn very quickly, by experimentation, and I think you would have to give it a great deal of deep thought, and you would have to have a lot of wisdom, but wisdom comes in an emergency of that sort. [Interviewer: When you said wisdom, that implied intellectual knowledge.] Not necessarily. I would say more a wisdom of the heart.

There is nothing mystical in the fact that one may react before having time to understand intellectually. We spontaneously catch a ball suddenly thrown to us without intellectually deciding on a course of action. Similarly, in the case of emotional relationships we frequently react in an appropriate way which is called "intuitive." It seems necessary to assume that the speed of emotional processes is greater than the speed of intellectual ones and that, in communication, emotional grasping of the feelings of another person is faster than intellectual grasping. Intellectual understanding may, however, enhance the relationship in which emotional understanding already exists. It may increase the effectiveness of the help offered because intellectual understanding may lead to useful suggestions which the recipient may be ready to accept.

READINESS TO HELP It is not by chance that expressions of sympathy are usually followed by some such statement as, "If there is anything I can do, let me know." Such readiness to help should be considered as much a part of the structure of sympathy as congruence of feelings and understanding. This is demonstrated when the injured inveigh against the "so-called sympathy which is nothing but words." For example:

> The good kind you try to do what you can for them to help them out. The bad kind they just say they feel sorry and let it go at that.

> Oh, absolutely [there is a good and bad kind of sympathy]. But it can be expressed through actions rather than through words—fidelity, sticking by you through thick and thin.

The kind of physical help which is acceptable is elaborated elsewhere.[5] In the sympathy relationship, we are especially concerned with emotional help in overcoming feelings of distress. Whether or not this type of help will be acceptable will depend upon whether the donor continues to be guided by the recipient's wishes and also upon his knowledge of the relative strength of the momentary tendencies toward and away from the distress area. The donor should be passive or active depending on these wishes and tendencies.

When the tendency to stay in the area of concern with loss is very strong, the recipient may want nothing more than assurance of concern, an understanding listener, or the comfort of bodily contact with a person with whom strong ties exist. The word "passive" should be taken very seriously. Expressions of concern which are uncontrolled and immoderate may be very disturbing. A few subjects give hints as to why demonstrative manifestations of sympathy are disturbing:

1. The injured person may be so keyed up emotionally in regard to the whole injury situation that additional emotionality is difficult to bear:

> Sympathy is disagreeable to the man because of the state of emotion he is already in.

2. Any strong emotional expression may make the man feel that his situation is even more unfortunate than he thought it to be. It can easily lead to a feeling of futility of his attempts to adjust:

> I don't want them to cry. It makes me feel sick. I can do anything anybody else can but when they do that I would have to feel that I would have to give up trying to do things.

3. The man does not know how to act when strong emotionality is shown. The situation tends to become unstructured. Embarrassment results:

> Sometimes a motherly old gal embarrasses you with how sorry she feels for you.

4. Strong emotionality may arouse feelings of guilt in the man at having caused so much distress:

> I don't want anybody to feel sorry for me. Sorrow isn't a thing to share.

Further, there are other important reasons why the injured objects to excessive emotionality. The injured may doubt the sincerity of the feeling, and any demonstration may convey to the injured that the donor is trying to make sure that his "goodness" is appreciated by the injured. We wish especially to stress the fact that excessive emotionality has also the danger of making the donor imperceptive to the shifts in feelings and changes in needs of the sufferer. It is important to note that in the opinion of the injured a deep positive feeling on the part of the sympathizer can be conveyed to them without any emotional display. They object to shallow sympathy, but shallow sympathy is not, of course, equivalent to sympathy that is manifested simply and without elaboration.

Active help requires that the donor be alert in watching for an occasion when he can strengthen the forces in the recipient in the direction of leaving the distress area without provoking resistance from the recipient. One injured subject identifies this as encouragement rather than sympathy, but the idea is essentially the same:

> You can always take encouragement. More than sympathy, it is the cheerful look, not a sorrowful look—a feeling of raring to go that kind of infects you—not the idea that the world has gone wrong.

Yet sudden or too strong or persistent urgings in the direction of leaving the area reflects on the genuineness of the donor's appreciation of the cause of distress. At the first sign that he has proceeded beyond the ability of the recipient to follow him, the donor must be ready to abandon any benevolent attempts. Because the emotions of the donor are not identical with those of the recipient, because he is not so depressed, he is already a step ahead in the struggle to overcome the distress. It is this discrepancy in feeling which gives the donor the possibility of shifting the recipient in positive directions. But the emotional change required of the recipient cannot be too great. Only small steps can be taken, the size of the allowable step being not infrequently smaller than the donor wishes would be possible.

The meaning of size of step may be grasped more fully if we consider the parallel case in the intellectual realm. A teacher may explain too quickly or may omit necessary intermediate points. The student is then unable to follow because the size of the steps taken by the teacher has been too great. In the emotional realm, we may take the case of a noninjured person who, wishing to overcome the brooding of his injured friend, suggests a joyful interlude. Though the injured friend *also* wishes to overcome his brooding, merrymaking requires too great an emotional change for him. It is interesting that when someone is deeply distressed a sympathetic person may suggest a cup of tea. This may represent not only concern for needs which the sufferer himself might neglect; it is also a shift from preoccupation with loss to an activity which is neutral enough not to seem incongruous. It will also not be seen as too great an emotional step if the donor gradually aligns himself with and strengthens those positive aspects which the recipient might express, for example that he has the fortitude or stamina required, or the hope of an eventually successful outcome.

SPONTANEOUS AND ETHICALLY DICTATED SYMPATHY—SINCERITY In the absence of spontaneous sympathetic feeling, there may still be strong social pressure to play the appropriate role.

Thus, besides sympathy based on genuine primacy of need of another person there is simulated sympathy—sympathy for the purpose of adhering to the ethical ideal that one *ought* to be a good person, which sometimes implies self-aggrandizement. Most people will be able to recall being at one time or another donors of both kinds of sympathy —that which is "ought-inspired" and that which is prompted by genuine concern. In some instances the former will be difficult to admit to oneself.

It is important that the dynamics of interrelationship between the donor and recipient is different in the two cases. If the sympathy is ought-inspired, the donor will do as much for the recipient as is required by the donor's need to be "good." We cannot help but suspect that he will be guided much more by what *he considers* good for the other than by the needs and wishes of the person he is sympathizing with. The recipient distinguishes between spontaneous and ought-inspired feelings of sympathy in the donor and speaks of them as "sincere" or "insincere." This does not mean that he always correctly detects them. But when the underlying feelings are seen as spontaneous and genuine they will be evaluated as positive, even though the recipient may not for other reasons welcome the overt expression of sympathy (for example, because of lack of knowledge or sensitivity in the donor or because of some conflict in himself). Positive evaluations of the genuine feelings are expressed in these terms:

> I don't mind [if old friends say they are sorry]. Being a friend I felt that his word was sincere, coming from the heart.
>
> Sincerity means a lot.
>
> Yes [there is a good kind of sympathy and a bad kind]. You can always tell the person who does actually have a feeling for you and is sincere.

Ought-inspired sympathy can be evaluated as proper when seen as a formal expression of politeness. The donor thereby conveys only a recognition of the seriousness of the event and his intention not to intrude further into the privacy of the recipient. A limited interaction of this sort is accepted, but it must be brief and does not bear repetition. The injured say:

> I think it is all right [for someone to say he is sorry on first meeting]. I think I would say the same thing. If he would let it go with saying he was sorry and not rave on about it.
>
> I don't mind anybody saying that. It's just like a person saying, "I'm sorry you are sick." Not if he just said it once. It's the same if you have lost a wife or relative or something; people offer their

condolences. That is the same thing. It is all right if you don't overdo it. That is just common politeness.

While this type of sympathy is less valuable to the recipient than is genuine sympathy, it bears no great dangers. Perhaps the only additional caution required is that overt expression of this sort of feeling should emphasize the event and not the man. To say, "I'm sorry it happened," conveys what is needed. "I'm sorry for you," may connote devaluation:

> A person can say he is sorry it happened, but I don't want him to say he's sorry for me. . . . It's in the time element. Sorry it happened refers to the past and it doesn't mean he keeps right on feeling sorry . . . and pity and being sorry *for* a person suggests looking down.

Though interactions of this kind are accepted, they are by no means considered necessary by the injured. But the injured know also that their acquaintances may feel embarrassed if they make no comment on first meeting the man after the injury. Hence, in addition to the evaluation of "proper," the same behavior may be regarded as *neutral or unimportant:*

> They don't really need to say it, but it's all right. If they say [casually], "It was hard luck," it's all right.
>
> I'd just as soon they wouldn't say it. If it's a friend of yours, you know anyway.

The evaluations become negative when the basis for the expression of sympathy is felt entirely to be a matter of obligation:

> Some people who are not so close to you feel they *should* give sympathy and say they're sorry you lost your leg.

> This sentimental stuff. It seems to be partly an act. Old people seem to think they are obligated.

The simulated sympathy which is feigned for self-aggrandizement or to satisfy some other need of the donor is rejected:

> Well, there's the crocodile type [of sympathizer]. . . . Cries, you know, like the crocodile. Then . . . the he-man type. He comes up and claps you on the back. All the time patting himself on the back.

Ought-inspired sympathy, when mistaken by the recipient for genuine feelings, provokes positive feelings toward the donor in return. When the recipient does reciprocate and later finds no real concern for his needs, he feels cheated or fooled—first because he was under false pretenses drawn into serving as a means of satisfaction of the needs of the other; second because he was ready to accept emotionally this person whom he now rejects as unworthy; and third because, believing himself secure with this person, he permitted himself to expose his private and sensitive feelings. Insincerity in such a case is therefore threatening; it is rejected and avoided.

DESIRE TO BE NONINJURED Sympathy may be unwelcome not only because of some failing of the donor but because of the recipient's own attitude toward his injury. To welcome sympathy means that the injured man must admit that the injury has made a difference to him, even if it is only in particular and confined ways. He must not only see himself in the sympathetic situation as an injured person but must also be willing to have the sympathizer see him as such. This is not easy to do if the man has negative emotional feelings toward being considered an injured man. The resistance against being regarded as an injured person may be seen in the man's resentment of sympathy when he says:

> Servicemen don't want their family to feel sorry for them. . . . Some people feel sorry but not around Utah. They see a lot of it. They treat you just as if you were another man.

The persistent demand by the injured to be treated like anyone else may be indicative of healthy attitudes when it reflects their resistance to being devaluated. But when it is a sign that the injured person doesn't want to share injury-connected matters because he is ashamed of them, that he wishes above all else to be considered a noninjured person, then he must of necessity remain troubled. When he reaches the point where he can face the fact of his injury, then he becomes able to receive the comfort which sympathy may bring.

SYMPATHY AND ADJUSTMENT The desire of the sympathizer is to help the sufferer to reach a happier state, to help him to adjust. The recipient, too, may wish sympathy not only because of the immediate comfort that it may give him but also because he hopes that the other will help him overcome emotional difficulties. But is there anything in the nature of the sympathy relationship as such which will assure better adjustment? Does it imply that the sympathizer will be better able to recognize intellectually or emotionally what leads to adjustment? Just as the recipient himself, the donor may err as to what is adjustive. He may lead in nonadjustive directions. One can say only that the sympathy relationship provides a favorable atmosphere for influencing the recipient, whether for better or for worse.

There is, however, another point to be considered, namely, whether sympathy, as an expression of we-group feelings, does not always have some adjustive value. Sympathy, as an expression of we-group feelings, gives assurance that one is of worth to another person. We shall see that adjustment may imply the overcoming of the feeling of worthlessness of oneself and meaninglessness of the world around.

Acceptance of Loss

We have spoken about the meaning which misfortune has for the noninjured and about his feelings toward the injured. We indicated that these feelings lead to difficulties and to attempts on the part of the noninjured to lessen the suffering of the injured. In his social relationship with the noninjured, the injured has to find a manner of living most satisfactory for him. He has also to overcome certain individual difficulties in addition to those produced by social relationships. He has to accept both personal loss and social loss.

The content of *personal* loss as felt by the injured may be conveyed by the following statement ascribed by us to a leg amputee:

> The leg which was a part of me and like the other is now detached from me. With it I felt free to move, to jump, to run, to play. I could move it, move with it; it moved me. I will be hampered. I will not be able to climb a mountain (even though I never climbed one before). I won't be able to dance or fight as well as before. I won't be able to take a job that requires standing for hours. The prosthesis can fail. I can slip and fall. I have to take care of the stump. When I look in a mirror I won't see a whole man; I will have to get used to seeing myself this way. I can't bound out of bed in an emergency. When I move I will think, "Is it worth the inconvenience and effort of getting up?" So much that I will do would have been so much easier; in a shorter time I could have done so much more. I will always be less able than I would have been. I was a better man when I had my leg and amounted to much more than now. I will never be what I wish I were, and ought to be—had I the leg.

In suffering from social loss, the individual suffers as a member of a group. He feels that he is not accepted as equally worthy. Other values which the group can offer, such as companionship, are made inaccessible.

The content of *social* loss as felt by the injured may be conveyed by the following statement ascribed by us to a leg amputee:

> I will be considered inferior by others. They feel that I can't contribute my fair share. I will be regarded as a burden. They won't want to associate with me. They might stand my presence but not

> accept me as they would a noninjured man. Girls won't want to go out with me. People will be repulsed by the sight of me.

One could consider each of these difficulties and see how each in turn could be overcome. This obviously is an endless task, for one could continue to enumerate specific sufferings involved in personal and social loss. Instead, it is more meaningful to try to see whether there are not some conditions common to diverse difficulties. Understanding of these conditions is actually a first step toward solving problems of adjustment, for only when they are clearly specified can we tell what it is that must be changed, and only then are we able to get some insight regarding the state to which it would be desirable to change and how to produce the change.

The desired state which we call "acceptance of loss" does not mean becoming reconciled to one's unfortunate situation. Instead, acceptance of loss is a process of value change. Before discussing value changes, however, we wish to describe those attempts at adjustment which seem promising to the injured, yet not only fail basically to overcome the difficulties but even create new ones.

MAINTAINING THE NONINJURED STANDARD The way in which the injured person tries to overcome difficulties is determined by the fact that his values are those of a noninjured person. A blow which damages a part of his body does not at the same time lead to changes within his value system. He may continue to maintain the noninjured position as *the* standard of comparison and direct his efforts toward reaching it. He may cling to the belief that the way to overcome his difficulties is to be, in his own eyes and in the eyes of others, a noninjured person. To achieve the end of being considered noninjured, he uses all means available, both realistic and unrealistic ones.

REALISTIC ATTEMPTS TO ACHIEVE THE NONINJURED STANDARD The realistic means used by the injured to be like the noninjured are strenuous efforts to perform certain tasks independently and to equal or surpass the success of the noninjured in certain roles. These attempts can be considered realistic because in certain limited ways they are successful. The injured can equal or surpass the noninjured performance on particular scales or in particular roles. But *if the sheer fact of being an injured person is a difference which makes a difference to the injured man, that is, if the noninjured remains the wished-for ideal, no matter how often he does as well or better than the noninjured he will still devaluate himself as an imperfect noninjured person.*

In their efforts to be noninjured, the injured impose upon themselves unnecessary strain. Whereas the noninjured person often readily accepts help when it is more convenient to do so than to perform a task alone, the injured person tends to be relucant to accept help if the help is not absolutely necessary.[5] Thus an injured man says:

> I wouldn't accept help except where absolutely necessary. Offers of help get me down unless I were in a real jam. [Interviewer: What do you mean by absolutely necessary?] Oh, something like an earthquake out here where I couldn't get my hands on my crutches in time.

And another says:

> You'd like to be a lot more independent than you were before. If somebody opened the door before, you never paid attention to it, but they do it now and you notice it.

In order to explain why the injured, in striving to be and behave like a noninjured person, is led to impose greater hardships upon himself, we must take into account that "help is necessary" has a double connotation. It means "Without help I will not reach a desired goal," and "I am not able." The latter implies comparison of one's own ability with that of another. "You cannot do it, but I can," is, in our ability-minded society, a most unwelcome comparison. For the injured person who wishes to be noninjured, the ability-comparison aspect of help has a greater weight than for the noninjured, and he wishes to deny that he *needs* to be helped. The necessity of the goal, therefore, has to be greater for the injured in order to overcome the resistance against being helped. This, we suspect, could be shown by a simple experiment.

A scale of the necessity of help is constructed. One end indicates "help is a pure matter of convenience" (that is, no great effort needed to perform the activity alone, but someone willing to share the effort), the other "help is absolutely necessary" (that is, an important goal completely inaccessible without the assistance of another). We can then determine the points at which help will be welcomed by injured and noninjured persons. Judging from the data we have, we would expect that the point of acceptance of help by those of the injured who wish to be as much like the noninjured as possible will not in general coincide with that chosen by the average of the noninjured subjects but will be nearer to the point of "help is absolutely necessary." Thus, when the injured person in speaking about help says, "Treat me like anyone else," he may not mean "Give me as much help as you would a noninjured person for whom a task is inconvenient." Instead, he may mean "Do not help me; a noninjured person would not require help in this situation."

UNREALISTIC ATTEMPTS TO ACHIEVE THE NONINJURED STANDARD The unrealistic means toward being considered noninjured are the attempts to deny that an injury makes any difference whatsoever, either to the person himself or to anyone else. The injured man should forget and others should forget; if both would forget there would be no difficulties:

> [Interviewer: How should a person go about adjusting?]
> I think he should forget about it.
> People should just forget what happened.
> If he doesn't think of it, it won't bother him.

Two reasons seem to support the belief in this literal kind of forgetting. First of all, in the highly emotional striving for adjustment, the aim and the means are not sharply distinguished. "I wish my injury would be forgotten," and "It can be done by actual forgetting," merge together in an emotional state which leads to primitivization in thinking. Second, the injured man does many things without feeling like an injured person. When he is in a bar, reading the comics, discussing political affairs, and so on, the thought that he is an injured person may not enter. In such situations he escapes the painful devaluative feelings associated with his loss. Temporary forgetting which the injured man does experience may make him believe that he can forget the injury most of the time.

Temporary forgetting may not be altogether valueless in the process of adjustment. Consideration of problems connected with the injury goes on at the emotional level with such intensity that temporary escape may be welcomed as a psychological rest from too much strain on the organism. But the injured person realizes in time that it is not only hard to forget what exists but that also so much happens which may "remind." Thus an injured man who said, "You can forget you are hurt if everybody ignores it," a few sentences later complained, "If you go out you can hardly go through a day without people asking you about it." And reminding is not due only to the incorrigibility of the noninjured. A person who wears a prosthesis, for example, has to put it on and take it off. The injured often has to enter situations in which other people are handicapped, and again he is reminded. Thus even if one could willfully forget, one would constantly be reminded by new occurrences. The wish and the impossibility of forgetting are brought out clearly in this statement:

> More or less forget about it is the best thing, but how are you going to forget when everybody keeps reminding you of it? I guess in time to come they won't be half as curious and will accept it. . . . I don't think about it unless someone speaks about it, or if I think about something I want to do and then I think, "Hell, I can't do that." You shouldn't worry about it, but you can't forget that one moment when you got hit. But it's about the future that you think.

The belief in the possibility of literal forgetting gives way, therefore, to the feeling that the injured and noninjured should behave toward each other *as if* the injury did not exist:

> I'd just act normal, as if nothing had happened.
>
> The happy and perfect thing is to have it ignored completely.
>
> [Forgetting?] That's hardly possible but we can all make believe.

It is evident that such behavior does not really mean that the man will be considered noninjured. On the contrary, it is implicit in acting "as if" that he actually is not noninjured.

As in the case of temporary forgetting, which has some positive aspects, so also "as if" behavior has its assets, though they may be limited. The injury may be considered a personal matter, and "as if" behavior serves the purpose of keeping others from intrusion into privacy. Thus, under certain circumstances, "as if" behavior may be appropriate, especially where strangers are involved. But "as if" behavior, again as in the case of the attempt to forget, brings about difficulties in the relationships between the injured and the noninjured. When the participants in a relationship are closely associated, persistent role-play has negative effects. First, if each feels that he can never relax his guard there will be a constant strain. But worse than that. It is characteristic of close relationships for the partners to share their feelings. If the formal surface behavior which is appropriate to stranger relationships persists, they will begin to feel like strangers to each other. Closeness, which is built upon easy communication, sharing of feelings, the warmth of sympathetic interactions, gives way to estrangement. Basic understanding between the persons cannot be reached. The injured person will continue to feel that he is not understood and cannot be understood.[8] Again, as in the case of help, the injured deviates from the actual behavior of the noninjured, for the noninjured does not ordinarily impose such restraint upon himself and does not in time of stress deprive himself of the comfort of sympathy.

SOME VALUE CHANGES INVOLVED IN ACCEPTANCE OF LOSS Denial that a difference exists, as we have seen, not only does not overcome difficulties; it may actually create new ones. But above all it hinders basic adjustment, for admission that a difference exists is a prerequisite for the further step of accepting the difference as non-devaluating. Most important for the process which we have called "acceptance of loss" is a process of revaluation. Although this process is too complicated to permit us at present to make more than a few statements regarding either observed changes or possible ones, we can present, as an incentive to further study, the advances we have thus far made in understanding it.

The first problem is why revaluation should be so difficult for the injured. Why, in the face of persistent difficulties, do they cling so strongly to those evaluations which hurt them? Two reasons may be mentioned. First, the injured seem to feel that, since abnormality of the body connotes psychological deviation or even mental abnormality to some people, they will only strengthen this impression should they maintain values which differ from the noninjured's viewpoints and ideals. Second, and most important, is the fact that to produce value changes on the emotional level is at least as difficult as to change the needs of the person. Though one may easily convince a person intellectually of the advantage of adhering to different values, their actual integration within the value system of the person is bound to meet resistance. This is understandable if we consider that single values are not independent from other values of the person, so that one change in the value system necessitates making changes in other values or giving them up.

Some of the value changes which we believe would do much to overcome suffering from loss may be examined in the light of certain considerations brought out in the discussion of devaluating misfortune. First, devaluation will be diminished to the extent that the values lost are felt to be nonessential for the evaluation of the person when the scope of values is enlarged to include other personal characteristics. Second, devaluation will be overcome when the values lost are regarded as asset values rather than as comparative values. A third possibility, viewing the value lost as a possession value rather than as a personal characteristic, doubtless has adjustive significance, but this will not be further elaborated here.

ENLARGEMENT OF SCOPE OF VALUES We may describe two examples in which enlargement of scope of values takes place.

The State of All-Inclusive Suffering. For the injured person to see the lost values in a larger setting of other values is of special importance in the case where he feels he has nothing more for which to live.

There are two characteristics of such a state which make the thought of suicide likely. First, the perception of only a single area which is characterized by suffering means complete devaluation of one's life. Moreover, the suffering seems to be boundless, not only in extent but also in time. If no other area is seen, then there is nothing to which one can hope to change. The only hope of escaping suffering is to leave life altogether.*

Fortunately, such black depression and despair does not persist in most of the injured who experience it. There is a gap in our knowledge as to just how it is overcome, but what is necessary is the perception of something besides suffering in life. It may be that, when the decision to commit suicide is made and when only execution of the plan remains, the injured may look back at what will be given up: suffering *and life*. When fighting against living further is no longer necessary, as it is before the decision is reached, life itself may be seen as a value. At such a moment this sudden experience of something else than suffering may be sufficient to give the first hold and with it the feeling of hope and strength which we have called the "stamina experience," so distinctive and easy to recognize when encountered, although difficult to convey, that it was named long before its place in problems of value change was seen.

Those who have had the stamina experience know that life is worth living again. They feel that "they have been all the way down to the last door and come back," that no other enemy will ever be so formidable. The realization that the essential value of life is regained means that the unbearability of the situation has been overcome. It means that the person is able to attend to what life holds for him, to begin to appreciate the fullness of meaning of having what he does have. As one very severely injured man put it:

> You gradually see that there is more to life than you thought possible. . . . They all think at the beginning that they are no good. Why there was a fellow here the other night who had a couple of fingers missing, and you would think there was nothing worse under the sun. And I said to him, "Well, son, you still have a pair

* In the present state of knowledge, we are not able to state whether those who consider or commit suicide after acquisition of a physical injury have had pronounced neurotic trends which prevent them from standing the additional stress of the unfortunate position or whether an otherwise stable individual but with an extreme evaluation of the fortunate position may consider or commit it.

> of arms, a good pair of legs, a good pair of eyes. Why just think of it! I would be glad to have a good pair of anything."

Another injured man stated:

> I have a sharper appreciation of things I valued before—health, happiness, comfort, friendship. I am a hedonist. I feel lucky for just being here.

And still another calls it a "conversion to life":

> Before, when I would try to analyze myself, I would come against a blank wall. For seven months I don't think half the time I knew what was going on. . . . Some things have become more important that before seemed so unimportant, and consequently less important the other things that seemed so important before. . . . I never had a clear conception of what it meant to live. In other words, I have come to the conclusion that most people go through life and never accomplish anything. They just live. They eat and sleep. . . . Cows I call them. . . . They just grow and disintegrate. . . . I feel that if I don't make a contribution what's the use of having come back alive. I don't want to waste my life now. . . . [Interviewer: It's almost a religious experience.] Well, it's a complete change . . . a conversion to life. Religion is another thing. . . . You have got to dance, to laugh, and have your fun, but also you can put your aims on a higher plane.

The injured frequently maintain that "It is up to the man himself," to overcome the depression in the acute suffering stage. In other words, perception by an outsider that something other than suffering exists is felt to be unconvincing to one who is within the area which seems all pervading. Some injured therefore state that the depressed one should be left alone. Others, however, try to overcome what they call "self-pity" in a friend by scolding and ridicule:

> That's all within the man himself. I have seen them when they haven't anything to live for after the injury. [One guy] wasn't eating, feeling so sorry for himself. I called him everything but a gentleman. I called him everything I could think of. After that he started eating.

The fact that the friend is hurt and feels these insults to his manliness means that he discovers at least pride as a remaining value. As different as the overcoming of depression by oneself or with this sort of "help" may be, they have in common the finding of a value at a time when every value is lost.

The method of hurting the injured man during depression should not be given as a recommendation to the noninjured. Such behavior on the part of the noninjured would simply intensify the feeling of being devaluated. When the injured use this method it means "He is not devaluating me for being injured but for being unmanly." At the same time, the injured friend is there as an example that one can be injured without feeling that everything has been shattered.

What the conditions are which give the values of manliness, of pride, the power to restructure the meaning of the lost values so that they no longer dominate the person's life needs further investigation. Though the lost values may retain their importance, the stamina experience brings with it the strength and hope which make the injured person feel that he is ready to live further *in spite* of difficulties. An important condition toward overcoming devaluation is thereby realized. The injured state is no longer regarded as an unadjustable one. At least in the sense of being able to make a go of it in spite of difficulties, the person feels he can adjust. But though the worst consequences of loss may be avoided through enlargement of scope of values, it does not mean that all suffering is overcome. It does mean, however, that the person has been faced with the necessity for revaluation. He has had to see the place of the lost values in his whole value system. In this way he is a step ahead, for adjustment, when the person is not in a depressed state, also entails value changes.

The Problem of Appearance. A person may be bothered by his appearance because he feels that it discounts his attractiveness to others. The injured person may believe, for example, that when someone looks at him his scar is seen and nothing else matters. We propose that devaluation due to damaged appearance will be diminished to the extent that surface appearance is felt to be nonessential for the evaluation of the person when the scope of values is enlarged so that surface appearance is included within personality appearance. Actually, the perception of the appearance itself may then change so that it is seen in light of the personality. Thus, whatever the objective condition of the surface appearance may be, when one reacts positively to the person the appearance may be felt to be attractive.

Of appearance, a man who was undergoing plastic surgery had this to say:

> Some people who can look at their picture and say that they are extremely homely and yet the people who know them will swear that they are good-looking. I heard that people used to think that Lincoln was very handsome. A man could not grow an awful lot homelier than Lincoln. . . . There are certain things in a man's face that are an indication of his character, and if those things are what you like they make him good-looking despite the fact that his features are a little irregular.

In this case the attractiveness of a person is determined not primarily by a smooth, unblemished surface appearance but more decisively by his personality, from which scars may not detract.

Many people quite naturally judge a person's attractiveness in terms of his personality. Under certain circumstances it seems that the influence of personality recedes to the background while that of surface appearance becomes the focus of attention. In the case of the injured, primacy of surface appearance leads to devaluation, so that the integration of surface appearance within the context of personality should diminish suffering. The conditions which determine the primacy of personality or surface appearance is a problem requiring special investigation.

We present below an excerpt from an interview with a person who has a severe facial injury. During the interview, the evaluation of the appearance or attractiveness of a person is seen to change from surface appearance to personality appearance:

> *Subject:* Undoubtedly at first it is a great shock to a person's family —their loved ones—when they see him with his features changed from what he was before. It is a great shock at first. They have to be around him for a while before they realize that fundamentally he is not changed.
>
> *Interviewer:* Do you think, actually, it is a big shock? I don't think so. I am speaking from my own experience, I am asking you, what do *you* see in a person you meet—a new person—what do *you* see?
>
> *Subject:* The first thing you see is his appearance.
>
> *Interviewer:* Why do you say that? The first person you saw here was John Hall. When he came in, what did you see?
>
> *Subject:* A fine looking young man—a gentleman.
>
> *Interviewer:* Now, has "gentleman" anything to do with a scar?
>
> *Subject:* No.
>
> *Interviewer:* Now let us say there is a new doctor on the ward. He comes in. What do you see?
>
> *Subject:* It is hard to say. If he has a strong personality, the first thing you see is his personality. Is he capable? How he approaches you.
>
> *Interviewer:* That is it. Myself, I think is it a nice person? Do you see? It is the kind of person. What kind of a nose? Do you remember the kind of nose John Hall has? What kind of mouth he has?
>
> *Subject:* Not distinctly. But if there had been something outstanding, for instance a bad scar, you would remember, wouldn't you?
>
> *Interviewer:* Now, for instance, when you look at the patients in the hospital, what do you notice about them?
>
> *Subject:* The boys, when you first see them, you notice first their scars.

Interviewer: The first moment?

Subject: The first moment. That is the hard part.

Interviewer: How long?

Subject: Until he says something. Then you start getting an idea about his personality, and once you start thinking of him as he really is, you don't think of his scars. You don't remember them.

Interviewer: You can see the nose of a person, but when you speak to a person you don't notice the nose. You notice the personality, because you see you looked at John Hall, and you only saw the personality.

Subject: The way I was impressed—that is the way I was impressed. That is new. I hadn't thought of that before.

In the above example, the attractiveness of a person is seen primarily in terms of the more inclusive personality appearance rather than in terms of surface appearance. If this is a lasting change, then we can expect that for this subject devaluation of the injured due to damaged surface appearance will be diminished.

CHANGE FROM COMPARATIVE VALUES TO ASSET VALUES Two situations involving a change from comparative to asset values may be described.

The Problem of Mourning. A person may mourn his loss because the personal satisfactions which the object of loss gave him in the past are now denied him. Overcoming of mourning does not require a lowering of the level of aspiration (being satisfied with less), nor does it require depreciating the object of loss. What seems to be necessary to overcome mourning is a change in relationship to the object of loss.

In the case of loss of a person, the one bereaved must recognize that, although further *interactions* with the person are impossible, a *relationship* nevertheless can still persist. Some of the values which they had formerly shared, and which, in his first grief, he may have seen as dependent upon the presence of the lost one, can be kept. He can do what the loved one would have done and wanted him to do. He can bring up his children to observe the traditions which his wife had begun. Then he can look back upon the past with tenderness rather than rejecting any painful reminders of it.

Some similarities may be found in the change of relationship to the lost object which is necessary in the case of the injured. An amputee, for example, has to feel that the most essential functions which the limb had formerly enabled him to perform can be carried on by the stump and the prosthesis. He has to feel that he is still an intact organism, a whole man. A change of feeling has to take place from that expressed by one subject:

> What does she see when she comes in? Half a man lying on the bed. . . .

to that expressed by another:

> I am a long way from worthless. I am still a good man without the leg.

Such a viewpoint implies that one turns to the satisfactions existing in the present and does not derive essential satisfactions or dissatisfactions from comparison with the noninjured state in the past. It means that a leg as a value has changed from a comparative value (without which one is inferior) to an asset value (a good thing when it is present). If such a change takes place on the emotional level, the past can be remembered without pain but with tenderness—with that tenderness which old people not infrequently feel toward the reminiscences of their youth.

The Problem of Disability. The change from comparative to asset values is indicated not only when the person suffers because of personal loss as described above but also when he suffers because of loss which is socially evaluated. As an example, we shall consider the disability aspect of the injury.

To call someone disabled implies that *performance* determines the evaluation of the person. In our society, people are frequently compared with each other on the basis of their achievements. Schools, for example, are predominantly influenced by the achievement or product ideology. High grades are given not to the one who worked hardest but to the one who performed best. Under certain circumstances, of two who reached the same performance level, the one who did so with greater ease is considered the better. He is seen as potentially a better producer than the one who had to work harder. Thus, effort is not always considered as a positive value but, paradoxically, sometimes as a liability.

If one would follow the maxim which also exists in our society to the effect that, "All that is expected of you is that you do your best," it would mean that the person would not be compared with others in regard to ability; it would mean that his own state matters and thus that it does not matter whether he lost or lacks ability. Actually, one wishes to say, a person does not lack ability; he can only *have* it.

The injured who applies himself with effort contributes the most that he can as a *person.* Though the unsatisfactory physical tools of his body may have limited his production, his personal contributions are at the maximum. As a *person* he is not different from the noninjured.

Effort as a basis for evaluation is observed in the injured. A bilateral amputee stated:

> Sorry is for someone who does his damnedest but still he is physically unable to accomplish what he does in the best way. Pity is for someone you feel like he isn't putting everything into it. Not up to standard, up to what you judge by. Maybe I am wrong but that's the way I think of it.

This man expresses the thought that, in addition to the scale of achievement ("accomplishing what one does in the best way"), there is another scale, that of effort ("doing one's damnedest," "putting everything into it"), and that devaluation ("pity") should be reserved for those who are lower on the effort scale. Only those who do not put forth sufficient effort should be judged as "not up to standard."

Why bring up the change from one comparative value (the product-achievement value) to what appears to be just another comparative value (effort) when we are discussing the change of comparative values to asset values? It is true that effort, in this case, is seen as a comparative value, but when effort becomes the yardstick by which a person judges himself, then the *values lost* are changed from comparative to asset values. Greater ability or achievement becomes a good thing when it exists, but not a loss, or a lack, or a disturbance when it is absent. Such a change is but one among others that are required for the person to perceive his existing state as valuable rather than as a crippled, noninjured state.

These differing evaluations of one's existing state have important consequences. The particular problem which we should like to discuss as an example is the effect of the two evaluations on the readiness of the person to improve wherever realistic improvements are possible and on his persistence in bettering his state.

It would seem at first glance that maintaining the noninjured state as the standard would have the advantage of leading the injured to increase his efforts, for example in dealing with the physical environment. The injured would desire the best prosthesis, try to improve in using it, and learn as many skills as he could in order to be able to perform the physical tasks which the noninjured can perform. But the desire to be able to handle the physical world does not stem only from the wish to be as much like the noninjured as possible. We even doubt that the desire to be as good as the noninjured is helpful. The injured person who emotionally desires to be noninjured will see even objective improvement over previous performance as still falling short of the goal and hence failure. The same objective improvement can be seen as success (in comparison with recent performance) or failure (in comparison with the noninjured). The following two examples illustrate the different feelings resulting from the different evaluations of one's present state. In the first, "always wondering whether I could have done better" indicates feeling of failure, in the second, "enjoying learning over again" a feeling of success:

> We'll be satisfied with less but there'll always be a little bit of doubt as to whether we could have done a little bit better without it. Maybe I'll be able again to play a good game of golf, but I'll always wonder whether I could have done better. . . . In some part of your mind you just have to check off the fact that you're missing something extremely valuable.
>
> The more you learn to use it the less it bothers you. If it's just hanging it will. . . . The more I learned the better off I was. . . . I figured it was gone so I might as well see what to do about it. . . . I enjoy learning to do things over again. It offers a challenge to you. I think, "What's the best way?" before I start fooling around.

It seems reasonable to expect that, if a subject feels he is improving, he will hopefully continue. If he is constantly frustrated by unsuccessful attempts, forces away from the unreachable goal and disruptive emotional effects will appear.[3]

Our discussion is of value for an important practical problem of the amputee. In trying out a new, technically improved prosthesis, some of the injured feel that it is an improvement and others do not. Besides the question of the physical fitness of the prosthesis for the individual, psychological conditions leading to the different reactions are important. It would be promising to study whether those injured who are dominated by the noninjured standard are more easily dissatisfied with the new prosthesis than are those who consider their postinjury state as valuable. We predict that the former group will more easily be disappointed because, in comparison with the noninjured standard, the results obtained with the prosthesis can be seen only as a failure. The latter group, however, will recognize any actual improvement and consequently will be encouraged to continue using the prosthesis. Those who maintain the noninjured as their standard require psychological adjustment before they will be able to accept an objective improvement as such rather than as a new indication of the unreachability of the noninjured state. We venture to say that only if the postinjury state is taken by the subject as a basis for comparison can he make valid judgments as to the advantages of the technically improved prosthesis.*

CONCLUSION Acceptance of loss is seen as involving changes in the value structure of the person. We have pointed out only some of the changes which may lead to acceptance of loss. Clearly there are others. Our statements have to be taken as suggestions for further research rather than at their face value. We discussed four kinds of situations: (1) overcoming all-inclusive suffering; (2) overcoming mourning; (3) overcoming devaluation produced by damage to appearance; and (4) overcoming devaluation produced by physical disability.

The kinds of value changes that may alleviate the suffering in these situations are closely connected with those value preconstructs discussed under *Misfortune and Devaluation*. The value change involved in (1) and (3) can be seen as one in which enlargement of the scope of values takes place. In the case of all-inclusive suffering, enlargement of the scope of values is the first step toward the possibility of acceptance of loss, since the main problem here is to regain, psychologically, values other than those lost. In the case of devaluating appearance, enlargement as such is not in itself an advantage unless with the enlarged scope of values the values lost are seen as relatively nonessential. In both cases, the person will maintain the noninjured standard and regard the values lost as comparative values. Thus, the person may still devaluate himself, for instance when a particular situation arises in which enlargement is made difficult.

The value change involved in (2) and (4) can be seen as one in which the values lost are regarded as asset values rather than comparative values. In this case, the person feels that his own state is a worthy one. When, instead of selecting unreachable states as a standard, he turns to what he has and can reach, life can be seen to offer more than he can possibly avail himself of. He frees himself from devaluating comparisons with a ghost ideal of a different but actually not better person, the noninjured. Thus, acceptance of loss seems to be more fully realized through the second type of value change.

ACCEPTANCE OF PERSONAL LOSS AND REACTION TO SOCIAL LOSS The injured person who has accepted his personal loss

* A similar practical problem is raised in a much more general area. If one's own state is felt to be valuable, should not comparison with oneself in performing activities be a better incentive than comparison with others and, if so, should not this guide our educational procedures?

will feel one way about the discriminatory attitudes of the noninjured. He who has not accepted his loss feels another. The social loss of the injured person—his feelings of nonacceptance as a group member—has a basis in reality. Whether or not the person has adjusted to his loss, therefore, he will experience difficulties in his relationships with noninjured people. But the reaction in the two cases will be quite different.

Where the person devaluates himself because of his loss, he will feel that his nonacceptance by others is largely justified. He will agree with the other group members that a noninjured person is more valuable, more likeable, more worthy. He will suffer keenly that he happens to be on the short end of this relationship, but he will see it as an unavoidable and natural fact, to be supported as morally valid. He will feel that no one can change this state of affairs—that one can perhaps try to behave "as if" he were noninjured but that emotional devaluation of him must prevail.

If, however, the injured person has accepted his loss, he will not devaluate himself. He will consider himself an equally worthy member of the group and thus feel that he should be fully accepted by the group and have access to the values which the group can offer. He will see that it is the maladjustment of the noninjured toward injuries which leads them to devaluate and reject him, a fact which hinders him from having access to the values of the group. He will see that the locus of the difficulties is not in the injured who adjusted to his personal loss, not in the natural, lawfulness of devaluation of the injured, but in the noninjured.

A considerable part of the suffering due to nonacceptance by others is thereby removed. Because the negative evaluations of others are seen as unwarranted, because the injured person does not blame himself, they hurt less. Instead, the person who holds them may in turn be devaluated and seen as ignorant or prejudiced. This counterdevaluation also may serve to diminish suffering from social loss.

Whereas the maladjusted injured person wishes to be accepted by the noninjured though he feels he ought not be accepted, the adjusted injured person will care less to associate with those whose values he does not share or respect. The adjusted injured person gains a considerable degree of emotional independence and freedom from the noninjured. This does not mean that the injured person does not and need not care about how the noninjured receive him. Even though he may not care to associate with a given person, he does wish to maintain close relationships with others. Moreover, in a world dominated by the noninjured, it is often the noninjured who determine whether the injured person can have access to important values such as jobs and group memberships of many kinds. Thus it is of vital interest to the injured that the noninjured become adjusted to injuries.

Acceptance of Loss by the Noninjured

Acceptance of loss is of great importance not only to the injured. Persons close to the injured (that is, those who are in the position of sharers), as well as the large number of noninjured who have little to do with injured people, have much to gain from healthy attitudes toward injuries. The sharer suffers not only because the injured person suffers (sympathy) but also because he too experiences a loss (personal and social loss). A wife may feel the loss of her husband's leg just as personally, just as deeply, as the husband himself. The sharer has, therefore, to accept the loss just as does the injured person before suffering may be overcome. It is of extraordinary practical importance for an injured man to realize that his closest sharers—his wife, mother, and so on—cannot be expected to accept the loss immediately. Just as he has to go through the struggle to accept the loss, so does the sharer.

For the nonsharer, adjusted attitudes toward injuries do much to free him from anxieties regarding bodily harm. He still will continue to regard body-whole as a value, but as an asset value and not as a comparative value. The loss, then, is regarded as an adjustable state and not as a catastrophe. Consequently, in threatening situations, he would not become careless about his safety, but the anxiety would be reduced to realistic fear.

Since acceptance of loss has adjustive significance for all persons, the question arises as to how the noninjured may be brought to face it as a problem. The need to attempt to accept the loss exists in noninjured sharers, for they also experience a loss. But what about nonsharers? In general, they do not feel the necessity of imposing upon themselves the problem of adjusting to injuries. Not only do they feel that real acceptance of this kind of loss is extremely difficult; what is more important, they do not feel that they should try to accept it. The general attitude may be described as, "Problems of visible injuries are special problems. They do not actually concern me."

At least two groups of people not in the position of sharing a loss with an injured person may consider more closely their feelings toward injuries. First, there are people who are bothered by social justice. When considering injured people, they may question their own attitudes, since negative feelings toward a suffering part of humanity are regarded as unjust and intolerable. As they puzzle, they may discover their own basic nonacceptance of injuries and struggle to see the loss as an adjustable and acceptable state. The second group consists of those people who have a general need for self-adjustment in whatever area anxiety is felt. Just as a person who is frightened when climbing a mountain may wish to ascend again in order to overcome the fear, so may a person who feels uneasy about body welfare wish to meet the problem of nonacceptance of loss.

Direction of Further Research

The study of adjustment of any kind, including acceptance of loss, requires the investigation of, first, the conditions c_1 and c_2 underlying the nonadjusted and adjusted states, respectively, and second, the conditions leading to change of condition c_1 to condition c_2, expressed as $ch(c_1 \rightarrow c_2)$. That is, two distinct tasks are involved: first, there must be determined *what* has to be changed to *what* and, second, *how* the change takes place. The study reported here deals only with the first task, that is, with the determination of conditions of nonacceptance (c_1) and acceptance (c_2) of loss.

For the determination of what has to be changed to what, manifestations of the two conditions c_1 and c_2 have to be observed. These manifestations, or events, which in our case were the statements by injured persons concerning nonacceptance and acceptance of loss, were the raw data on the basis of which the underlying conditions c_1 and c_2 were specified. Conditions c_1 and c_2 are always specified in terms of constructs and their interrelationships; the underlying conditions in our case are value statements on the conceptual level.

Once c_1 and c_2 have been determined, further research should take the direction of systematic search for and examination of the manifestations of $ch(c_1 \rightarrow c_2)$. As the result of our study, we know that conditions c_1 and c_2 involve different value structures. The conditions of value change could then be studied by designing experiments which would promote value change and permit the observation of its manifestations.

We will now suggest two examples of situations in which value change may be brought about. Both are designed to have the subject himself try to bring about the change.

First example: The injured man is asked to try for one day to accept the role he usually resists taking. namely, the injured role. The injured role does not mean one of overdependence and self-pity.

Rather, it means that the person does not go out of his way to appear noninjured. He is encouraged, for example, to take advantage of offers of special consideration by others which will make things easier for him. He may also be asked to discuss a personal matter related to his injury with someone to whom he feels close; this should be a matter which in the past he has refrained from bringing up. For that day he has to abandon the noninjured role as the ideal and accept the injured role as the one to strive for. He may succeed in changing, and report these changes, or he may fail and report the difficulties. In either case, a gateway is opened for analysis of the conditions of change.

Second example: An injured man is asked to note events, situations, and interpersonal relationships occurring during the day which are and are not injury-connected (that is, whether the event included any aspect of the injury). He is asked to consider further whether the injury entered in a positive, negative, or neutral way. Finally, he is to examine, for alternative interpretations which give them a more positive character, those events which he characterized as negative. For example, the events noted may have included a lift on the way to work (injury-connected, positive), staring by someone in the elevator (injury-connected, negative), or dictating letters (not injury-connected). Crucial for the study is the instruction given to the subject to search for a change in the character of the injury-connected negative events. In the elevator example, the subject may come up with the statement that not all staring needs to be staring at an amputation; someone might stare when he is in deep thought about his own personal concerns. In searching for a substitute for the negative character of the event, the injured person thus restricts the all-inclusiveness of the devaluating injury so that other values become available. As in the preceding hypothetical experiment, analysis of these attempts at changing values should lead us to the specifications of the general conditions of value change.

In returning to our study here reported, we want to mention a number of value constructs related in pairs to c_1 and c_2. These are: comparative values *vs.* asset values, personal properties *vs.* possessions, and all-inclusive value loss *vs.* partial value loss. The conditions of change from one member of a pair to the other, $ch(c_1 \rightarrow c_2)$, are yet to be determined.

These changes, we believe, are only a few of the necessary changes involved in acceptance of loss. One can be sure that acceptance of loss does not imply only the value changes mentioned above, nor only value constructs.

Although much further study of c_1 and c_2 is indicated, we feel enough is already known to encourage investigations of $ch(c_1 \rightarrow c_2)$. The knowledge to come from such investigations should provide a systematic basis for understanding and aiding the psychological adjustment of the injured.

NOTES*

1. D. Adler, G. Ladieu, and T. Dembo, "Studies in Adjustment to Visible Injuries: Social Acceptance of the Injured," *Journal of Social Issues,* 4 (1948), 55.
2. R. G. Barker, B. A. Wright, L. Meyerson, and M. R. Gonick, *Adjustment to Physical Handicap and Illness: A Survey of the Social Psychology of Physique and Disability* (rev.; New York: Social Science Research Council, 1953).
3. Tamara Dembo, "Der Aerger als Dynamisches Problem," *Psychologische Forschungen,* 15 (1931), 1.
4. L. K. Frank, "Time Perspectives," *Journal of Social Philosophy,* 4 (1939), 293.
5. G. Ladieu, E. Hanfmann, and T. Dembo, "Studies in Adjustment to Visible Injuries: Evaluation of Help by the Injured," *Journal of Abnormal and Social Psychology,* 42 (1947), 169.
6. Kurt Lewin, "Richtungsbegriff in der Psychologie," *Psychologische Forschungen,* 19 (1934), 244.
7. ———, *The Conceptual Representation and the Measurement of Psychological Forces* (Durham, North Carolina: Duke University Press, 1938).
8. R. K. White, B. A. Wright, and T. Dembo, "Studies in Adjustment to Visible Injuries: Evaluation of Curiosity by the Injured," *Journal of Abnormal and Social Psychology,* 43 (1948), 13.

---

* *Editor's Note* Because of a necessity for conserving space, several pages of materials painstakingly collected by Drs. Dembo, Leviton, and Wright and originally included in the form of three appendices have been omitted here. These appendices, entitled "Summary of Methods Other Than Interviews Used in the Study," "Record of an Interview with a Noninjured Subject," and "Records of Interviews with Injured Subjects," may be found in *Artificial Limbs, A Review of Current Developments,* Vol. 3, No. 2 (Autumn, 1956), the journal published by the Prosthetics Research Board, National Academy of Sciences–National Research Council.

BLINDNESS AND STRESS: CATASTROPHIC AND CONTINUING

Robert Lee Robinson

"Not blindness, but the attitude of the seeing to the blind is the hardest burden to bear." This statement attributed to Helen Keller[1] is most appropriate to our discussion.

In this article* three areas of research in adjustment to the misfortune of blindness are suggested. They are

1. Communication
2. Financial security
3. The role and image of agencies for the blind

COMMUNICATION

The previous paper, "Adjustment to Misfortune—A Problem of Social-Psychological Rehabilitation," presents valuable findings that may well be applied to the field of blindness research. However, the authors said, "Orthopedic cases and cases involving plastic surgery were chosen because the visibility of the injury is important in relationships with noninjured who are not close to the injured." Had blind persons been included as subjects, it would appear that perceptual or communication problems would have presented confounding variables in the study of the social problems.

The study we are discussing might usefully be replicated for blinded persons with respect to the problems of communication. The fact that most forms of communication are seriously impeded—if not completely thwarted—by blindness causes not a little stress to the blinded person and to those who interact with him. The social iso-

* Grateful acknowledgment is given to M. Robert Barnett for his helpful suggestions.

lation imposed by blindness was succinctly stated to MacFarland [2]: "In blindness no social use of the eye is possible."

For example, conversation with a blind person would seem to present at least two difficulties. The first is the strong emotional meaning blindness has for each of us. Looking into the blind person's eyes is a constant reminder of primal fears. Blindness has been described by some writers as symbolic of castration or death.[3,4] The other is that the blind person does not see the person with whom he is talking, who in turn feels his reality, his perception of himself, threatened because he is not visually perceived; his self-reality does not receive reinforcement. When an individual looks into the eyes of another person, he looks at a self-image. He validates the idea that the other is perceiving him as real and is focused upon him. In conversation with a blind person, the sighted person may unconsciously turn his gaze away from the other's face, not facing his fears, refusing to see the person who does not see him.

This problem of communication is, of course, compounded by the attitude constellation of the sighted toward the blinded and vice versa. Given the hypothesis that there are identifiable specific attitudes, would it be useful to isolate these attitudes so that a program might be structured to handle them?

Healthy family relationships are dependent upon effective interpersonal communications which are reflected in psychosexual adjustment. Both Fitting[5] and Cutsforth[6] have indicated that useful findings might result from further research in the area of psychosexual adjustment. In this connection, if blindness is symbolic of castration, then it can be hypothesized that a woman who marries a blinded man is not a punishing, castrating woman, but a woman who has deep feelings of inadequacy, who doubts her femininity, and who needs to be needed. If this is true, a man who has an area of physical inadequacy through blindness is marrying a woman who feels herself to be inadequate. And let me underscore the fact that I am distinguishing between a woman who *is* inadequate and one who *feels herself to be* inadequate.

In any case, if the hypothesis is true, both of the couple bring unclear role perceptions and role expectations into their marriage, and this will affect their psychosexual communication.

An article by Barnett suggests that the malady "blind man's wife" might apply.[7] The social distinction of being the wife of a blind man can cause frustration in the woman because, in addition to the daily problems of family living and community interaction, she must cope with the prevalent attitudes toward the blind.

FINANCIAL SECURITY

Another area needing study in relation to blindness and stress is financial security. Fear and depression are the natural result of a lack of adequate regular income. The disabled, as well as children and the aged, often live with this common human need unmet.

In the previous article one uninjured respondent stated clearly, several times, that there needs to be enough money if one is handicapped. He thus expressed the anxiety created when loss of financial security is threatened by physical disability. The absence of income is one of the primary factors causing devaluation of blind persons.

In the AFB-VA study,[8] "851 Blinded Veterans—A Success Story," 85 per cent of the blinded veterans claimed to be heads of households. This exactly equals the percentage of nonblinded U.S. veterans claiming themselves as heads of household.[9] The financial flooring provided through service-connected disability compensation may well be one of the factors enabling so many blinded veterans to have the self image of being heads of household.

When there is no financial security, the stress that ensues in the lives of blinded persons and among their family members is considerable. Lowenfeld states, "the blinded individual by reason of his handicap is more likely to be under nervous strain . . . to harbor feelings of insecurity and frustration which may produce a state of anxiety that is liable to interfere with his mental health . . .[10] The level of anxiety or concern on the part of society about loss of financial security for those persons who suffer the misfortune of blindness needs to be researched. That there is some degree of anxiety on the part of the uninjured was illustrated in the Dembo study. It would seem that financial security would lessen the stress, stigma, and devaluation involved in blindness.

Probably the biggest issue in the area of social welfare planning today is that of income maintenance. There is little likelihood that a universal "demogrant" will be enacted in the near future. Demogrant is defined by Schorr as . . . "universal payment to everyone in the country, without regard to income or status . . ." [11] We have, however, provided a partial demogrant to a large segment of the American population through the Social Security programs for the aged.

Extended partial demogrants for the aged and children would help to lessen the devaluated image that blind people have by grouping blinded persons along with children and aged who would receive a demogrant because need had been converted into a social right for these groups.

In our society economic well-being is a strong cultural value as was expressed by one of the injured subjects in the Dembo study. Yet, if there is not sufficient regular income the blind person is reduced to the role of infantile devaluated dependency. Some individuals might argue that this state of reduction is part of the rebirth process as a blinded person. It is my contention that it need be no such thing. Therefore, it is hypothesized that blinded persons, if provided adequate financial flooring as a right, can be rehabilitated psychosocially in a much fuller sense of that term.

ROLE AND IMAGE OF AGENCIES FOR THE BLIND

Why are so many blinded persons reluctant to go to agencies for the blind? This question continues to haunt professionals in the field. Are the so-called "hidden blind" really "hidden"—inextricably socially isolated—or are they simply "hiding"? An agency that is widely accepted for its sound programs and policies requested research into the number of blind persons not reached and found that a considerable number of blind persons in the area had not asked for its services and did not know it existed. As reflected in their report: "more than 2,000 blind residents were known to the agency but our pilot study suggested there may be at least half again as many blind persons who are unknown as such to local health and welfare agencies because the agencies have been unable to reach them, because they do not want or need to be reached, or because they do not know that they are blind . . ." [12]

The attitudes of workers for the blind is clearly expressed by Barker and colleagues[13]:

> Chevigny mentions the two extreme variations in attitude that he had encountered among workers for the adult blind: some workers seem to believe that the blind are maladjusted and incompetent, while others have only admiration and respect for their clients.
>
> These differences in the opinions of superintendents, teachers, and matrons in schools for the blind are not unexpected. They are undoubtedly due in some degree to differences in the experiences and values of the workers studied. But more fundamentally the diversity and conflict in the attitudes of those who work with the blind are doubtless based upon the ambiguous perceptual figure that blind

> persons present, viz. a partial devalued physique and a whole valued person. This ambiguity has been discussed in connection with other disabilities, but rarely does it appear so strikingly as in the behavior of professional people who work with the blind. On the one hand, they urge that the blind should not be isolated or considered a group apart but should be accepted and integrated into society; the unjust segregation of the blind and ways of overcoming discriminations and prejudices are frequent themes in their writings. At the same time, however, these workers justify special class legislation for the benefit of the blind on the ground that they are indeed a special group and not like other people, and vigorously promote the cause with appeals to pity and other emotions that devalue the blind.
>
> If this basic conflict is not resolved by individuals and groups concerned with the welfare of underprivileged, physically disabled minorities, severe tensions and serious inconsistencies in behavior become inevitable. It may be that the strong in-group forces prevalent in organizations concerned with the blind have their roots partly in this basic conflict. In any case, the social psychology of disability group organizations offers theoretical and practical problems of importance for research.

Scott[14] points up:

> Approximately 955,000 persons in the civilian, non-institutionalized population of the United States under the age of 80 are blind. There are a number of significant facts about the blind population. First, a majority of them are elderly. Sixty-six per cent are between the ages of 55 and 80; another 15 per cent are in the age group of 45–54; 17 per cent of all blind persons are in the age group of 18–44; and only 2 per cent are children under 18. According to these data, two-thirds of all blind persons are in age groups where retirement is either pending or a reality, and only a small minority of blind persons are in age groups where either employment or education is realistic.

What more has been done and what is being done by the agencies for the geriatric blind? They are considered unable to follow any gainful employment; they probably lack financial security; their savings—if any—are exhausted; and they are physically unable to maintain their own homes. All these factors, coupled with chronic conditions concomitant with old age, do not endear the elderly blind to agencies as "client potential." It is quite obvious that the definition of poverty mentioned by Graham[15] applies to these aged persons, and something might be done for them by the agencies if the "hidden blind" could be identified.

Experts in social change tell us that it is sometimes more difficult to modify an existing agency structure and function than to set up a new agency. Perhaps the new blind rehabilitation centers represent examples of an innovation which meets needs that, being newly identified, have not been met by the traditional agencies for the blind in the past.

Do we see this taking place in the National Institute for Neurological Diseases and Blindness?

Is a similar kind of social change occurring now in connection with the efforts to establish a new Eye Institute at the National Institutes of Health?

Are not the efforts traceable to the fact that the existing National Institute for Neurological Diseases and Blindness seems not to be stressing research on blindness so much as neurological problems?

The social problems of our day require imaginative investigation of traditional agency role and function.

NOTES

1. Phillip S. Platt, "Additional Factors Affecting the Blind," *Blindness,* ed. Paul A. Zahl (Princeton, New Jersey: Princeton University Press, 1950), 57.
2. Douglas MacFarland, "Social Isolation of the Blind: An Underrated Aspect of Disability and Dependency," *New Outlook for the Blind,* Vol. 60, No. 10 (December, 1966), 318–319.
3. Hector Chevigny and Sydell Braverman, *The Adjustment of the Blind* (New Haven, Connecticut: Yale University Press, 1950), 58–64.
4. Thomas J. Carroll, *Blindness, What It Is, What It Does, and How to Live With It* (Boston: Little Brown, 1961), 1–13.
5. Edward A. Fitting, *Evaluation of Adjustment to Blindness* (New York: American Foundation for the Blind, 1954), 71–75.
6. Thomas D. Cutsforth, *The Blind in School and Society, A Psychological Study* (New York: American Foundation for the Blind, 1951), 145–164.
7. M. Robert Barnett, "Hindsight," *New Outlook for the Blind,* Vol. 57, No. 5 (May, 1963), 180–181.
8. "851 Blinded Veterans—A Success Story," a study prepared by the American Foundation for the Blind, New York City (in press).
9. U.S. Department of Commerce, Census Bureau, *One-in-a-Thousand Sample Description and Technical Documentation, Census of Population and Housing* (Washington: Government Printing Office, 1960).
10. Berthold Lowenfeld, "Mental Hygiene of Blindness," *Selected Papers from the Proceedings of the University of Michigan Conference for the Blind,* 1947, eds. Wilma Donahue and Donald Dabelstein (New York: American Foundation for the Blind, 1950), 35–44.
11. Alvin L. Schorr, "Alternatives in Income Maintenance," *Social Work,* Vol. 11, No. 3 (July, 1966), 22–29.
12. Eric Josephson, "A Pilot Study of Visual Impairment," *Proceedings of the Symposium on Research in Blindness and Severe Visual Impairment,* May, 1964 (New York: American Foundation for the Blind, 1965), 41–104.

13. R. G. Barker, B. A. Wright, L. Meyerson, and M. R. Gonick, *Adjustment to Physical Handicap and Illness: A Survey of Physique and Disability* (rev.; New York: Social Science Research Council, 1953), 269–308.
14. Robert A. Scott, "The Selection of Clients by Social Welfare Agencies: The Case of the Blind," *Social Problems,* Vol. 14, No. 3 (Winter, 1967), 248–257.
15. Milton D. Graham, "What Good Are Statistics?" *New Outlook for the Blind,* Vol. 59, No. 7 (September, 1965), 229–232.

SESSION REPORT

John R. Swinton

Dr. Tamara Dembo responded to Mr. Robinson's paper:

> The questions which Mr. Robinson raises are extremely important. The first issue he discusses, communication, overlaps into the questions we were discussing during the session on interpersonal relationships. But, in dealing with communication between injured and non-injured people, he has raised a more basic problem which we have not discussed before.
>
> The second issue, which I am pleased to see raised, is the problem of financial security for the injured person. I think the stress Mr. Robinson places on it is very much to be supported. I think a demogrant would effect not only the actual financial security of the injured person but would also bring about better social relationships for him. In fact, this approach is now very prominent. We see it applied to other disabilities like poverty. It is important to notice the possibility that overlapping dual handicaps—physical and sensory kinds of handicaps plus simple poverty—can be imposed upon a person.
>
> Then Mr. Robinson also discusses the problem of agency relationships. And in this connection I would like to recommend an article by Eliot Freidson in the excellent book edited by Dr. Sussman,* which impressed me very much. It concerns rehabilitation and security and is especially informative with regard to the agency relationship. Freidson's account of how the agencies deal with the problem of deviancy can be highly commended to anyone who has not had the chance to read it.
>
> These are the three key problems. But Mr. Robinson raised a number of subsidiary problems. There is, for example, the question of whether blindness symbolizes castration or death. In fact, whether these comparisons are valid might be a fruitful research area. He also mentions the sexual relationship—what kind of person seeks a blind spouse?—which is a question worthy of our consideration.

Lee Lacey referred to Helen Keller's remark, cited by Mr. Robinson, and asked how one can modify the views of the seeing toward the non-seeing? Dr. Sussman suggested that no one can really change

---

* Marvin B. Sussman, editor, *Sociology and Rehabilitation* (1966).

people's attitudes; and, with this thought in mind, he suggested organizing programs of social action analogous to the Civil Rights protests. He advocated lobbies, action groups, and movements as much preferable to academic discussions of attitudes.

Dr. Dembo responded to Dr. Sussman's observation:

> I would agree that some action is important. Yet when Mr. Robinson mentions the necessity of instituting financial support for the blind, I think he has cited an equally valid approach; and there is no doubt that it would help blind people. It is true that psychological discussions do not change the laws of the country with regard to the minority groups, but I think it is extremely important to see that, along with organized action, they have a role to play. It is not right to say, "What is the use of talking about psychological problems?" While action and discussion cannot be interchanged, one should not take precedence over the other.
>
> What cannot be solved by action are the unsettling problems of the interpersonal relationships, community relationships, and agency relationships. These can be *influenced* by action but they cannot be completely changed. Even if financial security is arranged, and even if the person feels more secure, he would still have what we might call deviations which could, in turn, cause problems of frustration and stress. It is important to identify the attitudes toward the blind with which we want to deal, questioning why they exist; but we ought to concentrate more upon the reasons for their existence than upon the simple identification of them.

Here Dr. Sussman drew a distinction between the changing of attitudes and the enforcement of toleration. "The emphasis," he remarked, "should be upon the mobilization of as much power as we have to demand toleration rather than elicit love."

Dr. Dembo replied:

> I would say that Dr. Sussman has raised a very important issue: the idea that toleration, not change of attitude, should be pursued. His viewpoint is that action is important and my viewpoint is that *both* consideration *and* action are important. But relationships among people—not attitudes—is the topic under discussion.
>
> People have values and feelings, and these not only require study but are also necessary for the consideration of change. Much of the change that is going on in the world is based, after all, upon the existence of feelings and values. How do we bring a child to understand that difference does not imply evaluation? (We might watch children's reactions to a dog with only three legs, for example. Do they come to accept it? To love it?) Why is *devaluation* a part of the attitude of the noninjured person toward the injured person? We are approaching these kinds of conceptualizations in research with handicapped persons when we ask them how they believe noninjured persons should behave toward them—and I would agree 105 per cent with Dr. Sussman that it should be the injured person who is

> first consulted because his difficulties and his experiences are under primary consideration. Most injured people do admit that the attitudes of noninjured people are important and that more knowledge in this field would be welcome.
>
> A person who has lost a value can either regain it or adjust to the fact of its loss. Often he is faced only with the latter—there being no possibility of regaining the value. This value loss is obviously the source of some of the difficulty between injured and noninjured people. But we must remember that value loss can be dealt with. The regaining of the value (that is, locomotion, in the case of an amputee) is analogous to "bettering" the handicapped person. (It often takes on some of the characteristics of therapy in the field of mental health.)
>
> The approach is a difficult one. It involves noninjured as well as injured people, and noninjured people are liable to be the unconscious promoters of the secondary handicap—the social handicap. The secondary handicap is the devaluation which is ascribed to the value loss in *any* deprivation, and I am speaking just as much about the deprivations of the poor person, the mentally retarded person, or whatever the problem might be.

R. Paul Thompson then observed that the attitudes of seeing people seem to have changed only slightly over the years. In fact, according to Mrs. Mary K. Bauman, those attitudes have remained basically unchanged since Biblical times.

Dr. Sussman expressed agreement with Mr. Robinson's proposal to distribute demogrants. He envisioned the development as a substitute for counseling which, he suggested, may be costing up to $10,000 a year per blind person, when a simple grant of six or seven thousand dollars might actually be preferable.

Dr. Elena Gall suggested that the available resources in education have not yet been adequately tapped, and that they have not been given a fair chance in the realm of attitude changing.

Miss Yvonne Agazarian, to some extent, concurred. She pointed out that sighted children freely mix with blind children until adults vitiate the progress with their structuring of appropriate responses in children.

Loyal Apple attached no deep importance to eliciting the good fellowship of sighted people, but he did see the need to create the proper understanding among sighted people of the ways others become blind.

Miss Sophy Forward emphasized the importance of forcing those who are blind to face the fact not only that they are blind but that there are other concomitant disadvantages associated with the situation. She noted that the counseling methods currently employed are too often unimaginative and unappealing. (Miss Forward also noted, parenthetically, that there are many blind people who have access to extra funds yet fail to take advantage of them. They apparently experience feelings of degradation if they accept the money. This attitude might be worth examining.)

Mr. Robinson recognized that each blind person reflects his group, and that he therefore carries a certain responsibility. "Contagion of example," he remarked, "is a recognized phenomenon among any definable group, be it the blind, Negroes, or whatever." He continued: "I believe that if, as professionals, we are going to concern ourselves with a group of people and move forward, we are going to have to start thinking newer and fresher and more imaginative thoughts. Just as an example, the mature adult in our society is expected to pay his own way. It is my contention that a kind of financial flooring for any marginal group of people would be an ego supporter and that people with such a flooring could not be devalued to the extent that they are now."

Mr. Robinson stressed the word "extent." The more one handicap is alleviated, the less effect it will have, and the more attention might be paid to those handicaps remaining.

Dr. H. Robert Blank pointed out that, while it is not quite the same as attitude altering, removal of discrimination is nevertheless a potent educational force. He noted that the various agencies have a role in both education and social action, and that many agencies have minority group members serving as directors, helping to form policy. There is a growing attempt, according to Dr. Blank, among agencies to solve their ingrown blind spots; and unless they continue to try, the existing hostility toward them is liable to increase.

Dr. Blank remarked:

> Speaking as a psychoanalyst there is nothing that is as powerful a force acting on a person—with the possible exception of the loss of a young child—as the loss of a body part. One must face the fact that the part cannot be regained, and he must adjust to the fact that he has entered the class of handicapped people. Closely allied with this realization of loss is the subconscious fear that the loss will cause the individual's abandonment. The reaction to this fear is the most primitive of all reactions, rage. This rage is intolerable and is therefore liable to be turned against one's self and become suppressed.

Elaborating, at Dr. Sussman's request, upon the analogy between the loss of a young child and the loss of a body part, Dr. Blank explained that humans are automatically prepared for certain losses, like the loss of a parent, a spouse, or a friend. But the loss of a body part or of a young child so violates the sense of justice that humans are neither able to prepare for them nor to view them as logical.

Dr. Dembo interjected this observation:

> When someone, who is confronted with severe body loss, is in his deepest depression, he may often be confronted by another person who has had just as severe a loss but who has experienced the rehabilitative process. This second person often intentionally ridicules the person in injury, abusing him and calling him "cripple." The reason for it is good—though one must remember that only the injured should do it to the injured—because the depression keeps the injured person fixed in the present with no idea of the future and no plan for settling his difficulties. If the abusive injured person can cut through the depression and arouse ire, the focus is more upon the future than upon the present injury. Once the injured person sees he can go on, other people can begin to diminish the effect of the injury.

Dr. Dembo, Dr. Blank, and Mr. Lacey all emphasized the importance of recognizing the values of the evaluator. There is ample evidence that most people view blindness as the greatest disfiguration tragedy that could befall them, while at the same time they consider it not nearly so horrendous as, for example, major facial scars in a loved one.

Dr. S. C. Ashcroft desired information regarding the effect the actual event which caused loss of vision has upon the blinded person. Does a blind veteran, for example, enjoy more "status" than a blind civilian?

Mr. Apple replied that he thought it much less important where the accident happened than how it happened. A soldier, for example, might be blinded during a war while doing something foolish—like going AWOL—and with all his guilt feelings, he might have a more difficult time adjusting than someone who is blinded on his civilian job. An important thing to consider is how responsible you yourself feel for your difficulty.

Mr. Robinson did not quite accept this analysis. He felt that certain situations connote more "respectability" than others.

Miss Forward mentioned a relevant and irritating circumstance: "Everyone always asks when the accident happened; whereas, in many cases there was, of course, no accident at all. It seems more respectable to have had an accident. People don't like to think that other people are sometimes born blind."

Mr. Apple agreed with Dr. Leon Gorlow's summarization that it is useful to realize that the circumstances, whatever form they may take, do make a difference.

Responding to these remarks, Dr. Blank stressed the need for individual attention in all cases of blindness, after the accident; especially since problems of shame, futility, and abandonment may be even more serious than the loss.

"Let's not kid ourselves about the persons who take loss in stride," Dr. Blank warned. "They are actually exercising some kind of pathological reaction to loss, in this case probably *denial.* The *normal* reaction to loss is depression."

Dr. Sussman offered three variables to be considered in studies relating to reaction to loss:

1. A focus on the degree of impairment;
2. A focus on the career stage a person has reached when he suffers the loss; and
3. A focus on the age factor.

But Mrs. Bauman warned researchers against thinking of the circumstances surrounding the loss in terms of a single focus of attention.

Dr. Dembo reminded the participants that when one talks about a "loss" and when one talks about "depression" due to the state of affairs, one is discussing two separate things, and the difference ought to be kept constantly in mind.

Dr. Leon Gorlow, offered a partial summary of the potentially fruitful areas of study discussed: "We ought to be interested in the individual experiences of loss; the impact of the loss on various people; individual differences in grieving; the experience of loss; the prosperity of the handicapped person; individual adaptations; self-perceptions of individuals who suffer insult; the extent of the depression in individuals who suffer loss; the importance of social action; and the importance of funds, programs, and agencies."

COUNSELING

A CONCEPTUAL FRAMEWORK AND RESEARCH APPROACHES FOR EVALUATING COUNSELING

Donald H. Ford and Hugh B. Urban

In many respects it would be difficult to identify an integrated body of knowledge which has been acquired within the counseling domain, primarily because research in this realm has been effected in such different and unconnected ways and settings. In our view, the major factor contributing to the delay in coherent and substantive research in counseling has been the absence of a general conceptual framework to provide a context within which an integrated program of research could be developed. Ideally such a framework would not only represent a general conceptualization for describing and understanding complex human behavior, but also could foster the interrelationship among the behavioral sciences. Its major import for the field of counseling research and practice would be the organization of knowledge from several disciplines concerning complex human behavior, thereby providing a context within which ongoing research and practice in the professional and applied setting could effectively proceed.

A CONCEPTUAL FRAMEWORK

We have spent the last several years seeking to develop such a conceptual framework, since it has been our conviction that effective research in the counseling domain hinges upon a satisfactory conceptualization of the phenomena of concern. We presume this to be true, whether our concern is the modification of emotional problems, the assessment of behavioral efficiency, or the counseling of persons with various classes of motoric or sensory deficits; for the investigator's general theory must identify which of the myriad events to select for study; which relationships are presumed to be of significance; which dimensions he should choose to measure.

Several general themes have guided our efforts. We have sought a formulation which would accommodate the recent findings in areas such as brain function, the role of emotion, the development of language and thought, the human capacity to process and store information from his environment, and social psychology. But we also have been aware of the necessity for casting this information within a developmental context.

For example, in the realm of behavior disorders, it has become apparent that the form which the disordered syndrome eventually assumes is often very different from its origin; that a sequential analysis of this process is required in order to understand the course of pathogenesis. In the area of intellectual capability there is no escape from the recognition that man's subsequent capacity to achieve depends on his prior learning experiences, and that, in very important ways, this is tied in with the maturational schedule. It is therefore not just a question of what he learns, but also the order in which he learns it and when the significant learnings take place with respect to his pattern of development. Similarly, depending upon whether the defects occur in early childhood or in the adult years, differential impact of sensory and motoric disabilities would be expected.

It seems equally apparent that such a conceptualization would have to provide for the fact that human behavior occurs in an organized and integrated fashion. We need to recognize that important interrelationships do take place between man's thoughts and the way he acts. Conceptual frameworks which identify some of these without the others and which represent the human proceeding through time in terms of segmented and linear chains of responses, cannot serve as satisfactory vehicles for the representation of complex human behavior. To cope with these complex organizations of interrelated events, it is necessary to employ a systems framework and a method of systems analysis. For in systems approaches, explicit provision is made for the study of complex patterns of events occurring in organized relationships with one another.

There are, of course, all kinds of systems which surround us in the natural world: completely determined systems and probabilistic systems; open systems and closed systems; complex systems and simple systems. By and large, however, living systems are complex, open, and probabilistic and are capable of modifying their structures, posture, irritability, or movement, depending upon information and energy input from their surroundings.

The human being is a prime example. A satisfactory representation of his mechanisms of hunger, temperature regulation, respiration—in short, all of his vegetative functions—can be accomplished only in terms of feed-back systems. This is equally true of his sensory-motor coordinations, whether they involve the complex patterns of walking, standing erect, or manipulating objects with his hands. And, at the most complex level, the human being is seen as entertaining objectives, selecting courses of action to implement those objectives, obtaining information from his environment relative to the accomplishment of those objectives which is then fed back, permitting him to modify his actions so that they are more likely to achieve his purposes; and on and on it goes.

It seems appropriate, then, to view the human as a self-directing, self-guiding and self-regulating organization of interrelated component subsystems, shaping his environment as he is being shaped by it.

Some General Attributes of a System

What we will seek to do is to provide a grossly simplified overview of the major attributes of such systems in general; then we shall try to show how different aspects of complex human behavior may be considered in such a context. Such a system may be thought of as having five major functional components or subsystems.

1. *A goal setting, guidance, and regulating component.* Any system of this kind requires a component which defines the objectives that the system serves, guides the activity of the system, and evaluates and regulates its performance. A thermostat in a heating system performs these functions in a simple way. Its setting regulates the temperature to be maintained, while its mechanism makes possible some measurement of temperature and the production of electrical signals to adjust the operation of the furnace.

2. *A performance component.* To achieve the objectives of the system, some mechanism is required which can carry out operations related to the objectives of the system. A furnace and its heat distribution system might be considered a simple illustration of a performance element.

3. *An amplifying component.* In most complex systems, the rate and intensity with which the performance element functions must

be flexible to achieve the system objectives in varying circumstances. Variations in the length of time a furnace burns, or in the intensity of the fire, might be considered analogous to this element.

4. *An information collecting component.* To control its performance—and achieve its objectives—such a system must be able to collect information about the consequences of its performance. This information must then be fed back to the regulating element so that the performance can be adjusted in relation to the results being achieved. In a thermostat, this function is frequently performed by a piece of metal which expands or contracts as temperature changes. Within the limits established by the thermostat setting (the objective), this expansion or contraction will turn the furnace on or off.

5. *A domain of consequences.* For every objective of a system, there is a domain of consequences toward which the performance of the system is directed. The eliciting of appropriate consequences provides the information which guides the system's future performance. To continue our simple analogy, the air temperature in a room might be thought of as the consequence toward which the functioning of a heating system is directed.

Every system is composed of a set of structures, interrelated with one another, which provides the basis on which the five functions previously described can be performed. In a furnace, such structures would be illustrated by fuel, a fire box, pipes, and so on. Since the focus of this paper is primarily on functional attributes, little attention will be given to structural considerations, though they are a prerequisite.

Complex Human Behavior as an Open System

With this rather sketchy overview of systems and system components, let us examine the extent to which such a view can be applied to complex human behavior and the degree to which it can render human behavior more intelligible.

GOAL-SETTING, GUIDANCE AND REGULATION—THE COGNITIVE SYSTEM It is not necessary to be a scholar to recognize that man is constantly aware of events which go on around him and the effects of his actions. He analyzes, plans, evaluates, dreams, or loses himself in a stream of reverie. He makes decisions; and he plans and executes complicated courses of action. He communicates information and ideas to others in speech, in writing, and in various forms of artistic expression.

Such complex and varied activities may be extended over long periods of time. They involve actions not only in terms of events present at the moment, but also in terms of past and future events; and they require some kind of behavioral functions which can organize and control, and collect and store information; and which can subsequently retrieve the information and employ it in the guidance of later behavior. These events are ordinarily thought of as falling within the cognitive realm. It is legitimate, therefore, to think in terms of a cognitive system.

Innumerable elements go to make up such a rich and elaborate system of events; so, it will be useful to think in terms of various kinds of cognitive subsystems. Some of these subsystems have to do with the processing, storage, and retrieval of information, often referred to as memory. A good deal of evidence exists, at present, to support the notion that humans innately develop categories of concepts which influence the way future information becomes stored. The utilization of such categories is probably one of the most elementary forms of cognition. It has the advantage of rendering it unnecessary to record each discrete experience separately.

The initial categories are not language categories, but probably represent perceptions which organize sensory information from multiple sources. Obviously, the absence of a particular kind of sensory information (for example, vision) will have a major influence on the concepts formed. In data processing terms, they may be thought of as analogous to a simple program for handling large masses of data. The categories undergo constant revision, with new ones evolving through discrimination and old ones combining through generalization. The general developmental trend seems to be toward increasingly differentiated categories subsumed under larger organizing categories. Soon, further categories become elaborated, representing not merely aggregates of individual units of things, but categories which reflect the interrelationships between things—what leads to what or, more generally, what is related to what. Finally, the role of language becomes involved. Labels become attached to these varying categories, facilitating the individual's capacity to manipulate them in his thinking. He communicates them to others, acquiring new categories through the medium of language and the like.

Some of these categories become organized as symbolic representations of anticipated events. They may be simple or complex. This category of thoughts is of basic importance because it represents the directing element in human behavior. What people represent to themselves as desirable become the objectives toward which they aspire. And it is in terms of such objectives that they will subsequently evaluate their performance. A special group of such thoughts are those self-defining conceptions which characterize the kind of person one wants to be. These seem to have a special controlling force in eliciting behaviors directed toward developing or maintaining that representation of one's self.

A third category of thoughts can be regarded as primarily evaluative. The thoughts in these categories perform a regulatory function because they carry the task of judging the difference between the initial goal-setting criterion and the information from the person's efforts which indicates how close to the goal he actually has succeeded in arriving.

Of particular note with regard to these self-evaluative types of thought is the way in which they are so intimately related to emotional patterns. Judgments of oneself as able or ineffectual, competent or worthless, tend to engender powerful emotional patterns in the person himself—patterns which are especially significant in the business of counseling.

We should emphasize that the impact upon the person's cognitive capability (the categories of thoughts he has acquired, the strategies of thinking he has developed, and the evaluative attitudes he has already developed) of a significant physical handicap such as blindness or cerebral stroke, will vary tremendously depending on the point in his developmental course when the deficit takes place.

PERFORMANCE—THE TRANSACTIONAL SYSTEM It seems obvious that man's capacity to move around in, and physically to manipulate, his environment is fundamental to his survival and to his entire social structure. Because of his motor capabilities he is not solely dependent upon conditions as he encounters them, but can actively shape and modify his physical environment to render it more favorable to himself and his objectives. One of man's most important capabilities is his capacity to communicate information to others through speech and writing. The reverse is represented by the living helplessness of the human in whom this capability has been eliminated. This is apparent in persons who have suffered some cerebral assault—a stroke, for example—which has destroyed the functioning of the motor systems. Such a person survives through the efforts of others to keep him alive by protecting and feeding him, and, in effect, substituting their motor capabilities for his.

The developmental course of the growing human can be represented in terms of increasingly elaborate and increasingly protracted patterns of motor performance—the aroused habit patterns whose subsequent articulation is guided by the cognitive system as it organizes and utilizes information collected by the senses.

AMPLIFICATION—THE AROUSAL SYSTEM Human behavior is characterized by an impressive variability in degree of arousal and level of activity. A person may be lethargic or excited. These varying degrees of emotionality and physical activity would appear to be a pervasive and fundamental element in human behavior and are often recognized as having great adaptive significance. It is supposed that these two major factors—emotional arousal and activity level—may well rest upon some common physiological substratum; but from a functional standpoint they seem to operate somewhat separately and thus are often thought of as somewhat distinct patterns of events.

A great deal of relatively new information has been acquired in recent years concerning the operation of what are typically called "the emotional states." First of all, habits of emotional responding seem to be acquired only in an alerted organism. In many respects, emotional patterns represent, on the one hand, an amplification or augmentation of an existing state of awareness or, conversely, a diminution or attenuation of that state of awareness. The elevation and depression of other sets of behaviors by the operation of emotions can be seen in many ways. There is considerable evidence to suggest, for example, that moderate emotional arousal facilitates performance (as when a football team is "up" for a game) and renders the person more alert, sharpens his attention and increases the efficiency of his processing and storing of experiential events (that is, his learning).

There is also evidence, however, that in excessive emotional arousal (such as in panic states or explosive anger) there tends to be a general disruption of cognitive activity and an interference with smoothly coordinated and controlled learning and motor performance. Moreover, different emotional states appear to have differing consequences. Some, such as fear and anxiety, augment and amplify signal and motor output; others, such as depression and apathy, serve to diminish or to attenuate these factors. Interestingly, there appears to be major individual differences at birth in the biological systems which sustain these emotional patterns; and the excitation or restriction of a particular response is strongly modified by learning.

Much evidence has been accumulated to demonstrate that whether a person responds emotionally will be determined by the construction he puts upon the situation which he encounters—whether he sees it as dangerous, attractive, disgusting, or thwarting. The occurrence of these patterns depends upon the meanings a person attaches to events and his perceptual interpretation of them. Thus they are importantly tied in with his cognitive structures.

As a person develops, he gradually becomes less sensitive to stimuli which earlier elicited emotional patterns. As a result, a given situation may no longer arouse any emotion, or may arouse only an abbreviated pattern. Thus, development normally leads to an increasing mastery of situations, a lessening of their emotional impact, and increasing control over emotions. On the other hand, people can acquire exquisite sensitivities to certain sets of events or situations; and the nature and extent of certain kinds of emotional arousal tend to grow as these persons develop. Deficient patterns of control over such emotional states, or inappropriate methods of coping with them once they have become instigated, often lead to the need for the counselor's services.

We spoke earlier of the factor of varying levels of energy expenditure. We can remind ourselves that, from hour to hour, the amount of physical effort which we expend can vary considerably. It is supposed that such variations result from a behavioral arrangement in which the level of activity necessary is determined centrally by our intentions as to what we want to perform (objectives) and our perceptions as to what will be involved. The degree of activity (arousal) is determined by the degree of effort required by the situation as *interpreted* by the individual. This is humorously exemplified by the person who tries to lift a heavy box and nearly falls over backward because the effort exerted turns out to be entirely inappropriate to raise what proves to be an empty box. Of course, variations in the amplitude of response (whether the person speaks, calls, or shouts) will be dictated by the integrity of the physiological substratum upon which the behavior depends. If underlying biochemical and metabolic processes have gone awry (as in thyroid deficiency, or in an attack of influenza) the degree of amplification which is possible will have been considerably attenuated.

INFORMATION COLLECTION—THE SENSORY SYSTEM None of the foregoing systems are completely self contained. Their successful functioning depends upon continual inputs of energy and information from outside the systems. Just as the vegetative subsystems cease to function in the absence of the relevant inputs of oxygen, water, or food, it can now be demonstrated that the human behavioral systems will slowly subside and come to a halt if they are deprived of a continuous sensory input.

This informational supply, however, is not only necessary to maintain the operating capability of the systems in general, but also —and particularly—to permit the completion of goal-directed behavior. The motor subsystems cannot function without feedback information about their performance. In any motor activity, there must be steady feedback in order to maintain the coordination and direction of that activity. Feedback through the eyes guides the hand in its efforts to pick up a desired object. Feedback through the ears tells the pianist when he "strikes a sour note." Feedback through the kinesthetic and vestibular sensory mechanisms are necessary to maintain body balance and to coordinate postural movements.

Successful transaction with the environment, then, requires systems to act upon the environment; but in addition it requires information collection systems to provide the data for judging the performance. Sensory reception is a key element in the selection and guidance of a line of behavior an organism may follow. It provides the current news which can be "compared" with stored information resulting in further modified effort.

DOMAINS OF CONSEQUENCES—THE ENVIRONMENTAL SYSTEMS Behavior does not occur in a vacuum. Behavior is a function of the situations under which it occurs. In the past, efforts have been made to account for human behavior purely in terms of the traits the person might have acquired, the type of personality which he appeared to represent, or the need structure which he seemed to have developed. In a number of respects, however, the interrelationships between situational occurrences and the individual's behavior are so importantly operative that a satisfactory account of the situational factors is essential to the understanding of human functioning.

Studies of stimulus deprivation reveal that, if an individual is deprived of all external stimulation for an extended period of time, cognitive functioning declines toward disorganization, impoverishment, and frequently complete suspension and sleep. And the arousal system, whose variability is controlled by the cognitive system, obviously depends upon external stimulation.

The situational events which take place in relation to our selected lines of action represent a set of consequences which influence how we subsequently perform. They provide the circumstances which dictate whether the actions are retained within our repertoire as an effective way to accomplish the objective, or whether they become discontinued and others are selected in their place. Most of the present theories of learning assume that it is the situational consequences of behavior which influence the acquisition and maintenance of certain behaviors in preference to others (for example, the concept of reinforcements).

It is useful to think of situational events in two categories. The first represents the physical environment within which a person behaves. Most attributes of the physical environment tend to be relatively stable and predictable and, therefore, somewhat easier to cope with, though eliciting what one wants from the physical environment may be quite difficult. The second category is the social environment. The family context, the extended family, the neighborhood, schools, churches, and clubs illustrate the growing variety of social contexts which exercise socializing forces as an individual develops from infancy to maturity to old age. In particular, the social attitudes—the evaluations by other people—have a special force in shaping a person's behavior, and some theorists (for example, Carl Rogers) have been so impressed with this that they have seen self-evaluations learned from others as the root of all emotional disorder.

While the physical environment is reasonably predictable, the human environment is highly unpredictable. Denied adequate data through some sensory deficit like blindness, the person will find the usual unpredictability of the social environment compounded by his inability to collect what data are available for judging what is happening.

Situational consequences function to produce variability in behavior patterns as well as to create stable habits. Behaviors acquired in one situation may not be effective in another. For example, a child may have learned that by screaming, crying, and pounding his head on the floor, he could get his parents to do what he wanted at home. In school he is likely to utilize this same behavior pattern on a new adult figure. However, it will probably prove ineffective, thus disrupting an old behavior pattern and requiring the development of a new one. Changing situational contexts are one of the major forces in the development and modification of behavior patterns as the individual matures and ages. Human behavior is constantly changing, both because an individual's response capabilities change, and because the situational contexts which confront him change.

Complex Behavior in Natural Settings

We shall complete this sketchy summary view by emphasizing that the various components of human behavior operate in carefully interrelated fashion in their natural settings. Here is a simple example: The objective of a good performance on a science examination tomorrow may temporarily dominate a student's behavior. Between now and tomorrow, that objective may influence the amount of time he spends with his friends, what he eats and when he eats, how much and how well he sleeps, what he reads, what he listens to, and what he talks about. Every realm of behavior may be coordinated toward the goal of achieving a good grade on the examination. Therefore, a counselor and a researcher concerned with complex human behavior must understand not only the components of an individual's behavior patterns but also how these components are coordinated and what objectives that coordination is serving in particular kinds of situations.

The complicating factor in accomplishing this kind of understanding is that complex human behavior may be, and usually is, directed toward several consequences simultaneously. It is a characteristic which contributes to the great efficiency and effectiveness of human behavior. A given behavior pattern, therefore, may achieve some but not all of the consequences toward which it is directed. An important function of the cognitive system is its role in determining what proportion of the consequences sought will be accepted as complete performance. This concept of multiple determination is present in a variety of psychological theories and was a fundamental psychoanalytic concept. It explains why a behavior pattern may continue in the face of apparent failure. Complex human behavior must be thought of as occurring through time. The person's behavior is reshaped through successive approximations toward the consequences which it seeks.

Blindness as a Deficit and its Consequences

Blindness is only one behavioral deficiency that human beings can experience. In that sense, the study of blindness and its consequences should be seen in the context of the general study of behavior disorders in human beings. Some of the effects of blindness on behavioral systems have much in common with effects produced by other kinds of deficiencies.

DEFICIT IN AN INFORMATION COLLECTION COMPONENT In its simplest terms, blindness represents a deficiency in only one component of human behavioral systems. Its significance is that it denies the person certain kinds of informational feedback essential for guiding behavior, and that it requires a search for substitute or correlated sources of information. We might expect such a deficit to have an impact on every other component in the behavioral system and we shall seek to trace what those impacts might be.

It should be noted that blindness as a deficit may vary in degree from total blindness to partial sightedness, and the degree of deficit may be a factor in the coordinated functioning of the system components. Also, it is important to recognize that this information collection component is an integrated part of the total system, and blindness may be correlated with other deficits such as neurological damage and cerebral palsy. The consequences of blindness may be multiplied if coupled with another sensory deficit.

Finally, it must be emphasized that the developmental stage in which the deficit occurs probably makes a major difference. A person who is blind from birth never has had any visual imagery. In contrast, the person who is sighted until the age of thirty years and then loses his vision will have a very rich store of visual imagery available from his past learnings. He will have ideas about himself and his competencies which may require major changes because of this new deficiency. On the other hand, the person who is blind from birth must initially build a concept of himself and his competencies which acknowledges the deficiency with which he was born.

IMPLICATIONS FOR THE COGNITIVE SYSTEM A person who has acquired some degree of visual imagery before the loss of sight probably has considerable advantage over a person with no visual imagery, because he can think in terms of his remembered representations of events and situations, rather than having to think by analogy in terms of auditory imagery or tactual imagery. Such a deficit will have an influence on the thoughts which a person develops about the goals that may be feasible for him to seek. Since such thoughts are a guiding force in the behaviors a person will seek to perform, their formation is crucial. Similarly, the thoughts and styles of thinking that a person develops about how to achieve goals are likely to be influenced by blindness. The recognition that certain kinds of informational feedback are not available, that certain kinds of situations are too unpredictable without such feedback, that people react differently to blindness, and so forth, will place definite limitations on the kinds of plans that a person evolves to achieve his objectives. Self-evaluations may be powerfully influenced.

The attitudes and expectations that the blind person acquires concerning the reactions of others also are important cognitive developments. Does he come to believe that others see him as inadequate, prefer not to be in his company because they are embarrassed by his deficiency, are laughing at him behind his back, are unwilling to give him an opportunity to do significant work? Expectations of the attitudes of other people and how they will react, powerfully control the way a blind person chooses to perform in social situations.

IMPLICATIONS FOR THE TRANSACTIONAL SYSTEM As was noted earlier, performance or instrumental behavior is guided by sensory feedback. Denial of visual feedback may prohibit some performances, such as playing baseball, and will reduce proficiency in many other performances. A person may have motor capabilities and even the habits from past learnings for carrying out certain kinds of activities. Unless appropriate informational feedback can be arranged in the kind of situation in which he will have to perform, he cannot utilize those capabilities. A problem for a blind person, therefore, is not only the acquisition of skills but, perhaps more importantly, the development of sources of information with which those skills can be used in practical situations.

Spatially oriented behaviors are among the most important transactions that blindness reduces in efficiency. The ability to travel alone is a motor capability highly valued by blind people and not easy to acquire. It is relatively easy to develop this capability in an environment which is stable and predictable, such as the living room of his home. However, traveling outside the home places the blind person in an environment filled with people, making that environment highly unpredictable. For a blind person to be able to travel alone, he must develop substitutes for information collection in order to observe and predict relevant changes in the environment. Dogs and canes are the most frequent substitutes; but their limitations are well known.

The performance of work skills is significantly influenced by the lack of visual feedback. For example, eye–hand coordination appears to be essential for a person to work with a moving object if the movement is not in a standard and routine sequence of patterns. It is difficult, therefore, for a blind person to compete with a sighted person in some work skills, although compensating feedback may make possible effective competition in others. For example, a blind person would have difficulty becoming a skilled surgeon; with appropriate talents, however, he might equal a sighted person in musical accomplishments. Probably the reason why blind people emphasize the value of getting a good education is that education decreases the importance of visual motor activities and increases the importance of cognitive and verbal skills which, in their performance, are not so seriously handicapped by the lack of visual feedback.

Social relationships with others are formed and regulated by the reactions of others. What people say and what they do, do not always coincide. It is difficult for a blind person to evaluate his impact on others—and his own appearance—without information about the other person's expression, gestures and the like. This lack also hinders some kinds of shared activities or at least makes them seem more difficult for blind persons.

IMPLICATIONS FOR THE AROUSAL SYSTEM The absence of vision will deny a person certain kinds of information which would lead to emotional arousal in a sighted person. If a person cannot see the car bearing down upon him, he can have no fear reaction. If he cannot see the smile of approval, he cannot experience the satisfaction of acceptance in response to it. Thus, emotional reactions to environmental emergencies and rewards may be seriously attenuated.

Furthermore, the absence of appropriate information may be a source of unfounded fears. This has been found to be true in a great variety of human disorders and certainly seems appropriate in blindness. When a person cannot see what is happening around him, he must interpret what he hears and feels; and he may fear that a mistake in interpretation will lead to dire consequences.

On the other hand, positive emotions and hope about the future are essential for constructive activity in accommodating a deficiency such as blindness. Positive emotions are related to the way a person thinks about himself, his deficiency, the consequences of his efforts, others' reactions and the like. Emotions affect thoughts as thoughts affect emotions.

IMPLICATION FOR INFORMATION SYSTEMS When a person loses one kind of sensory information, he tends to become more skillful at noticing and utilizing other information that sighted people often ignore. This skill is probably trainable, as illustrated in the training of blind people to read through touch.

The alternative is to develop technological devices which extend the capabilities of the modalities remaining intact. The cane, the dog, and the tape recorder all illustrate such extensions. It might be possible to use radar or laser technology (or technologies not yet developed) to pick up information about spatial arrangements and other complicated environmental activities and translate them into vibrations or sounds which a person could use to guide his behavior. As knowledge of brain functions advances, it may not be unreasonable to think of devices which can stimulate visual images in the brain despite the fact that the visual apparatus itself is inoperative.

IMPLICATIONS FOR ENVIRONMENTAL SYSTEMS The blind person's environment is not the same as that of a sighted person although his physical environment is generally the same. Much more could be done, we believe, in the design of our physical environment to make it serve both handicapped and non-handicapped persons.

It is the blind person's social environment that is definitely different from that of a sighted person. People react differently to a handicapped person, such as a blind individual, than they do to an ordinary person. A variety of studies have revealed that this fact is of major importance to blind people. They must struggle to overcome the curiosity, overprotection, or rejection of those around them. Thus, effective efforts with a blind person may require working with the significant people in his social environment, such as his family members.

COMPLICATIONS CUMULATE IN A SYSTEM It is important to emphasize again that the various components described above function in interrelated fashion. This means that a development in one component may have consequences for the interrelated functioning of all other components. For example, a blind person may develop certain kinds of thoughts about his deficiency and about his capability for future achievement. These thoughts may arouse anticipatory fears about future activity, produce loss of hope and, in turn, lead to a restriction of effort to accomplish tasks and to learn new things. This restriction will produce consequences which tend to confirm the blind person's view of himself as inadequate and incapable of accomplishment—consequences such as the loss of friends who become discouraged at his unwillingness to become involved in shared activities. These consequences may produce further thoughts about how unsatisfactory the world is, and how helpless he is within it. These thoughts may further decrease his hopes for the future and produce a growing unwillingness to try new things; and so the cycle continues.

The other side of the coin is that a change in one component in the total system may have consequences for the operation of the total system. If a counselor can help a person change the way he thinks about himself, the person's fears may decline, his hopes may increase and he may begin to try new activities and seek to learn new things; and then he will produce different reactions from his environment which further encourage him. Also, a counselor may attenuate a person's fears and elict more positive emotions which, in turn, will influence the way he interprets things, changing what he tries to do, and so forth.

Counseling the Blind

By now it should be apparent that counseling the blind, or anyone else, requires careful specification of the counseling objectives. Different counseling procedures are appropriate for different objectives. There is an unfortunate tendency to assume that counseling is one thing when, in fact, it is a great variety of things. Without careful specification, the differences will be obscured and the impact of counseling efforts attenuated. Some illustrations of differences in objectives may be useful.

COUNSELING OBJECTIVES VARY A frequent focus in counseling is to help a person change his self-evaluations. Among things which can keep a person from living a full life are the judgments he has acquired about himself. For example, he may think he is a failure, that the things he does are unimportant, that he is unlikable, or that he is incapable of improving in the future. In contrast, the person who lives a full and rich life usually has confidence in himself. He evaluates himself positively, he expects to do worthwhile things and expects others to see him the same way. Very often these self-evaluations are related to emotional responses: a fear, or anger, or affection which may interfere or facilitate certain kinds of behavior. The nondirective counseling procedures developed by Carl Rogers are focused primarily upon the modification of such evaluative habits.

Changes in attitudes toward, and relationships with, others is another focus of some counseling efforts. The formulation of educational objectives and the development of plans for acquiring certain knowledge and skills through education frequently is the focus of educational counseling. The formulation of career objectives and plans for obtaining employment are usual focuses of vocational counseling. These illustrations should suffice to show that counseling can have a variety of objectives and that research on counseling must carefully specify its goals.

COUNSELING PROCEDURES VARY Moreover, counselors use a variety of procedures that may have varying effects. For example, talking to a person in certain ways may affect the way he thinks about things. This is a major tool in counseling. It is important, however, to recognize that conversation has, as its direct effect, changes in the way the other person thinks and talks. It does not directly produce changes in other response capabilities such as motor skills. On the other hand, if the way a person thinks is changed, he may begin to act differently. Social imitation, social modeling, or demonstration also are procedures that have some value. The ordinary person has always known that children imitate their elders, and that a good way to teach is to demonstrate. To some extent, counselees model their behavior after that of their counselors. This may be why the counseling of blind persons by blind persons can have a greater impact than counseling by a sighted person.

"Reinforcement" is still another way to affect behavior patterns. This term simply means the manipulation of the consequences which follow behavior. The basic strategy requires identifying the behavior pattern desired and then identifying the existing behavior pattern that might be shaped in that direction. It involves a set of consequences that can be applied when behavior moves in a desired direction and the sequence in which the shaping of the behavior pattern can be accomplished. People utilizing these procedures sometimes call themselves behavioral counselors or behavioral therapists.

One way to influence behavior patterns is to place a person in a completely different environment. This may elicit a different pattern or a new one; or, possibly, an old pattern may return which works more effectively. Placement in a different school or a foster home or even "taking a vacation" illustrate common procedures for effecting behavioral changes. "Rehearsal" is still another procedure. It requires the person to practice a behavior pattern, progressively trying to contribute to the consequences that he wishes to achieve. Rehearsal is usually combined with some other procedure such as social modeling. Then the behaviors practiced are illustrated by someone else.

COUNSELING DIFFERS FROM TEACHING AND TRAINING It may be important to recognize certain distinctions between counseling and teaching or training. Counseling focuses primarily on interrelationships among cognitive and arousal systems. The assumption is that the way a person thinks and feels guides and regulates how he behaves. But effective behavior often requires training in performing the responses as well as in developing plans—and a willingness to do so. Effective performance usually requires certain kinds of knowledge, tools of learning and skills whose acquisition requires procedures and learning settings characteristically thought of as related to teaching and training rather than counseling. The counselor should be able to help people determine how to arrange for such teaching and training.

Research on Counseling the Blind

Our purpose here is to discuss only research that is related to counseling the blind. This perspective suggests several generalizations which might serve as guides.

USE GENERAL RESEARCH ON HUMAN BEHAVIOR First, it should be apparent that research on counseling the blind can and should build upon a much broader base of research. We should not look at research on blind people only; research on many other samples of behaviors and subjects have considerable relevance to the understanding of work with the blind. For example, research on attitude change, self-concept formation, the reactions of amputees to their handicaps, and so forth, may have much to say which will help us understand blind people and their efforts to lead a meaningful life.

The most effective research will be accomplished by recognizing the relevance of the work going on in a variety of settings. An example from social psychology on the development of attitudes may help illustrate this point:

Evidence is accumulating that the determinants of positive versus negative evaluation of an object, event, or behavior are significantly related to the attitudes a person forms in relation to his objectives. If an objective is viewed positively, things related to or instrumental in achieving that objective tend also to be viewed positively and vice-versa. By extrapolation, we might suggest that blindness is a barrier —a real barrier—to the accomplishment of certain classes of objectives. Therefore, it should follow that a blind person would be expected to have a negative attitude toward his blindness since it is a real obstruction. Moreover, this negative attitude may become related to anything the person views as correlated with his blindness—certain behaviors of those around him, for example. In addition, blind people, like other people, may over-generalize; and the blind person may not only develop a rejecting attitude toward his blindness, but may come to develop a rejecting attitude toward himself entirely. A book by Goldstein, Heller, and Sechrist, *Psychotherapy and Psychology of Behavior Change* (1966), represents one of the few serious attempts in recent years to go through a variety of literature and abstract those ideas and findings which might be relevant to the modification of human behavior using counseling and psychotherapeutic procedures. Much more of this work needs to be done by persons seeking to do research on counseling in all settings, including counseling of the blind.

CAREFUL SPECIFICATION ESSENTIAL Clearly, research on counseling requires careful specification of the events being studied. As we have illustrated, the term "counseling" can refer to a great variety of procedures with a great variety of objectives. Research focused on questions such as whether the client has "improved" or "not improved" will be of little use. Research focused on specific changes that can be accomplished and specific procedures for that purpose is likely to be of long-term significance. The researcher must also specify the counseling procedures used to accomplish the counseling objectives.

CRITERIA The researcher must also specify the criteria which he will use to evaluate whether the consequences have been achieved and whether the procedures identified were the source of the change. If these criteria are not carefully selected so that we can be sure they are related to the behavioral changes sought and the procedures used, the research will be of little consequence. This kind of research is very complicated, and, too often, it may become shaped by the use of readily available criteria and measures rather than through the selection of the most important ones.

RESEARCH METHODOLOGIES Finally, we see no need for developing special types of research methodologies. It seems to us that methodologies evolved for use in similar settings, such as the evaluation of psychotherapy or the study of speech and hearing problems, should be readily applicable, with minor modifications, to research on counseling with the blind. Of course, there may be special measurement problems involved in this research; but the kinds of designs that can be used—the principles of statistical analysis which are most applicable, the "rules of the game" that need to be observed—are not specific to research on the blind. Since most workers in this domain are unlikely to be highly sophisticated theorists in experimental design and mathematical statistics, we recommend that they use statistical consultants to help them insure that the design and method of analysis which they have selected is appropriate to their data. Such consultants should be used in the planning stages of the research, not after the data have been collected.

RESEARCH APPROACHES TO EVALUATING COUNSELING

In the first part of this paper, a conceptual framework for evaluating counseling was summarized. This second section will examine some examples of such research and discuss some of the methodological problems involved.

The person interested in research on counseling and psychotherapy will find four books very helpful in illustrating a great variety of research designs, variables, measurement procedures, statistical analyses, and rationales. In addition, they identify many of the theoretical and methodological problems involved in such research. Goldstein and Dean[12] included 63 papers in their book. The papers are divided into eleven groups; research philosophies, ethical issues, problems of experimental design, measurement, criterion problems, spontaneous remission, time dimensions, therapist or counselor variables, patient or client variables, relationship variables, and interview and verbal conditioning models.

Stollak, Guerney, and Rothberg[27] focus on articles that appear to have particular value for stimulating future research. In addition, they include articles representing a variety of approaches such as individual and group counseling, child treatment, family therapy, client-centered and behavior therapy and they try to illustrate the various experimental designs and methodologies that represent current research approaches. Gottschalk and Auerbach[14] present 34 different papers. After discussing general goals and problems of research, they present several papers discussing theoretical and practical problems associated with the process of data collection (for example, the use of sound films). This is followed by a section in which several papers discuss problems of data analysis and various theoretical models that may be used to guide such research. Finally, they present seven papers which discuss the effects or outcomes of treatment procedures. Ford and Urban[10] reviewed the literature on counseling and psychotherapy published between April 1965 and April 1966. These four publications, which present or summarize nearly 300 relevant articles and books, provide a good starting point for anyone considering doing research on counseling psychotherapy. In addition, the *Journal of Counseling Psychology* published by the American Psychological Association is the best single journal for relevant articles.

Careful Specification of Variables Is Essential

Far too much research on counseling and psychotherapy does not define the variables involved in terms specific enough to make evaluation possible. Two recent studies are illustrative.

Volsky and colleagues[28] report a ten-year project which is a model of careful design and psychometric sophistication, but it yielded few differences arising as a function of counseling and psychotherapy interviews. They studied 100 subjects—80 in an experimental group and 20 in a control group. All subjects experienced a sophisticated program of pretesting before counseling began. The experimental subjects were counseled and the control group was placed on a "waiting list." All subjects received post-tests 30 days after the experimental group completed counseling. Then the "wait" group was offered counseling.

There were no significant results. Why? Several typical faulty assumptions were made. Implicit was the assumption that all clients received the same treatment—"counseling." This is undoubtedly not true. Each counselor-client pair probably talked about different things in different ways, in different sequences, and for different lengths of time. Studies of actual protocols of interviews in many other studies consistently reveal such variability. Even where careful attempts are made to train counselors to provide the same treatment, considerable variability remains.[2] Second, it was assumed that the same changes would occur in all clients. The three major dependent variables were manifest anxiety, defensiveness, and problem-solving effectiveness.

Counseling was expected to reduce anxiety and defensive behavior, and to increase the ability to solve problems in all subjects. But clients' problems and characteristics are different. One client may be very anxious and another not concerned enough. The effect desired might be to decrease the anxiety in one and increase it to motivating levels in the other. If counseling proved effective, the subjects' scores would move in opposite directions and if averaged, the changes would cancel one another out, obscuring the changes that actually occurred. Third, they assumed that the changes would manifest themselves in the same way in all clients. For example, their measure of anxiety was a self-report inventory. However, clinical experience and some research indicate that different persons reveal their anxiety in different ways.[19] Changes in manifest anxiety may occur in a particular person, but may not be revealed in a self-report inventory. This critical analysis is not intended to minimize the efforts of this group of able scholars. Their study is one of the most sophisticated reported in the literature. But it serves to illustrate several rather telling faults which are found in much of the counseling literature. Much more careful specification is essential if counseling research is to be worthwhile.

Another long-term expensive study by Stieper and Wiener[26] on male veterans treated in a clinic in Minnesota demonstrates even more the glaring deficiencies which stem from inadequate specification. Their sample included a wide range of clients with a great diversity of problems which were lumped together in the study—a heterogeneity of counseling or therapy approaches which were unspecified and ignored in the study—and these approaches were aimed at producing a great variety of changes in the clients which were also unspecified. They were interested in "improvement," an impossibly vague criterion.

Kinds of Variables on which Counseling May Focus

Krumboltz[20] argued that the goals of counseling should be stated as those specific behavior changes desired by each client, compatible with the counselor's values, and which are also externally observable. His listing of examples is useful in illustrating how one can become far more specific about the goals of counseling. Without such specification, one cannot select the counseling approach most effective in achieving the desired result. Hill and colleagues[16] studied observable variables (grades and graduation rates) but made the mistake of assuming all the counseling was focused on these objectives. They compared 479 counseled students with matched controls. They found no differences. Probably some of the counseling focused on grades; some probably focused on emotional disturbances; some focused on difficulties with parents; and some focused on interpersonal problems —to cite only a few of the probable concerns. One should expect a particular counseling procedure to affect only those behaviors on which it is specifically focused.

Moreover, in complex situations, many factors are simultaneously operating, and it is difficult to attribute changes to one factor out of many. For example, Ford and Urban[9] present data to show a major decrease in the number of students dropped for poor scholarship, and an increase in the number achieving Dean's list averages during an eight-year span following the implementation of an extensive counseling program in a major university. But, they point out, one cannot attribute these changes solely to counseling. Many other changes took place in the same period. The university underwent a major academic reorganization. The academic calendar was changed, requiring most courses and examinations to be rewritten. The admission standards changed. Such multiple causation is probably the rule in individual cases as well as in programmatic evaluations.

Finally, we would suggest that when a researcher decides to study a particular counseling approach as it affects specified kinds of responses, he should familiarize himself with what is known about that category of behavior. Good applied research can build upon basic knowledge. For example, counseling research focused on affective behavior can draw considerable background knowledge from a book by Cofer and Appley.[5] Graham's book[15] on visual perception and Dember's book[7] on the psychology of perception are useful resources for the counselor concerned with such behaviors. A book by Cohen[6] on attitude change and social influence provides a useful review of research on attitude change. Goldstein, Heller, and Sechrest provide a useful example of how hypotheses for research on counseling and psychotherapy may be drawn from the basic literature of social psychology.

If examined closely, much counseling research can be seen to be implicitly focused upon one of several response systems which go to make up complex human behavior. By making such objectives explicit on the one hand, and more specific on the other, it becomes possible to identify more precisely (1) those aspects of behavior which are being dealt with, and (2) the range of research in the basic disciplines which becomes immediately relevant. A few examples will be cited to illustrate this point, and to exemplify some of the problems.

COGNITIVE RESPONSES Cognitive responses form the realm upon which more counseling research has been focused than any other. The way people think about themselves, their self-concepts and habits of self-evaluation, the plans they make, the decisions they reach, and the explanations they give themselves for their own and others' behavior, have been of great interest to counseling researchers since these seem to be responses which guide other behaviors. Goldstein[13] summarized many studies concerning the role of the client and the counselor's expectancies in the progress of psychotherapy or counseling. In general, he concluded that what clients anticipate will happen influences what they do and how they interpret what does happen. Confirmation or nonconfirmation of their expectations affects subsequent affective and cognitive behavior. His review is instructive for anyone interested in counseling focused on this category of responses.

Hills and Williams[17] reported a study focused on client self-evaluations. Their clients received brief educational-vocational counseling. Forty-five clients received written interpretations of a battery of test results after their first interview. Forty other clients did not receive such information. Client self-descriptions were obtained before and after counseling. The investigators concluded that the effect of receiving test information in this context appeared to be either negligible or detrimental depending on the degree of consonance between the test findings and the client's expectations and goals. However, no evidence is provided as to the relative permanence of this change or its effects on other behaviors. Still another example of a focus on cognitive responses is reported in a study by Ryan and Krumboltz.[23] Their subjects were 60 male college students, randomly assigned to two counselors and three treatment groups. They were interested in increasing the frequency with which clients weighed alternatives, considered possibilities or deliberated about outcomes in terms of probability of success with reference to educational and vocational planning, and the extent to which clients made decisions about a course of action, or eliminated some alternative. The counselor sought to increase deliberation responses in one group by saying things which would lead the client to consider such questions. Decision responses were encouraged in the second group by raising questions about decisions to be made and related contingencies. In the third group, no such focus was provided. They found they could increase such responses in clients by focusing on them. This same phenomenon was demonstrated by Rogers[22] almost two decades ago within a different theoretical rationale. A client will think about and talk about the topics to which the counselor directs his attention, even when the client is not particularly aware of the bias the counselor is giving to the conversation. There is relatively little evidence, however, about the extent to which such temporary changes in the counselor's office carries over into other life situations.

Dreiblatt and Weatherley[8] examined the relative effects of discussing client symptoms (implicitly confirming their role as an ill or handicapped person) in contrast to talking with them as people with human problems and human concerns. They reported consistent superiority for the latter techniques in producing positive changes in self-concept, among other things.

As indicated by a survey study reported by Bauman,[4] the way blind people think about themselves and their competencies, their self-evaluations, their expectations about the reactions of other people, the goals they establish for themselves, and the way they go about planning to achieve those goals, are all questions of considerable importance in the adjustment to blindness. Such thought patterns apparently influence the education they will seek, their employment preferences and the jobs they will accept, their willingness and ability to travel, their recreation patterns, and their social activities.

TRANSACTIONAL BEHAVIORS The ways in which people behave toward their natural and social environment to achieve their goals and satisfactions is another category of behavior on which counseling may focus. For example, Williams[29] sought to eliminate tantrum behavior in a small boy. The child enforced some of his wishes, especially at bedtime, by unleashing this behavior to control the actions of his parents. The child would scream, cry, and fuss unless the parents stayed in the bedroom and paid attention to him. These transactions often lasted for two hours at each bedtime. By changing the procedures used in preparing the child for bed and for putting him to bed, the pattern of tyrant-like behavior was fairly rapidly extinguished. Adults use more sophisticated procedures to control others, and a handicap is frequently a person's greatest asset in getting others to do what he wants. Our culture shows great sympathy for individuals who are ill or handicapped. Study of such patterns and how they can be changed could be of considerable importance.

Another kind of transactional behavior that receives a good deal of attention is school performance. A study by Winkler, Teigland, Munger, and Kranzler[30] is illustrative. They were interested in the effects of selected counseling and remedial techniques on underachieving elementary school students. They selected 121 fourth grade students whose grades were lower than one would expect of them on the basis of IQ scores. They were randomly assigned to one of five experimental conditions: individual counseling, group counseling, reading instruction, Hawthorne-Effect, and control. The counseling was done by six male counselors, each with at least a master's degree. They concluded that none of the approaches produced a significant improvement in grades and that underachievement is not a surface phenomenon which is easily modified. Similar results have been found in studies at the secondary school level.[25] To put it differently, the reasons students do poorly in school will differ from student to student. No single counseling procedure can cope with all of these varied conditions. Careful diagnosis and selection of appropriate procedures is essential. Social behaviors are transactional patterns of considerable importance, and researchers interested in this topic will find the work of Bandura and Walters[3] of considerable interest.

AFFECTIVE SYSTEM Moderate degrees of affect seem to facilitate many kinds of behavior. Excessive degrees seem to interfere. Counselors are concerned with these phenomena in two ways. The emotions which occur during counseling interviews may facilitate or interfere with the counseling itself. Moderate positive emotions seem to be related to increased trust in the counselor, a willingness to try harder to deal with the questions under consideration, and greater frankness in discussing all the factors involved. Mild negative emotions may have some of the same effects. However, intense positive or negative emotions may occur and must be modified as a step in the counseling process. Second, emotional reactions in life situations such as school, work, or family may be a barrier to more effective functioning. Thus, some counseling is focused on helping clients learn how to control their emotional reactions in such situations.

Anderson[1] reports a detailed study of one case counseled with client-centered procedures. Changes in heart responses were used as his measure of emotionality. He found that there were positive and significant relationships between the trends in a client's emotional and cognitive behavior during client-centered psychotherapy. Isaacs and Haggard[18] report a group of studies which suggest that the development of a certain level of affective capacity is a significant prerequisite for participation by patients in insight therapies.

Phobias are generally considered to be avoidance response patterns. Elimination of a phobia seems to involve the elimination of a fear response to the phobic stimulus. Thus, counseling may be focused on changing a fear pattern in a situation outside the counseling setting. Patterson[21] presents a detailed report of the treatment of a seven-year-old boy in whom a school phobia was eliminated in ten hours of counseling time. Each of these three studies illustrates that where affective changes are a focus of counseling, or are a condition for effective counseling, direct attention to them is important.

ENVIRONMENTAL SYSTEMS A person's behavior is a function of the circumstances under which it occurs. Sometimes the easiest way to change a person's behavior is to change the circumstances which relate to, or are antecedent to that behavior. For example, change a student's teacher and the student's school performance may change. Shift a person from one job to another and his work productivity may improve. In the counseling interview itself, the counselor's behavior is not only a determinant of, but is effected by, the client's behavior. For example, Schuldt[24] reports a study of counselors' approach-avoidance responses to clients' expressions of dependency. They found that each counselor had a relatively consistent pattern of approaching or avoiding dependency statements by clients, and that clients tended to express feelings of dependency when counselors responded to them. Whether or not clients talk or act in a dependent way in counseling depends in part on how the counselor behaves. Gamsky and Farwell[11] report a related study of counselor verbal behavior as a function of client hostility. They used client-actors who portrayed different amounts of hostility in interviews with 30 school counselors. They found that client hostility directed toward the counselor evoked greater negative reactions than hostility directed toward others. Untrained or partially trained counselors tended to avoid responding to hostile behaviors. Experienced counselors showed somewhat less avoidance. People in our culture are often made uncomfortable by angry behavior. Counselors who are uncomfortable in the face of client hostility will tend to avoid it and tend to create interview conditions in which clients are less likely to reveal it. Clearly, research on counseling cannot ignore the setting provided by the counselor, and its impact on the client behaviors on which the counseling is focused.

Research Design and Methodology

The problems associated with accomplishing effective research on complex human behavior in the naturalistic social context (which is what counseling practice represents) are extremely intricate and difficult. All the considerations involved cannot be represented here. An effective review has recently been provided by Goldstein, Heller, and Sechrest, who note the inevitability of practical constraints upon the satisfactory investigation of treatment effects. Their discussion of this fact and various research designs which can be employed to cope with such contingencies can be considerable help to researchers in this area.

An added problem, however, stems from what appears to us to be unsatisfactory differentiation between various kinds of research which are possible on the human situation. This is a point which we have developed elsewhere[10] and which can only be touched upon here. In our view, there has been a tendency to think of research approaches in terms of their approximation to a single hypothetical ideal. Studies have been judged relative to a single yardstick, the classic experiment; and they have been squeezed, cramped, and consequently prejudiced by efforts to render them consonant with the experimental model. It is our feeling that rather than a single model for empirical research, there should be at least three models, and possibly more.

First, there is *experimental research,* in which artificially contrived situations and arbitrary controls are used, arranging for as homogeneous a set of conditions as possible so that only specified factors are allowed to vary, and randomizing the uncontrolled sources of variance so that they exert no systematic effect. There is, second, a brand of investigation which might be termed *field research,* where the investigator begins with a group of subjects in circumstances which can be only partly controlled. He can exert control over some of the conditions he employs, but cannot control other relevant events occurring in the person's life, or the behavioral events the client will present. In this type of research, a significant dimension of control is lost; but it is offset by coming one step closer to the real human situation. The third type one might call *field trials.* Using knowledge gained under more controlled conditions, the counselor applies the ideas with real clients under natural conditions. The counselor does not select the problem nor does he control the factors which govern its occurrence in the practical counseling setting. The welfare of the individual is of paramount importance. The counselor cannot treat any two clients precisely alike. Careful description of such trials (for example, studies) can be quite enlightening, however, particularly when viewed in the context of other research.

These categories of designs not only are conceptually distinct, but would lead to essentially different investigatory procedures because they are designed to answer essentially different sets of questions. Investigators need to reconsider the empirical procedures which they have been using in the past, and to evolve more differential, and hence more powerful, patterns of research.

NOTES

1. Robert P. Anderson, "Physiological and Verbal Behavior During Client-Centered Counseling," *The Investigation of Psychotherapy,* eds. Arnold P. Goldstein, and Sanford J. Dean (New York: John Wiley and Sons, Inc., 1966).
2. J. D. Ashby, D. H. Ford, B. G. Guerney, Jr., and L. F. Guerney, "Effects on Clients of a Reflective and a Leading Type of Psychotherapy," *Psychological Monographs,* 8 (1957), 1–32.
3. Albert Bandura and R. H. Walters, *Social Learning and Personality Development* (New York: Holt, Rinehart and Winston, 1963), Print 329.
4. Mary K. Bauman, *Adjustment to Blindness* (Harrisburg: State Council for the Blind, Department of Welfare, Commonwealth of Pennsylvania, 1954).
5. Charles N. Cofer and Mortimer H. Appley, *Motivation: Theory and Research* (New York: John Wiley and Sons, Inc., 1964).
6. A. R. Cohen, *Attitude Change and Social Influence* (New York: Basic Books, 1964).
7. W. N. Dember, *The Psychology of Perception* (New York: Holt, Rinehart, and Winston, 1960).
8. I. S. Dreiblatt and D. Weatherly, "An Evaluation of the Efficacy of Brief-Contact Therapy with Hospitalized Psychiatric Patients," *Journal of Counseling Psychology,* 29 (1965), 512–19.
9. D. H. Ford and H. B. Urban, "College Dropouts: Successes or Failures," *The College Dropout and the Utilization of Talent,* eds. L. A. Pervin, L. E. Reik, and W. Dalrymple (Princeton, New Jersey: Princeton University Press, 1960).
10. ——— and H. B. Urban, "Psychotherapy," *Annual Review of Psychology,* Vol. 18 (Palo Alto, California: Annual Reviews, Inc., 1967).
11. Neal Richard Gamsky and Gail F. Farwell, "Counselor Verbal Behavior as a Function of Client Hostility," *Journal of Counseling Psychology,* 13 (1966), 184–190.
12. A. P. Goldstein and S. J. Dean, *The Investigation of Psychotherapy* (New York: John Wiley, 1966).
13. ———, *Therapist-Patient Expectancies in Psychotherapy* (New York: Macmillan, 1962).
14. L. A. Gottschalk and A. H. Auerbach, *Methods of Research in Psychotherapy* (New York: Appleton-Century-Crofts, 1966).
15. C. H. Graham, ed., *Vision and Visual Perception* (New York: John Wiley and Sons, Inc., 1965).
16. Arthur H. Hill and Laurabeth Grieneeks, "Criteria in the Evaluation of

Educational and Vocational Counseling in College," *Journal of Counseling Psychology,* 13 (1966), 198–201.

17. D. A. Hills and J. E. Williams, "Effects of Test Information Upon Self-Evaluation in Brief Educational-Vocational Counseling," *Journal of Counseling Psychology,* 12 (1965), 275–281.
18. Kenneth S. Isaacs and Ernest A. Haggard, "Some Methods Used in the Study of Affect in Psychotherapy," *Methods of Research in Psychotherapy,* eds. Lois A. Gottschalk and Arthur Auerbach (New York: Appleton-Century-Crofts, 1966).
19. Peter H. Knapp, ed., "Expression of the Emotions in Man," *Proceedings of the American Association for Advancement of Science Symposium,* 1960 (New York: International Universities Press, Inc., 1963).
20. John D. Krumboltz, "Behavioral Goals for Counseling," *Journal of Counseling Psychology,* 13 (1966), 153–159.
21. Gerald R. Patterson, "A Learning Theory Approach to the Treatment of the School Phobic Child," *Case Studies in Behavior Modification,* eds. Leonard P. Ullmann and Leonard Krasner (New York: Holt, Rinehart and Winston, 1965).
22. C. R. Rogers, *Client Centered Therapy* (Boston: Houghton-Mifflin, 1951).
23. T. Antoinette Ryan and J. D. Krumboltz, "Effect of Planned Reinforcement Counseling on Client Decision-Making Behavior," *Journal of Counseling Psychology,* 11 (1964), 315–323.
24. W. John Schuldt, "Psychotherapists' Approach-Avoidance Responses and Clients' Expressions of Dependency," *Journal of Counseling Psychology,* 13 (1966), 178–183.
25. M. C. Shaw and J. Grubb, "Hostility in Able High School Underachievers," *Journal of Counseling Psychology,* 5 (1958), 263–266.
26. D. R. Stieper and D. N. Wiener, *Dimensions of Psychotherapy: An Experimental and Clinical Approach* (Chicago: Aldine, 1965).
27. G. E. Stollak, B. Guerney, Jr., and M. Rothberg, eds., *Psychotherapy Research, Selected Readings* (Chicago: Rand McNally, 1966).
28. T. Volsky, Jr., T. M. Magoon, W. T. Norman and D. P. Hoyt, *The Outcomes of Counseling and Psychotherapy: Theory and Research* (Minneapolis: University of Minnesota Press, 1965).
29. C. D. Williams, "The Elimination of Tantrum Behavior by Extinction Procedures," *Case Studies in Behavior Modification,* eds. Leonard P. Ullmann and Leonard Krasner (New York: Holt, Rinehart and Winston, Inc., 1965).
30. R. D. Winkler, J. J. Teigland, P. F. Munger and G. D. Kranzler, "The Effects of Selected Counseling and Remedial Techniques on Underachieving Elementary School Students," *Journal of Counseling Psychology,* 12 (1965), 384–387.

COUNSELING THE BLIND

Douglas C. MacFarland

The excellence of the organization and the smoothness of the writing of Drs. Ford and Urban in the previous paper leave one with the feeling that they have provided us with a conceptual framework of beguiling simplicity. This paper will attempt to apply their approach of systems theory to counseling.

They list five components in any system: (1) A goal-setting, guidance and regulating component; (2) a performance component; (3) an amplifying component; (4) an information-collecting component; and (5) a domain of consequences. If we organize our consideration of research related to counseling on the basis of this model, we have the following:

1. The goal-setting, guidance and regulating component would include at least:

(*a*) All types of facts about the client, including studies of his environment including his family background, present home and family, and significant community influences; his educational and work histories; his medical history; the history of his visual loss, with present and probable future status from the point of view of the ophthalmologist; evaluation of his mobility and communication skills; and complete psychological evaluation results.

(*b*) On the part of the counselor, a thorough knowledge of the present labor market and predictions for the future; and of the content of a wide variety of jobs which might be appropriate to the client. Obviously the counselor must be familiar with many jobs in order to judge which are appropriate to this particular client.

(*c*) A thorough knowledge of where to find and how to arrange for the training necessary to bring this client into readiness for the chosen job, and ultimately a knowledge of how to place the client, which means how to find the appropriate employer and sell him on hiring a blind client.

These might be described as cognitive elements, knowledges necessary before any real action can be taken, and it is a minimal list.

2. The performance component may be identified as the counseling process—not merely the interplay between counselor and client, but work with the family, with other agencies needed to achieve the client's goal, work with schools and colleges used in preparing the client for his goal, and work with employers until a satisfactory placement has been consummated.

3. The amplifying component would appear to relate to the less factual elements in the counseling relationship. Here one must consider the nature of the counselor himself, and the nature of the client in those less objective areas described as motivation, attitudes, and inner drive. It would seem that in this component, feelings, rather than cold facts, would have their place.

4. The information-collecting component appears to be the immediate feedback from the counseling and placement activity. Here we would identify the placement itself which, in vocational rehabilitation, is often regarded as the significant measure of the success of counseling. Short-range measures of the satisfaction of both the client and the employer might also be listed here.

5. In the domain of consequences, we might consider more long-range evaluations of success in training and placement, follow-up studies done after some years have passed. We might also consider the impact of blind workers upon the attitudes of employers and the community and, indeed, the shaping of legislative policies, research grants, counselor training programs, and so on. This component might also include evaluations of agencies and standards set for professional functioning.

First, I want to agree very strongly with Dr. Ford's statement that, between disciplines, there is great need for more communication which would hopefully lead to an integrated approach toward research. Even within our own small field, the tendency is to work with your own discipline, seldom crossing disciplinary lines. We will have little really effective research in counseling until we accept everyone on a research team who can make a contribution.

Indeed, when one is asked to present a paper on "counseling," one is immediately faced by an interdisciplinary question: Does "counseling" include psychotherapy? Patterson[59] says:

> it appears impossible to make any clear distinction between them. If experts in counseling and psychotherapy were asked to list the theories which should be considered under each heading, there would probably be great overlapping in the lists. . . . The definitions of counseling would in most cases be acceptable as definitions of psychotherapy, and vice versa. There seems to be agreement that both counseling and psychotherapy are processes involving a special kind of relationship between a person who asks for help with a psychological problem (the client or the patient) and a person who is trained to provide that help (the counselor or the therapist).

Perhaps the question is an academic one. If the content of this paper is to be limited to mention of research studies, no space is required to list formal research on psychotherapy with blind people; for none has been done. For years we have quoted such psychoanalytically oriented concepts as those expressed by Chevigny[21] or the quite negative picture painted by Cutsforth.[28] Such writers as Cholden[22] and Blank[14] have contributed concepts which have had a significant impact upon the understanding of blind people and the psychodynamics of adjustment under the stress of blindness, while other workers, such as Carroll,[20] have carried these concepts into programs of training and counseling. Yet research evaluating the influence of these concepts is lacking.

Let us briefly review some of the more significant or recent research which fits into our conceptual framework. In some cases, when it seems to have special meaning for work with blind people, we will touch upon research not specific to blindness.

GOAL-SETTING, GUIDANCE, AND REGULATING

Although many articles have been written concerning the importance to counseling of the client's background, family, and community influences, the major research in this area is the work of Teare,[66] who has developed weights for significant facts in the client's history and has related his system to job success through very sophisticated procedures. The relationship of educational and work histories was developed in both the original study of *Adjustment to Blindness*[3] and its followup,[10] and in Bauman's studies of visually handicapped people at work.[11,12] One of the most complex studies relating education, training, and employment was done by Dauwalder[29] at the Western Pennsylvania School for Blind Children, including consideration of local employment practices, sheltered as well as competitive employment, and the local economy at the time. Fitting[35] and Buell [18,19] did smaller studies in Michigan and California. Specific studies of the relationship of medical history to rehabilitation are lacking, although some of the work on the multiple-handicapped blind child might be interpreted under this heading. In the training of the rehabilitation counselor, the implications of secondary handicaps are given consideration, but we have no formal studies of blind persons with additional handicaps.

The history of the client's visual loss is, on the other hand, given frequent consideration. Drs. Ford and Urban mentioned the difference between counseling with a congenitally blind person and counseling with one who has been adventitiously blinded. They likened the human being to a system with a number of complex sensory inputs, amassing data from these inputs and utilizing feedback from these data on which the behavior of the human being will depend. Blindness, of course, severely limits or entirely destroys one major channel for information reception and consequent reaction. Quite obviously, the person blinded in later life would have a considerable storehouse of information gained through visual means which he could adapt after he learns to make full use of other sensory modalities. The child blind from birth must be given a rich background of information through the remaining senses. Concepts which are normally obtained through sight must be stimulated without any visual memory on which to build. It is extremely important that he have a visual orientation toward things since he must make his livelihood and construct his social life in a sighted world. Counseling with the congenitally blind client constitutes a real challenge and requires a depth of knowledge in the large area of deficit which Drs. Ford and Urban discussed. Suffice it to say that a higher degree of competency in counseling techniques is not enough unless the counselor thoroughly understands blindness—what it is, what its effects are on the human being, and to what extent these effects can be overcome. This is much more easily said than acquired. A number of excellent discussions relate to age of visual loss, but the very small amount of research appears chiefly as part of larger studies.[3,5,12]

One of the important aspects of counseling a blind client that is very often completely overlooked is residual vision and the part it can play in the client's total social and vocational life. Any counselor who hopes to be successful in this field must learn a great deal about partial vision; and under medical supervision learn how, and to what extent, the remaining sight is functional. We are all too familiar with the partly sighted child or adult who is treated and trained as a totally blind person. Great frustrations result, but it can be equally disastrous to treat a person with a small amount of residual vision as though he were fully sighted. A person with partial vision must be encouraged and trained to use his sight to the maximum, but also he must be cautioned about his limitations—when to rely on other sense modalities or other people. Here, again, significant research is lacking or very nearly so.

Studies related to mobility and communication skills are few, involve small numbers of subjects, and usually lack acceptable criteria, clear control of procedures, and control groups. Most of the literature in this field consists of opinion, advice, and defense of whatever mobility or communication procedure the writer represents. On the other hand, when an effort is made to establish firm controls over a program, the complexity of the task makes it almost unmanageable.[24,49,51,74,75,76]

In the area of psychological evaluation, a small but steady stream of reports has appeared since the early work of Samuel P. Hayes.[38–44] Bauman developed or adapted measures of manual dexterity[4,8] and developed personality measures for adults and adolescents.[9] Through the study of *Adjustment to Blindness*[3] and its more recent followup,[10] and through smaller studies,[2,6] Bauman has given added meaning to these tests by showing how they relate to employment and general life adjustment or to the nature of physical handicap or the nature of schooling. Studies of adjustment, using both new and familiar measures have been done by a number of workers, including Sommers,[63] Dean,[31] Fitting,[34] and Jervis.[47] Studies of young blind children include the excellent work of Maxfield [50] in her development of a social maturity scale at the preschool level, and the work of Norris, Spaulding, and Brodie as reported both in their *Blindness in Children,*[57] and in their followup of the school-age child.[56] An unusually broad and sophisticated study of the adolescent blind child was done by Cowen, Underberg, Verillo, and Benham,[25] including the development of several scales and similar measuring instruments. Unfortunately, these instruments were so directly related to their study that they have not been very useful to psychologists in other settings.

It is not feasible to list here all of the varied efforts to develop specific tests for blind children and adults, but two areas have been and continue to be active: (1) Numerous efforts have been at least initiated to develop projective measures of personality in some form not requiring vision. Unfortunately, most of these have been dropped short of completion, although the work of Palacios[58] may be regarded as an exception. (2) A number of studies have shown that the Wechsler Verbal Scales have significant predictive value for the success of blind persons in education and work;[65] but in recent years a number of efforts have been made to develop a suitable performance measure. Work has been completed on the Haptic Intelligence Scale,[62] the Vocational Intelligence Scale for the Adult Blind and the Tactual Reproduction Pegboard,[37,48] and one evaluative study of these was done by Bauman.[7] Suinn, Dauterman, and Shapiro[64] have recently reported on an adaptation of the Ohwaki-Kohs Blocks, and Anderson[1] has begun an adaptation of the Raven Matrices in tactual form. There continues to be a very significant lack of performance measures of general ability for children under the age of 16 years since all of the work completed at this time is designed for persons over that age. This means that in the many cases of educational deprivation below the age of 16 years, no appropriate measures are available.

We have already indicated that the counselor needs a thorough knowledge of the labor market. It is inconceivable that he can intelligently discuss applicable jobs and requisite training unless he has a full understanding of the current world of work and can relate this complex store of knowledge to the limitations that blindness may impose. Fortunately, research on the labor market is rather well covered by both governmental and private services and is of course not the responsibility of work with the blind. We have already noted some studies of the employment of blind persons in our earlier discussion of work histories. To these might be added the study of graduates of The Seeing Eye[73] and of war-blinded veterans.[72] Over a period of some years, the Vocational Rehabilitation Administration has published descriptions of jobs done by blind people, and this literature has been significantly enriched in recent years by the studies of blind workers in the professions,[11] and in clerical, industrial, and service jobs.[12]

The final item in Component 1 is knowledge of training and placement opportunities, both of which are inevitably local and difficult subjects of "research." Fortunately, a section of this conference will be devoted to placement and will consider needs in this area in detail.

THE COUNSELING PROCESS

Obviously a great deal of training has been done and a great deal has been written concerning the counseling process, but it is difficult to single out studies specific to blindness. It is probably fair to say that rehabilitation counseling has been most influenced by Williamson and the Minnesota school of thought, largely because they concerned themselves more with *vocational* counseling than do most other counseling theorists. The thinking of Carl Rogers has come in for much discussion but rare use, although we have borrowed the phrase, "client-centered," and bent it rather freely to our own interpretation. There is a great need for well controlled studies which might disclose the usefulness of other theoretical-practice approaches to counseling, such as the "psychological counseling" of Bordin, with its quite different approach to the use of tests, the reciprocal inhibition of Wolpe, the use of learning theory and reinforcement.[59] Bauman and Yoder raise significant questions concerning the possible utility of the "behavioral approach to counseling and guidance" in their *Adjustment to Blindness—Re-Viewed.*[10] The Cummings[27] make a strong argument for work as therapy with which the whole rehabilitation movement must be deeply in sympathy. In addition, their design for role relationships within a therapeutic (rehabilitative) milieu suggests exciting possibilities for the rehabilitation agency and its set with regard to staff responsibilities as well as client relationships.

While, in work with the blind, we do not have studies with highly theoretical orientation to our credit, some very practical work on the process of counseling has been done—such as the development of a structure for counseling at the professional level by Crawford and Lirtzman.[26] Other examples can be found in such publications as *Vocational Counseling of Blind Students,*[60] *Guidance Programs for Blind Children,*[30] and *Vocational Rehabilitation Counseling with the Blind Through the Use of Social Casework Methods.*[23]

Although not directed toward blindness alone a good bit of other work includes concern for blind people and their counseling, especially studies done at the universities which offer training for rehabilitation counselors. An example of this would be the work of Marceline Jacques[46] on critical counseling behavior, or the various publications by Muthard and his group which will be mentioned again under our next heading. The work of Muthard and Jacques seems to be spurring others to studies of the counseling process, such as Benedict's[13] report on counselor efficiency and Moses' [53] concern with counselor's roles—although the latter obviously has other precedents, such as the work of Hoffman[45] on counselor sub-roles. Currently a study is in process at the Johnstown Research and Training Center concerning the effectiveness of democratic, autocratic, and leaderless groups in counseling and therapy. The Arkansas Center is doing related studies of sensitizing counselors to the counseling process. All of this is extremely valuable in counselor training, and much more needs to be done in these areas.

THE NATURE OF THE COUNSELOR RELATED TO THE NATURE OF THE CLIENT

The nature of the rehabilitation counselor is well defined by Usdane:[71]

> Rehabilitation counseling subscribes to the hard core counseling requirement of all the counseling professions: a face to face relationship enabling the individual to internalize an awareness of his problems and his potentialities toward a program of adjustment and self-improvement. But there is a cluster of skills which provides the rehabilitation counselor with a distinctive focus. He works with the physically or emotionally disturbed, including the mentally retarded. There is primary emphasis upon the vocational aspects of the total rehabilitation process which includes medical, personal and social adjustment. Vocational planning as well as implementation of the individual's occupational goals, are indigenous to the counseling interaction. Vocational counseling as it is professionally practiced by trained rehabilitation counselors with the handicapped becomes the distinct focus, and as a member of the professional team, the counselor also recognizes his several quasi- and non-counseling roles. With this recognition, furthermore, he is able to differentiate administrative from professional duties, quasi- or non-counseling from counseling interaction, and the major contribution of this distinct professional role from that of other members of the rehabilitation team.

Drs. Ford and Urban alluded to the fact that blind persons are sometimes considered better fitted to counsel with the blind. Perhaps some research needs to be done in this area, but at the moment there is very little fact on which to base such a conclusion. Somewhat similar studies with general counselors might suggest that there is no relationship. For example, Branan[16] found that the use of self-experience examples did not improve the counseling relationship with graduate students. Brayfield[17] points out that research on the counseling process is largely trivial or completely missing, but studies by Truax,[67] Brams,[15] and Schwebel[61] suggest that the most important characteristic in any counselor is the ability to communicate, the ability to relate to the client. Unfortunately, many of the reported studies of the qualities of counselors are actually studies of counselors in training. There are obvious difficulties in observing the counselor at work so that one can describe his qualities; but tape recordings offer some opportunities for analysis.

If we study the nature of the counselor by asking him about himself, his attitudes, his goals, a number of studies are available. Goldin,[36] for example, reported on Vocational Rehabilitation counselors in New England and concluded that this was a profession "in a state of flux, struggling to define its role while its practitioners suffer from feelings of inadequacy relative to other professions that enjoy more clearly defined roles."

As noted previously, some of the best studies of this type come out of those universities where rehabilitation counselor training is offered. It is impossible to list all of these, but the varied publications of the University of Iowa group are a good example. They have been concerned with the roles and functions of the counselor, with job satisfaction among counselors, and with criteria for counselor performance.[52,54,55] A section on the qualities and attitudes of counselors is also included in the report on blind workers in clerical, industrial, and service occupations.[12]

Although counseling is usually thought of as a one-to-one relationship, we must recognize that the degree of success depends on the understanding and cooperation of many persons. The counselor will carry the major responsibility, but he will have very little effect on the client's real goals unless he makes use of persons who affect the immediate environment. It is almost axiomatic that very few clients achieve a high level of competency without the full understanding and cooperation of their families. While this is very important with most counselees, it is essential with the blind person. Unless the family fully understands the problems, various methods for solving them, and ultimate goals and how they relate to the family as well as the client, it is almost certain that the counselor will fail. Handling of the patient during the initial convalescence can be extremely important in shaping his attitudes toward himself and his acceptance of counseling therapy.

This brings us to the second element in Component 3—the nature of the client. Periodic efforts are made to predict rehabilitation potential. Dishart,[32,33] for example, has been concerned with this, and many studies involving test development, or applications of batteries of tests, have actually been efforts to measure rehabilitation potential. A weighted index to predict job success also was developed as part of the followup of the study of *Adjustment to Blindness*.[10] Under the recent amendments to the rehabilitation law, permitting longer diagnostic study, use of shelter shops and rehabilitation centers, such predictive measures seem less significant.

IMMEDIATE FEEDBACK THROUGH PLACEMENT AND JOB SATISFACTION

In vocational rehabilitation, successful employment is the ultimate yardstick for measuring the counselor's success; therefore, interpreting to employers or helping the client assess his own strengths and weaknesses so he can "sell" himself becomes a major counseling objective. However, placement is a special area of discussion on the agenda of this conference and it seems inappropriate to enter this very complex subject here.

LONG-RANGE EVALUATION OF COUNSELING SUCCESS

Although almost any of the studies of employed blind persons mentioned above might be regarded as to some degree an evaluation of the success of their counseling, none of these are well controlled studies from that point of view. The Adjustment Study followup[10] might also contribute to thinking in this area but is far from having been devised for this purpose. Thus, while there have been a number of these longitudinal studies in general counseling, we can point to very little in work with the blind. There is real need for a project which follows all of some relatively unselected group, not just those who attend college, obtain jobs, and so on. It is important that this should be a group with rather common background in terms of the way they were handled—the way they were evaluated psychologically, counseled, and given opportunities for development. Truax has pointed out that many studies of the results of counseling have yielded little, but he suggests that this is because, to get large enough numbers for study, the work of good counselors, and the work of poor counselors has been lumped together. Naturally, it came out to just about zero. Indeed, Truax[68,69,70] makes the disturbing suggestion that our clients may be injured, as well as helped, by the counseling relationship.

One might also list in this component, which Drs. Ford and Urban call the "domain of consequences," the agency's concern with itself, a very lively concern reflected in the present accreditation activity in work with the blind. None of this is a matter of "research," however. Equally lacking is any research evaluation of attitudes of employers, the community, legislators, all of which fall into the domain of consequences.

Finally, although I have implied a number of research needs in the previous pages, I would like to list the following for special consideration:

1. Further refinement of existing test instruments and the development of some new techniques, for example, a couple of good projective tests and tests using thematic material.

2. We need a good deal more work on family attitudes toward a blind person, both the successful and unsuccessful, from the vocational standpoint. There are a growing number of us who believe that the degree of success in rehabilitation is directly related to understanding of the family.

3. We could profit by a longitudinal study of congenitally blind adults specifically designed to uncover kinds of data they have stored and analyzed and how these are used to deal with a sighted society. This study should be designed to include what the congenitally blind person feels are gaps in his own knowledge and sensory input system.

4. A selective study of highly intelligent and successful blind persons to determine some of the major frustrations that are manifest to these subjects and what, if anything, can be done to reduce them.

5. A study in depth of the functional use of severely impaired vision, though I recognize that this is entering the medical field, an area which is not to be covered by this conference. Nevertheless, true success in counseling will depend in a large measure on an understanding and a factual appraisal of this important aspect of our work including the use of optical aids.

6. Since the question has been raised by Drs. Ford and Urban and many others, perhaps a study should be conducted to determine whether blindness is a substantial asset to a counselor who is working with blind clients.

7. An attitudinal study of a random sample of sighted persons might determine the attributes they feel a blind person must have in order to be fully accepted in society,

8. One of the most pressing needs for all of us at present is the completion of a national census of the blind which will include not

only pertinent medical data but as much social information as possible. Such a study in fact is now underway, sponsored by the National Institute of Neurological Diseases and Blindness. It is imperative that this study be completed as quickly as possible; for it is difficult to conceive realistic planning during the next ten years without a solid demographic base from which to work.

NOTES

1. R. P. Anderson, *Final Report, Raven Progressive Matrices for Presentation to the Blind* (Lubbuck, Texas: Texas Technological College, 1964).
2. Mary K. Bauman, "A Comparative Study of Personality Factors in Blind, Other Handicapped, and Non-Handicapped Individuals," *American Psychologist,* 5 (1950), 340–341.
3. ———, *Adjustment to Blindness: A Study as Reported by the Committee to Study Adjustment to Blindness* (Harrisburg: Pennsylvania State Council for the Blind, 1954).
4. ———, *Manual of Norms for Tests Used in Counseling Blind Persons* (New York: American Foundation for the Blind, 1958).
5. ———, *Characteristics of Blind and Visually Handicapped People in Professional, Sales and Managerial Work* (Harrisburg: Pennsylvania Office for the Blind, 1963).
6. ———, "Group Differences Disclosed by Inventory Items," *International Journal for Education of the Blind,* Vol. 13, No. 4 (1964), 101–106.
7. ———, "Performance Tests for the Adult Blind," *Blindness 1965* (Washington: American Association of Workers for the Blind, 1965).
8. ——— and Samuel P. Hayes, *A Manual for the Psychological Examination of the Adult Blind* (New York: Psychological Corp., 1951).
9. ———, H. Platt and Susan Strauss, "A Measure of Personality for Blind Adolescents," *International Journal for the Education of the Blind,* Vol. 12, No. 1 (1963), 7–12.
10. ——— and Norman M. Yoder, *Adjustment to Blindness—Re-Viewed* (Springfield, Illinois: Charles C Thomas, 1966).
11. ——— and Norman M. Yoder, *Placing the Blind and Visually Handicapped in Professional Occupations* (Harrisburg, Pennsylvania Office for the Blind, Department of Public Welfare, 1962).
12. ——— and Norman M. Yoder, *Placing the Blind and Visually Handicapped in Clerical, Industrial, and Service Occupations* (Harrisburg: Pennsylvania Office for the Blind, 1966).
13. T. C. Benedict, "Enabling the Counselor to Increase His Efficiency," *Journal of Rehabilitation,* Vol. 21, No. 17 (1965), 57–59.
14. Robert H. Blank, "Psychiatric Problems Associated with Congenital Blindness Due to Retrolental Fibroplasia," *New Outlook for the Blind,* 53 (1959), 237–245.
15. J. M. Brams, "Counselor Characteristics and Effective Communication in Counseling," *Journal of Counseling Psychology,* 8 (1961), 25–30.
16. J. M. Branan, "Client Reaction to Counselor's Use of Self-experience," *Personnel and Guidance Journal,* 45 (1957), 568–572.
17. A. H. Brayfield, "Counseling Psychology," *Annual Review of Psychology,* 14 (Palo Alto, California: Annual Reviews, Inc., 1963).
18. Josephine Buell, "Rehabilitation Status of Former Students of the Cali-

fornia School for the Blind," *New Outlook for the Blind,* 49 (1955), 166–173.
19. ———, "Employment Status of Former Pupils of the California School for the Blind," *Exceptional Children,* Vol. 23, No. 3 (December, 1956).
20. Thomas J. Carroll, *Blindness—What It Is, What It Does and How to Live with It* (Boston: Little, Brown, 1961).
21. H. Chevigny and Sydell Braverman, *The Adjustment of the Blind* (New Haven, Connecticut: Yale University Press, 1950).
22. L. S. Cholden, *A Psychiatrist Works with Blindness* (New York: American Foundation for the Blind, 1958).
23. Frances Clay, ed., *Vocational Rehabilitation Counseling with the Blind Through the Use of Social Casework Methods, Proceedings of an Institute for Vocational Rehabilitation Counselors* (Memphis, Tennessee, 1959).
24. M. Cotzin and K. M. Dallenbach, "Facial Vision: The Role of Pitch and Loudness in the Perception of Obstacles by the Blind," *American Journal of Psychology,* Vol. 63, No. 4 (October, 1950), 485–515.
25. E. Cowen, Rita Underberg, R. Verillo and F. Benham, *Adjustment to Visual Disability in Adolescence* (New York: American Foundation for the Blind, 1961).
26. F. L. Crawford and S. Lirtzman, *Counseling and Placement of Blind Persons in Professional Occupations: Practice and Research* (New York: The New York Association for the Blind, 1966).
27. J. Cumming and Elaine Cumming, *Ego and Milieu* (New York: Atherton Press, 1962).
28. T. D. Cutsforth, "Blindness as an Adequate Expression of Anxiety," *Research Bulletin,* No. 12 (New York: American Foundation for the Blind, January, 1966).
29. D. D. Dauwalder, *Education, Training and Employment of the Blind* (Pittsburgh: Western Pennsylvania School for the Blind, 1964).
30. C. J. Davis, ed., *Guidance Programs for Blind Children* (Watertown, Massachusetts: Perkins Publication No. 20, 1959).
31. S. I. Dean, "Some Experimental Findings about Blind Adjustment," *New Outlook for the Blind,* 25 (1958), 182–185.
32. M. Dishart, "Testing the Blind for Rehabilitation," *New Outlook for the Blind,* 53 (January, 1959), 1–14.
33. ———, "A Study of the Effectiveness of Psychological Services for the Blind," *New Outlook for the Blind,* Vol. 54, No. 9 (December, 1960), 351–356.
34. E. A. Fitting, *Evaluation of Adjustment to Blindness* (New York: American Foundation for the Blind, Research Series, No. 2, 1954).
35. ———, "Rehabilitation Status of Former Students at the Michigan School for the Blind," *New Outlook for the Blind,* Vol. 49, No. 1 (January, 1955), 21–26.
36. G. J. Goldin, "Some Rehabilitation Counselor Attitudes Toward Their Professional Role," *Rehabilitation Literature,* 27 (1966), 360–364.
37. A. Gruber, "Testing the Psychomotor Skills of the Blind: The Development of a Measure of Tactual Perceptiveness and Gross Manipulative Dexterity," *Correlates of Adjustment to Vision Loss: A Symposium* (Wichita, Kansas: University of Wichita, 1963).
38. S. P. Hayes, *Report of a Preliminary Test of the Reading of the Pupils of the Pennsylvania Institution for the Instruction of the Blind at Overbrook, April, 1918* (Philadelphia: The Institution, 1918).
39. ———, *Mental and Educational Survey in Seven Schools for the Blind* (Washington: American Association of Instructors of the Blind, 1920).
40. ———, *Ten Years of Psychological Research in Schools for the Blind*

(Philadelphia: Pennsylvania Institute for the Instruction of the Blind, 1927).
41. ———, *Twenty Years of Research: Aims and Achievements* (Washington: American Association of Instructors of the Blind, 1936).
42. ———, "Mental Measurements of the Blind: History, Inventory, Criticism," *Teachers Forum,* 13 (1941), 42–52, 60.
43. ———, *Contributions to a Psychology of Blindness* (New York: American Foundation for the Blind, 1941).
44. ———, *Vocational Aptitude Tests for the Blind* (Watertown, Massachusetts: Perkins Institution, 1946).
45. A. E. Hoffman, "An Analysis of Counselor Sub-roles," *Journal of Counseling Psychology,* 6 (1959), 61–67.
46. Marceline E. Jacques, *Critical Counseling Behavior in Rehabilitation Settings* (Iowa City, Iowa: State University of Iowa, 1959).
47. F. M. Jervis, "A Comparison of Self-concepts of Blind and Sighted Children," *Guidance Programs for Blind Children* (Watertown, Massachusetts: Perkins School Publication No. 20, 1960).
48. W. R. Jones, "Development of a Non-verbal Intelligence Scale for the Adult Blind," *Correlates of Adjustment to Vision Loss: A Symposium,* (Wichita, Kansas: University of Wichita, 1963).
49. Roseanne Kramer, "Personality and Attitudes of Blind Teen-Agers Learning Cane Travel," Research Bulletin, No. 2 (New York: American Foundation for the Blind, 1957).
50. Kathryn E. Maxfield and Sandra Buchholz, *A Social Maturity Scale for Blind Preschool Children* (New York: American Foundation for the Blind, 1957).
51. J. Mickunas, Jr., and T. B. Sheridan, "Use of an Obstacle Course in Evaluating Mobility of the Blind," *Research Bulletin,* No. 3 (New York: American Foundation for the Blind, August, 1963), 35–54.
52. L. A. Miller and J. E. Muthard, "Job Satisfactions and Counselor Performance in State Rehabilitation Agencies," *Journal of Applied Psychology,* 49 (1965), 280–283.
53. H. A. Moses, "A Rationale for Providing Counseling for Handicapped Students," *Journal of Rehabilitation,* 32 (1966), 14–15.
54. J. E. Muthard and L. A. Miller, "Perceptions of Rehabilitation Counselor Behavior," *Personnel and Guidance Journal,* 44 (1966), 519–522.
55. ——— and L. A. Miller, *The Criteria Problem in Rehabilitation Counseling* (Iowa City, Iowa: State University of Iowa, 1966).
56. Miriam Norris, *The School Age Blind Child Project* (New York: American Foundation for the Blind, 1961).
57. ———, Patricia J. Spaulding and Fern H. Brodie, *Blindness in Children* (Chicago: University of Chicago Press, 1957).
58. ———, May H. Palacios and John Palacios, "Clinical Use of the Sound Test with Blind Adults," *Correlates of Vision Loss: A Symposium* (Wichita, Kansas: University of Wichita, 1963).
59. C. H. Patterson, *Theories of Counseling and Psychotherapy* (New York: Harper & Row, 1966).
60. N. J. Raskin, *Vocational Counseling of Blind Students,* A Study sponsored by The Committee on Relationships Between Rehabilitation Agencies and Schools For the Blind of the States Vocational Rehabilitation Council (New York: American Foundation for the Blind, 1955).
61. M. Schwebel, L. Karr and H. Slotkin, "Counselor Relationship Competence: A Unifying Concept Applied to Counselor Trainees," *Educational and Psychological Measurement,* 19 (1959), 515–537.
62. H. C. Shurrager and P. S. Shurrager, *Haptic Intelligence Scale for the Adult Blind* (Chicago: Technology Center, 1954).

63. Vita A. Sommers, *The Influence of Parental Attitudes and Social Environment on the Personality of the Adolescent Blind* (New York: American Foundation for the Blind, 1944).

64. R. M. Suinn, W. L. Dauterman and Bernice Shapiro, "The Stanford Ohwaki-Kohs Tactile Block Design Test for the Blind," *New Outlook for the Blind,* 60 (1966), 77–79.

65. ———, W. L. Dauterman and Bernice Shapiro, "The WAIS as a Predictor of Educational and Occupational Achievement in the Adult Blind," *New Outlook for the Blind,* 61 (1967), 41–43.

66. R. J. Teare, "Vision and Vocational Achievement: an Early Experience Approach," *Correlates of Adjustment to Vision Loss: A Symposium* (Wichita, Kansas: University of Wichita, 1963).

67. C. B. Truax, "Effective Ingredients in Psychotherapy: An Approach to Unraveling the Patient-therapist Interaction," *Journal of Counseling Psychology,* 10 (1963), 256–263.

68. ———, *et al.,* "The Therapist's Contribution to Accurate Empathy, Nonpossessive Warmth, and Genuineness in Psychotherapy," *Journal of Clinical Psychology,* 22 (1966), 331–334.

69. ———, *et al.,* "Therapist Empathy, Genuineness, and Warmth and Patient Therapeutic Outcome," *Journal of Consulting Psychology,* 30 (1966), 395–401.

70. ———, *et al.,* "Toward Explaining Success and Failure in Interpersonal Learning Experiences," *Personnel and Guidance Journal,* 44 (1966), 723–728.

71. W. M. Usdane, "Rehabilitation Counseling," *Handbook of Counseling Techniques,* E. Harms and P. Schreiber (New York: Macmillan Co., 1963).

72. United States Veterans Administration, *War Blinded Veterans in a Postwar Setting* (Washington: Government Printing Office, 1958).

73. R. Whitstock, Study Director, *The Employment of Graduates of The Seeing Eye, Inc.* (Morristown, N.J., 1960).

74. Philip Worchel, "Space Perception and Orientation in the Blind," *Psychological Monographs: General and Applied,* Vol. 65, No. 15 (1951).

75. ——— and K. Dallenbach, "Facial Vision: Perception of Obstacles by the Deaf-Blind," *American Journal of Psychology,* Vol. 60, No. 4 (October, 1947), 502–553.

76. H. N. Wright, *Use of Auditory Cues by the Blind for Travel,* Yearly Progress Report, Contract No. RD-510, Office of Vocational Rehabilitation (Washington: Department of Health, Education and Welfare, February 1961).

SESSION REPORT

John Aboud

During the discussion on motivation, several problems were presented. While there was general agreement that the motivational problems were troublesome and that there is need for new or further research, suggestions were not forthcoming as to the conduct of the research with respect to each problem. The first issue that was raised was the reason for the considerable lag in the time between the onset of blindness and the desire for vocational rehabilitation. It was noted by Dr. Douglas C. MacFarland that often the lag is so pronounced that the blinded person's attitudes and spirits sink to the point where he will not respond to vocational rehabilitation. It was recognized that this motivational problem was so complex that much research is required before any answers can be proffered.

A second problem, susceptible to research, is that of short-term counseling. Dr. Donald H. Ford noted that in practice the counselee and counselor have, on the average, from ten to twelve sessions in which to work on the subject's problems. It was agreed that this was indeed representative of short-term counseling, and that research is needed to determine how a counselor can be most effective in such a brief period.

A third potential area of inquiry is that of the individual motivation of the blind person. The general discussion centered on the fact that some blinded persons seem to lack the motivation to help themselves. It was later brought out that the nonmotivated person really does not exist. Rather, there may exist incongruencies between the values and goals of the counselor and/or the rehabilitation program and the blind person. Subsequently, the participants agreed that the solution to the problem lay in redirecting the motivation of the blinded person. However, a great deal of research would be needed to effect this redirection.

The first question that this research must answer is: What goals are the blind person's behavior serving? For example, in the case of persons who seem totally unmotivated, the probability is that they are engaging in some sort of avoidance behavior; but again, research should be done before this generalization is acted upon.

On this same issue, the application of learning theory was explored. If the first aspect of a research program were to uncover an individual's goals, then the problem would become how to use these immediate goals as motivators in guiding the individual into constructive rehabilitation. Further discussion centered around the concept of goal gradients and their utility for achieving these ends.

Research is also needed on the relationship between the expectations and values of the counselor as possibly reflected in his success with the client. Rather than shaping each individual to society's stereotypical concept of the well-adjusted blind person, the counselor equipped with knowledge of his own set of values may be more effective with people of different socio-economic classes.

The question was raised whether blind counselors are more effective in dealing with the blind than are sighted counselors, and it was agreed that although this is a persistent and popular notion, empirical evidence is needed before firm conclusions can be drawn.

A second broad category for research with the blind is that of the environment. Especially important are the family attitudes toward the blind person, the attitudes of the blind person toward himself, and the relationship of the family constellation in general. One question asked was: what kind of attitudes are conducive to optimal adjustment for the blinded person? Another question was: what differences exist in the adjustment of blinded persons coming from "warm" versus "cold" home environments? A further suggestion for research was an investigation into the adjectives used by parents to describe their blind children and those not afflicted. Also there was a discussion of what kinds of family constellations make for optimal adjustment.

The third area of research on counseling with the blind focused upon the technology of the counseling process itself. There was a discussion of just what the objectives that should be worked toward in counseling are, and it was suggested that this should be a matter for negotiation between the counselor and the counselee. They should agree between themselves upon what type of therapy is to be used. However, it was felt that research should be conducted to determine just how this negotiation ought to be accomplished with different kinds of people. In addition, research is needed to determine the best procedures for achieving these goals once they are agreed upon.

It was felt that, depending on the desired outcome of counseling, different approaches to the counseling process, such as Behavior

Theory or Rogerian Theory, could be employed. More research is needed to determine in what ways these different theories produce different results.

The problem of assessment is related to this problem of applying the preferred theory. How does one measure, for example, the outcome of these therapies? New instruments are needed or at least new procedures should be instituted, and this is strictly a research problem area.

In summary, the consultees decided with some narrow reservations that progress in counseling the blind was dependent upon progress in counseling in general, and that most of these problems were not peculiar to counseling work with blind people.

THE AGENCY AND THE PERSON

THE AGENCY: AGENT OF CHANGE

Yvonne M. Agazarian

This paper analyzes the relevance of selected research in social science to the relationships between the agency of rehabilitation and the client. Systems analysis provides the frame of reference for the approach to the subject and the organization of the paper.

In this study, the agency is viewed as an agent of change. It performs this function, in part, through matching its client to the appropriate organization or organizations. It also seeks to provide, at any given stage in the attempted process of change, the orientation that is most congruent with the next step. Furthermore, it seeks to effect the conditions which, in turn, direct the change toward the adopted goals.[1]

This study postulates that the agencies have a basically social purpose; that their central goal is social change; and that, as far as their dealings with the individual client are concerned, their task is to contribute to social change by increasing the social mobility of the client. Hence, at any given stage in the change process sought for the client, the immediate goal is to orient "next step" conditions toward increased social mobility for the client.

FACTORS IN AGENCY-PERSON CHANGE RELATIONSHIP

The first condition of change exists when the client contacts the agency. That very contact implies a potential for change in which the client is in the role of someone who wishes something changed, and the agency is in the position of potential agent of that change. The simplest condition of change is seen in the stimulus-response model. The agent does something which acts as an input stimulus and which results in an immediate output response that is different from previous responses. Change success or failure can then be determined by the criteria of the output behavior.[42] This change can take place without implying purpose or motivation.

A more complex model is introduced when change is intentionally directed, purposeful, or goal oriented. Goal orientation demands that the stimulus input be intentionally related, in some way, to the stimulus output. Success or failure can be measured by correlating the intention with the result. Because attempting to influence change in the human condition is complex, the match between intention and result is rarely simple. At times the outcome appears to be a mismatch, and the output behavior appears to correlate more highly with some postulated intention other than that set for the initial change process. But this does not necessarily imply that there *was* some other intention. It is at this point that confusion between output behavior, which is a function of input, and output behavior, which is a function of system goal, can arise. It is important to discriminate between the goals of the change agent, the stated goals of the client, and the system goal of the client.[49]

Locus of Change Energy

Goals can be established by the agent for the client, by the client, or by the client and the agent in interaction.

When a change agent functions in such a way that he independently determines both the goals of change and the path to the goal—when he independently makes all the relevant decisions about when, how, and where the change is directed—an important factor in change success will be the locus of the change energy.[15] If the source of that change energy lies with the agent, change will occur when he can apply sufficient pressure on the client, for a long enough period of time, to move the client towards the goal.[70] Once the goal is reached, however, the change agent will have to continue to apply enough pressure to keep the client near the goal, unless the client himself adopts the new level of equilibrium or continues to direct the new output behavior towards the agent's goal.

A different condition exists when the client can invest some change energy of his own. Then, provided both the client and the agent are investing their energy in the same direction, the work of change becomes an interdependent phenomenon. In other words, the change input is no longer directed from the environment towards the system, but becomes, instead, functionally related among components of one and the same system. When change influence becomes an interdependent phenomenon, the system under analysis is the agency-person system.[77] It is at this point that the conditions in which change takes place, as well as the way change energy is invested, can function either as restraining forces or driving forces towards the goal of change.[77]

Communication in the agent-and-person group is an important variable in influencing change.[3,27,57] To the extent to which individuals participate in the decision to change, resistance to change is reduced, and the driving forces towards change are increased.[15,29] A further important variable, then, becomes participation in goal setting for change, and participation in the determination of the path to the goal.[57] Finally, research suggests that when the group goal of change is seen as congruent with, and facilitating, individual goal achievement, driving forces towards the goal of change are increased, and restraining forces are reduced.[45] It is logical to conclude that the goal of change is a function of the goals of both the client and the change agent. As postulated for this study, the change agent, by virtue of his role in a social change agency, implicitly has change goals that are social.[78] Therefore, in the broadest sense, the goals of the change agent and those of the client are congruent with the goals of society.

Relevance of Social Goals

Social goals are implied by social norms and are explicitly stated in the literature of social service.[28,48] Some recent literature states that the goals of social change are oriented away from isolation and towards independence;[8,59] and away from passive fantasy gratification towards active, goal oriented, problem solving.[24] Social agency goal setting is, therefore, predicated on the view that the goals fall within the boundaries of the norms that the culture possesses, and point toward those changes society appears to desire. (Here *society* and *culture* are treated as equivalent.) The concept of cultural norms is useful here. On the one hand, it implies behavioral prescriptions for the social role of the individual, and, on the other hand, it implies the boundaries of role behavior that can be achieved, supported, and reinforced. At this point in cultural time, the stated goals of socialization, independence, and interdependent problem solving, though set, have limited means for general implementation. Not only is there no clear path to the goal, but there is also as much interdisciplinary competition as there is cooperation in mapping alternative paths to the goal.

In the rehabilitation field, there are many remarkable examples of a particular theory being put into practice, with the methods of practice refined and mapped in step-by-step approach to the goal. Reinforcement therapy[46] applied in a disciplined program has obtained results with such recalcitrant problems as the mute, echolalic, and autistic child; the severely retarded and the Mongoloid child; and the chronic mental patient. Another example is the "neurological organization" [38] approach, which results in the rehabilitation of children with symptoms as prognostically grave as a dominant hemispherectomy.

Possibly one consideration helping to keep these treatments ungeneralized is the lack of detailed planning of change-agent behaviors in a step-by-step process. Compared with the tight match between theory and procedure that is demonstrated in the cases cited above, more usual change agent behaviors appear to be applied almost at random, and can include behaviors as incongruent with the change goal as using dependency coercing behavior towards a goal of independence.[65]

Another factor helping to keep these treatments ungeneralized may be the isolation between theory and empirical research. Results in one discipline are often not related to existing theory in another that would permit their generalization to an allied discipline. For example, Vroom's research described in his *Work and Motivation*[5n], revealed some useful methods of influencing goal achievement; but these findings are rarely related explicitly to goal gradient theory[51] upon which they could have been predicated, and from which they might be generalized to other human phenomena. Thus, the practitioner's attention is not drawn to a clear underlying concept from which he can derive change agent behaviors that might be congruent, on the one hand, with theoretical knowledge about human behavior and, on the other, with the particular human behavior in which he is involved: "freedom of movement and of communication between systems is quite as important as it is within a system." [71] This quotation, although taken from a discussion of the context of an organizational system, applies equally to all social systems, whether they be systems of thought or of practice.

Potential Resources for Change

Research and analytic literature focusing on the problems of social change today raise three major issues. These issues are implicit in the following points:

1. Research is continually yielding information about methods of practice that increase the likelihood of influencing a match between intention of change (input) and result of change (output); but this

information is not being integrated into the practical methodology of agency practice.[6,9,12,23,26,27,68,73,74,81]

2. Research is continually yielding information about the types of organizational models that can influence the match between the stated purpose or function of the organization and the type of product or payoff that is the goal of the organization; but this information is not being integrated operationally into social agency structures.[1,2,32,35,39,48,73,82]

3. Research itself needs a conceptual framework that will allow for interdisciplinary generalizations at both theoretical and practical levels.[59]

The inferences are not only that the cultural goals imply prescriptions for operational behavior which cannot, at this point, be implemented; but also that information about variables which are relevant to the problem is accumulating faster than it can be organized, integrated, and applied.[51]

SYSTEMS ANALYSIS AS A CONCEPTUAL RESOURCE In the face of this exponential escalation of information, systems analysis seems to offer a framework which allows some generalization from the literature in the comprehensive field of social science.

First, the components of the system under analysis are defined by their relevance to the particular system under analysis and are functionally related, so that change in one implies a change in the relationships among all the components.[40] Second, change in the response of the system (output) is a function of change in the system of equilibrium, extraction of information from an environmental input, or both.[40] Third, the particular level at which the equilibrium is maintained in the system (the system goal) can be described without references to whether human desires or motivation are reflected in any way.[40] Finally, a component of one system can be a component of two or more different systems, and every system is functionally related either as a subsystem component in a larger system or as a system with its environment. Thus, all "behavior" in the universe can be conceptualized as an interaction of parts of systems among themselves, or of systems with their environment of subsystems.[40]

This approach provides, for the agency and the person, a model that allows broader findings in the social science field to be generalized to the blind person system and to the agency system. It also allows generalization to apply to the client and to the cultural system.

DISCRIMINATION OF CHANGE FOCUS It thus becomes possible to analyze the particular components that are relevant to the system "blind person," and differentiate them from components that are relevant to other systems to which "person who is blind" belongs. This separation becomes particularly relevant when the change agent is influencing change in a person who has components both in the system "blind person" and in the system "dependent person." Components relevant to the first system are different from those relevant to the second. This difference carries *different* implications for effective change agent behaviors. Influencing change in the system "blind person" implies a focus upon the sorts of input from which information relevant to a blind person's social mobility can be extracted.

One of the most crucial differences between blind and sighted people is the way in which they abstract information from their environment. To the extent that the person who is blind cannot obtain adequate information, his social mobility is curtailed. For example, a subsystem (component) in the learning system is eye-brain-hand coordination. One of the functions of this system is to provide trial-and-error experience. The blind person has to modify this system so that information processing is maintained by substituting the sound-touch function for the sight function. Theoretically, if the sound-touch function were as efficient as the sight function, the gap between the mobility—both social and physical—would not exist. Thus, change agents concerned with the goal of mobility for the blind person must have a primary concern about methods of re-visualization information through sound and touch. Consequently, appropriate change behavior should be focused on types of input from which information relevant to the re-visualization process can be abstracted.[5]

Influencing change in the system "dependent person," however, implies input with a different goal; and, therefore, with a different information input content. It is the system goal, or level of equilibrium, that must change, in the learning process, from a dependent system that behaves as if its only mobility potential is passively other-directed, to a system that behaves as if its mobility potential can be actively self-directed. Thus, Rieff implies that a primary goal for agents working with dependent people is the goal of self-determination, which carries with it the orientation of problem solving and the integration of new skills in a problem-solving approach.[59]

Rieff's contribution has implications for the change agent attempting to influence a person whose system equilibrium is "dependent." Unless the change agent's behavior is focused upon a change in the functional relations among the components of the system "dependent person," there is no guarantee that information about revisualization skills will be extracted from any input. If information is extracted, it may be that the output behavior will be subordinated to the system goal of maintaining a dependency equilibrium, not directed towards the social goal of independence and problem solving. Any new behavior in a "dependent" person's repertoire will probably be used to consolidate his dependent position unless the variable of dependence is also modified towards independence.

CONDITIONS OF CHANGE AS A DRIVING FORCE It is at this point that the change agent must effect an explicit match between the primary goal of change and the type of conditions that are most likely to influence that change—to match the goals of the change to the type of organizational structure that provides optimal conditions for change in the desired direction[43]—and "there are the ideological differences in the more usual sense—values, goals and styles of life—between the low-income patient and the professional himself which affect communication between the two." [58]

Scheff [74e] talks of four basic types of social agency systems of orientation. Each of these systems can be assumed to function with a different effect, each sets up conditions for change that serve as driving forces towards some goals and restraining forces towards others.

Wesson offers a paradigm consisting of possible organizational postures—"passive," "committed," "defensive," and "engaged,"—each reacting differently to the goals of the social movement. These postures can be used to classify the orientation and practices of rehabilitation agencies in a manner similar to the cataloging of organizations by use of stereotypes, as suggested by Scheff [74e]: (1) there is a need for agencies to furnish "heavy duty" care, the tried-and-tested treatment, training, and placement (passive posture); (2) there is a need for others to seek new advantages and opportunities to improve the rehabilitation of the disabled (committed posture); (3) there is a need for a few to be resistant to new and innovative practices, questioning their utility and demanding recognition of their priorities in reordering service (defensive posture); and (4) still others must hold to an experimental and innovative stance and practice, continuously searching for new and improved management in rehabilitation (engaged posture).

The meaning for the client or patient of the posture of an organization structure is that it affects his access and utilization of the rehabilitation facility and his rehabilitation outcome. The discussions by Friedson,[74b] Scheff [74e] and Scott[74f] suggest a similar conclusion. The disabled individual's rehabilitation outcome is affected as much by the organization structure of rehabilitation as by his medical or physical deficiencies. It may even be affected more by them.[74]

It is obviously inappropriate for a "passive posture" system to become strongly invested in "revisualization" input since the product of such a system would probably be restricted not only in the range of service orientation and model, but also in the range of service methods and resources.

In interaction with the person, a "passive posture" system could be expected to reflect the equilibrium of the system. Interpersonal communication between the change agent and the person, will reflect hierarchical status, one-way communication, dominant-submissive role relationships, and rigidly delineated role functions.* The locus of responsible change energy will most likely be maintained within the organization itself.[2] Although predictably dependency coercing, a passive posture or a defensive posture organization might operate with high efficiency when the appropriate change influence is directed towards the highly dependent person. If the change goal encourages the dependent blind person to move from a passive, isolated home existence into a sheltered workshop, the dependency-coercing conditions of change might well be the most efficient.[54] The change influence, in this case, would be directed towards the passive system goal of the person, and the change of equilibrium would be congruent with what is possible for that person at that particular time. Thus the agency-person relationship might be operating at optimal efficiency. However, this type of agency would obviously be inappropriate if the change goal involved was one of influencing the person to change from a role in a protected workshop to an industrial work role.

---

* ". . . Readers, and especially practitioners, should be reminded that the model of the organizational structure purports to understand all organizations who use, at the outset, a pyramidical structure. Thus, for example, churches, families, schools, and scout troops tend to coerce dependency long before people become employees of industrial companies [or interact with social change agencies]." [27]

The goal of change influence would include a change both in the dependent system goal of the person and in the revisualization skills of the output. The agency whose organizational structure offered conditions that facilitated an interdependent role relationship in the decision making would be much more likely to match successfully conditions of change to the goal of change; and in this case, an agency whose organizational structure typifies the committed or engaged type of posture would be more likely to include interdependent problem solving as well as methods of service in its spectrum of change influence behaviors.

Thus, it becomes clear that part of the responsibility of a change agent is to choose his client in two separate ways. First, he must determine "where the client is" and whether the change need is located in the goal of system equilibrium change, or system output change, or both. Then he should match the agency influence conditions (derived from the agency goals and organizational structure) to the goals of change determined for the client. Thus, there must be a match not only between the agency-person goals of change but also between the agency-person structure for change. Implicit here is the need to recognize the subsystem component of the person involved in the goal of change. A person who is blind does not automatically fall under the aegis of an agency whose goal is to rehabilitate "the blind." (This claim becomes clear when the blind person's goal of change is to have a broken bone knit. Here, the agency for the blind would not be likely to see subsystem "blind" as a primary goal, with "skeletal system" secondary.)

So far, the focus of this discussion has been upon the match between the person's goals of change and the agency's goals of change, and upon the structure both of the agency's system goal and of the person's system goal as a driving force in the direction of the goal of the agency-person interaction. It has also been emphasized that the goals of change for the given process are subgoals of the social goals of change. Success or failure can, therefore, be measured by the changes in the person's potential mobility. Thus, the "behaviors" of change can be discussed in terms of social roles; and social roles can, in turn, be conceptualized as components of the social system.

Relationship Among Person, Change Agent, and Society

It is here that change agent influence is directed not only toward the person but also toward the society of which that person is a part.

Change agent influence is concerned with the role in the family system, in the social-groups system, in the formal-organization, in the work-group system, and ultimately in the social system.[73]

Productive output can be matched conceptually to the input-output relationship between the system and the environment; whereas productive living can be matched to the output that is a function of the system goal, or level of equilibrium within the system.[84]

The change agent function, therefore, is concerned not only with changes in the potentiality for productive living and productive output in the person who seeks change, but is also concerned with influencing opportunities for practicing productive living and productive output in the social subsystems in which the person moves.[84]

Thus, the agency influence has two directions: (1) influencing the person, his state and his skills, (2) influencing the different formal and informal groups in which the person plays an active role.[78] On the one hand, the agency influences the components of the person's potential performance of a role, and, on the other hand, it influences the environment, which in turn will be the system of which the person's role is a component.

The change agent influences change in the person's environment simply by influencing the person's output into his environment. More directed influences take into account a congruent influence of the components of the person's potential role performance and the system itself in which the person's role will be a component.

This connection is simple when the match is between a person and a learning institution. The change agent, in this situation, influences the person so that he can learn in the institution and also influences the institution so that it provides materials and an environment relevant to learning. More complex is the coordination of influence towards change of the person, on the one hand, and change in the primary and secondary groups which are the environment of the person, on the other. To ignore the second focus is to ignore a major force in social role mobility.

Mismatch is again the simpler aspect to illustrate. It is a mismatch when the potential of a person's output is in a system environment that cannot utilize that potential; for example, the situation in which a blind person whose potential output is the role behaviors of a lawyer is placed in a protected workshop system whose required role behaviors are mechanical skills.

Matching a person and an environment is less simple. Logically the more professional the role requirements, the less the component "handicap" is a criterion. For example, a blind person who has a system equilibrium of problem-solving and the revisualization skills that fulfill the output requirement of paperwork will be well matched in a component role of a university system where problem solving behaviors are part of the role prescription for both students and teachers. His output as a student or as a teacher would probably be congruent with the goals of output of the university system, which in turn are postulated as congruent with the goals of the social system.

The change agent's function is not only to match the person to a relevant organization so that the person's output matches the organization's goal, but also to influence the organization so that it utilizes that person's output in terms of the appropriate goal.[34]

This may well mean that the change agent focus is on influencing behaviors that belong to a cultural stereotype rather than to cultural role relationships.[36] It is a simple matter to match a person to a job, using these criteria of role behaviors required. It is not a simple matter to influence the interaction between the person and the people around him so that the needed role behaviors are encouraged (reinforced) and used productively (integrated into the organization's productivity).

Right now there are certain stable stereotype roles that have their matching organization and person-role relationships. For example, the person in a dependent, passive role has behaviors that match a component role in the D. P. A. system. Again, the person in the role of "dependent worker" has output behaviors that match the goals of the "protected workshop" system. Predictably, role behaviors that are congruent with the stereotype are reinforced, and behaviors that are incongruent are not.[14] In both cases the structure of the organization and the component role relationships can be matched to rehabilitation roles; however, the congruence is problem oriented rather than problem-solving oriented. Once the person's role behaviors match the problem *solving* role, then the appropriate match is no longer a problem *oriented* system.

Stereotyping as a Change Influence

Incongruence of match between role relationships and organizations appears when the output behaviors that are congruent with organizational work are not the behaviors that are primarily integrated into the system. A major mismatch occurs when a worker, hired by an organization to do a job, is in a position where his success or failure is not primarily determined in terms of his output, and when the behaviors that are reinforced are not those that fit the work role.

It is at this point that change agent influence needs to focus on the system goal of the organization that is offering job placement and to concentrate on defining the subsystem of which the person is actually to be a component. If the subsystem is not the work system but the "hiring handicapped persons" system, the role requirement will probably be different. In other words, the component of the person hired will not be "worker" but "handicap."

Two very different sorts of goals might be implied by the line "typed by a blind typist" on a sheet of stationery. When the stationery is an output from the Office of the Blind, "typed by a blind typist" carries information about kinds of work output of which the person who is blind is capable. There is congruence between this sort of information and the change agent goal of influencing conditions in the environment that will facilitate the goal of social mobility for the person who is blind.

However, when "typed by a blind typist" appears on the stationery of an industrial firm, congruence with the profit-making system-goal of the organization is less clear. Here, clearly, the "blind typist" is hired as a component of the "public relations" subsystem of the industrial system. And the component of the person system that is the subsystem is "*blind* person who can type" rather than "*typing* person who is blind." (It is perhaps indicative that industry rarely advertises other rehabilitated employees. One finds no subscripts "typed by an ex-convict.")

It is clear from the literature that behavioral output is valued to the extent that it is perceived as congruent with the group goal.[78] For the typical worker in an industrial system, behavior that is congruent with social and work norms of production is rewarded at a peer level, and behavior congruent with expectations of production is rewarded hierarchically.[64,80] All organization results in a certain role stereotyping, and to the extent that stereotyping is rewarding, behaviors that match the stereotype are rewarded. Thus it is that output antithetical to the norms of production may be negatively reinforced in industry.[21,81]

It can therefore be hypothesized that when the primary role requirement is "handicapped," behaviors that are congruent with the stereotype of handicapped people will be reinforced, whether or not they are also congruent with productive work. The stereotypic behavior of the handicapped is "passive, dependent, grateful, and conformist." This is not behavior that is congruent with any output that requires anything more than routine work. It is highly incongruent with a role that is problem-solving, innovational, and independent.

This analysis has relevance for change agent function, for the potentiality for a serious mismatch is implicit. The change agent can interact with a person so that the person's equilibrium changes from dependent to self-determining. The person's output can change from inefficient revisualization to highly efficient revisualization; the person's social mobility potential can rise. If, however, the work role carries with it the behavioral prescription "handicapped person," then precisely those behaviors of dependency which are antithetical to the goal of change will be reinforced, because dependency behavior will fit the stereotype of the work goal, and work output will be a secondary reinforcement criterion.

Thus, the change agent functions are: (1) to discriminate among the change issues at the level of the system equilibrium of the person (the variable of self-determination); (2) to evaluate the output from the system of the person into the environment (revisualization); (3) to match the appropriate change agent influence behaviors to the goals of the interaction; (4) to determine the type of agency organization that offers optimal conditions for facilitating the goals of change; (5) and to match the person's potential output of social mobility with the organization in which the person can make social mobility a reality. The change agent must also be able to discriminate among the output goals that the organization has for the individual which are congruent with the social goals (self-determination, problem-solving) and the output goals which are incongruent (dependency coercing) so that the social role behaviors that are rewarded are consistent with social goals.

The final point to be made here is that, although stereotyping of behaviors expected from the "handicapped" may be incongruent with the goal of social mobility and may be as much of a handicap to the blind person's social mobility as blindness itself,[55] this stereotyping is also incongruent with the *public* goal of social mobility.[36]

Robert Theobold raises some relevant issues here. Rehabilitation is most frequently discussed in terms of handicapped people, where the handicap itself means that the person must achieve social mobility by modifying the way in which he relates to the world and by selecting a role that can be appropriately rewarding both to himself and to society. Theobold observes that if we are to educate for the future, we must find ways to develop creativity.[76] He continues:

> The best way to achieve this is to change our educational system from being discipline-oriented to being problem-oriented. . . . We may reasonably hope to change the educational process so that those still within it will understand that toil is unnecessary and will accept

> the freedom made possible by cybernation. It will be far more difficult to bring an older generation that was raised within the Protestant ethic to this point of view. Will we have to develop political policies to preserve jobs for the older members of society while challenging the young to work in nonstructured situations? And if this is indeed necessary, what social norms can we develop to prevent a profound generational split?

The concept of rehabilitation, in Theobold's view, has come to include a concern with people who have no immediately identifiable handicap: high school dropouts, draft rejectees, automation casualties. In these situations, a person's mobility is handicapped by his relationship to the culture. Social mobility then becomes no longer a rehabilitation problem of the obviously handicapped but a general social problem.[48]

Social Issues in Change

The role prescription implied by the social goals of self-determination, socialization, goal oriented problem solving, and productive living cannot yet be implemented. The equilibrium in the culture as a whole is not functioning at the level of creative problem solving that is necessary in order to integrate existing information input and to provide productive output. But most Americans do not want to be mere cultural spectators, and look forward to fulfilling some social role.[76]

Practical operational methods are not yet generally available; and, therefore, no general, practical steps can be taken towards the goal. Methods of influencing conditions for productive *living* are still at the theoretical, question-formulating stage. What is more, relevant information that is already available from research, analysis, experience, and theory has yet to be organized so that it can be extracted and integrated into the cultural system and placed into the environment effectively in terms of change.

If goal attainment depends both on the factors of clarifying the goal and also on mapping out operational, alternative paths to the goal, it is now appropriate for change agents to focus on the cooperative, operational skills required in doing both. In the service of these two aims, perhaps it is not enough to recognize the discrepancy between the way things are, and the way the social literature conceives that they might be. Perhaps it is more important to focus directly on the skills of clarifying the change agent role and on improving the skills that are needed to perform that role. In the problems of rehabilitating the handicapped, retraining the handicapped, and influencing the social mobility of the handicapped to a more productive output in terms of productive living goal, all the issues crucial in social change are present.

NOTES

1. Chris Argyris, *Interpersonal Competence and Organizational Effectiveness* (Homewood, Illinois: Richard D. Irwin, 1962).
2. ———, "Organizational Leadership," *Leadership and Interpersonal Behavior* (New York: Holt, Rinehart and Winston, 1961), 326–354.
3. Jean M. Arsenian, "Young Children in an Insecure Situation," *Journal of Abnormal and Social Psychology,* 38 (1943), 225–249.
4. E. M. Bass and M. Faye-Tyler Norton, "Group Size and Leaderless Discussion," *Journal of Applied Psychology,* Vol. 35, No. 1 (1951), 397–400.
5. Mary K. Bauman and Norman M. Yoder, *Adjustment to Blindness Reviewed* (Springfield, Illinois: Charles C Thomas, 1966). The following references were used in the *Bauman* and *Yoder* chapter on motivation:
   - 5*a*. L. Festinger, *A Theory of Cognitive Dissonance* (Evanston, Illinois: Row, Peterson, 1957).
   - 5*b*. R. N. Filer and D. D. O'Connell, "Motivation of Aging Persons," *Journal of Gerontology,* 19 (1964), 15–22.
   - 5*c*. S. L. Fink, Rainette Fants, and J. Zinker, "Relevance of Maslow's Hierarchy to Rehabilitation," *Rehabilitation Counselors' Bulletin,* 7 (1963), 41–48.
   - 5*d*. M. Grayson, Ann Powers, and J. Levi, "Psychiatric Aspects of Rehabilitation," *Monograph II,* Institute of Physical Medicine and Rehabilitation, New York University—Bellevue Medical Center (1952).
   - 5*e*. Nancy Kerr and L. Meyerson, "Motivating Working Behavior in Workmen's Compensation Clients," Paper read at Convention of the American Psychological Association (September, 1964).
   - 5*f*. H. Levinson, "What Work Means to Man," *Menninger Quarterly,* 18 (1964), 1–11.
   - 5*g*. T. Linde, "Techniques for Establishing Motivation Through Operant Conditioning," *American Journal of Mental Deficiency,* 67 (1962), 437–440.
   - 5*h*. S. Lissitz, "Motivating Geriatric Hospital Patients," *Geriatrics,* 17 (1962), 301–308.
   - 5*i*. J. Michael and L. Meyerson, "A Behavioral Approach to Counseling and Guidance," *Harvard Educational Review,* 32 (1962), 383–402.
   - 5*j*. C. H. Patterson, *Counseling the Emotionally Disturbed* (New York: Harper and Brothers, 1958).
   - 5*k*. M. J. Reichel, "Understanding in Rehabilitation of the Severely Disabled," *Archives of Physical Medicine and Rehabilitation,* 38 (1957), 307–310.
   - 5*l*. L. E. Schlesinger, "Staff Authority and Patient Participation in Rehabilitation," *Rehabilitation Literature,* 24 (1963), 247–249.
   - 5*m*. ———, "Staff Tensions and Needed Skills in Staff-patient Interactions," *Rehabilitation Literature,* 24 (1963), 247–249.

5*n*. V. H. Vroom, *Work and Motivation* (New York: John Wiley and Sons, 1964).
5*o*. Marshall C. Youvitz, George T. Jacobi, and Gordon D. Goldstein, *Self-Organizing Systems* (Washington: Spartan Books, 1962).
6. George W. Bartholaw and Bulent Tunakan, "Rehabilitation of the Chronic Patient," *Occuptional Mental Health Notes* (August, 1966), 0700029607999.
7. Robert C. Behan and A. H. Hirschfeld, "Disability Without Disease or Accident," *Occupational Mental Health Notes* (October, 1966), 0700032801999.
8. Warren G. Bennis, "Changing Organizations," *Journal of Applied Behavioral Science,* Vol. 2, No. 3 (1966), 247–263.
9. Leonard Berkowitz, *Studies in Group Norms: The Perception of Group Attitudes as Related to Criteria of Group Effectiveness* (Lakeland, Florida Air Force Base: Air Force Personnel and Training Research Center, November, 1954).
10. J. H. S. Bossard, "Law of Family Interaction," *American Journal of Sociology,* 50 (1945), 292–294.
11. Leland P. Bradford, J. R. Gibbs, and Kenneth D. Benne, *T-Group Theory and Laboratory Method* (New York: John Wiley and Sons, 1964).
12. Dorwin Cartwright, "Achieving Change in People: Some Applications of Group Dynamics Theory," *Human Relations,* 4 (1951), 381–392.
13. ——— and Alvin Zander, *Group Dynamics* (Elmsford, New York: Row, Peterson and Company, 1960).
14. Mark A. Chelser, "Ethnocentrism and Attitudes Toward the Physically Disabled," *Journal of Personality and Social Psychology,* Vol. 2, No. 6 (1965), 877–881.
15. L. Coch and R. P. French, Jr., "Overcoming Resistance to Change," *Human Relations,* I (1948), 512–532.
16. Hardin A. Collins, "Counseling the Retarded—Factors in Predicting Success," Abstract in *Occupational Mental Health Notes* (August, 1966), 0700030717999.
17. "Earning a Living in Today's Anxious World," *Occupational Mental Health Notes* (October, 1966), 0700032788999.
18. L. Festinger, *A Theory of Cognitive Dissonance* (Evanston, Illinois: Row, Peterson and Company, 1957), 32–347.
19. ——— and E. Aronson, "The Arousal and Reduction of Dissonance in Social Context," *Group Dynamies: Research and Theory,* eds. D. Cartwright and A. Zander (Evanston, Illinois: Row, Peterson and Company, 1960), 214–231.
20. ———, A. Pepitone and T. Newcomb, "Some Consequences of Deindividuation in a Group," *Journal of Abnormal Social Psychology,* 47 (1952), 382–389.
21. ——— and J. Thibaut, "Interpersonal Communication in Small Groups," *Journal of Abnormal and Social Psychology,* 46 (1951), 92–99.
22. Ned A. Flanders, *et al., Helping Teachers Change Their Behaviors,* U.S. Office of Education project numbers 1721012 and 7-32-0560-171.0 (University of Michigan, Ann Arbor, April, 1963).
23. Fred H. Frankel, "Emotional First Aid," *Occupational Mental Health Notes* (August, 1966), 0700028066999.
24. Mervin B. Freedman, "The Post-Industrial Generation," *The Nation* (June 14, 1965).
25. William Furst, "Homogeneous Vs. Heterogeneous Groups," *Group Psychotherapy and Group Function,* eds. Max Rosenbaum and Milton Burger (New York: Basic Books, 1963), 407–411.

26. J. R. Gibbs, "Defensive Communication," *Journal of Communication,* Vol. 11, No. 3 (September, 1961).
27. ———, *Factors Producing Defensive Behavior Within Groups* (Boulder, Colorado: Group Process Laboratory, University of Colorado, August, 1956).
28. Eli Ginzberg, "Psychology and Manpower Policy," *American Psychologist,* Vol. 21, No. 6 (1966), 549–554.
29. Robert T. Golembiewski, *Behavior and Organization* (Chicago: Rand McNally, 1962).
30. ———, *The Small Group* (Chicago: University of Chicago Press, 1962).
31. William Gomberg, "The Trouble With Democratic Management," *Trans-action,* Vol. 3, No. 1 (1966), 30–35.
32. Philip G. Hanson, Paul Rothaus, Dale L. Johnson, and Francis A. Lyly, "Autonomous Groups in Human Relations Training for Psychiatric Patients, Houston, Texas, Houston VA Hospital," Paper read at the 72nd Annual Convention of the American Psychological Association, Los Angeles, California (1964).
33. Paul A. Hare, *Handbook of Small Group Research* (New York: Macmillan, 1962).
34. Lawrence C. Hartlage, "Receptivity of Employers to Hiring Mentally Retarded and Ex-mental Patients," Abstract in *Occupational Mental Health Notes* (August, 1966), 0700030740999.
35. Georgina Hotchkiss and Curtis T. Prout, "Use of the Community in the Rehabilitation of Patients," Abstract in *Occupational Mental Health Notes* (August, 1966), 0700030720999.
36. William S. House, "Effects of Group Cohesiveness on Organization Performance," *Occupational Mental Health Notes* (October, 1966), 0700032775999.
37. "How Do You Like Your Job?" *Today's Health,* Abstract in *Occupational Mental Health Notes* (August, 1966), 0700029657999.
38. Carl Delacato, Robert Doman, Glenn Doman, and Eugene Spitz have founded a center in Philadelphia (Institute for the Development of Human Potential) where a new system for the treatment of children with severe brain injuries is used. The concept, based on neurological organization, is aimed at the injured central nervous system rather than at the resultant peripheral symptoms. The project consists of permitting the child normal developmental opportunities in areas where the responsible brain level is undamaged, externally imposing the bodily patterns of activity which were the responsibility of damaged brain levels, establishment of hemispheric dominance and early unilaterality, respiratory improvement as measured by vital capacity, and sensory stimulation to improve bodily awareness and position sense. The center also sponsors the Institute for Language Disability. Aphasia, delayed speech, stuttering, retarded reading, poor spelling and writing, and reading below mathematical ability are approached from the point of view of neurological organization. Doman Reading Exposure Materials are available as educational aids for teaching reading to children as young as 18 months of age.
39. Robert L. Kahn and Elise Boulding, *Power and Conflict in Organizations* (New York: Basic Books, 1964).
40. Alfred Kuhn, *The Study of Society* (Homewood, Illinois: Richard D. Irwin and The Dorsey Press, 1963).
41. Leonard Krasner, "The Translation of Operant Conditioning Procedures from the Experimental Laboratory to the Psychotherapeutic Interaction," Paper prepared for the American Psychological Association Annual Meeting (September, 1966).

42. John D. Krumboltz, "Behavioral Goals for Counseling," *Journal of Counseling Psychology,* Vol. 13, No. 2 (1966), 153–159.
43. Martin Lakin, "Human Relations Training and Interracial Social Action: Problems in Self and Client Definition," *Journal of Applied Behavioral Science,* Vol. 2, No. 2 (1966), 139–147.
44. Harold Leavitt, J. Ronald, A. H. Mueller, "Some Effects of Feedback on Communications," *Human Relations,* 4 (November, 1951), 401–410.
45. Kurt Lewin, *Field Theory in Social Science* (New York: Harper and Row, 1951).
46. O. I. Lovaas, *et al.,* "Reinforcement Therapy," Smith, Kline & French Laboratories, Film Supplement (1966).
47. Helen B. Lewis and M. Franklin, "An Experimental Study of the Role of the Ego in Work, and the Significance of Task-Orientation in Work," *Journal of Experimental Psychology,* 31 (1944), 195–215.
48. John Maciver, "Behavioral Sciences in Occupational Health," *Occupational Mental Health Notes* (October, 1966), 0700032789999.
49. David Marlow and Robert Frager, "Commitment to Action Taking As a Consequence of Cognitive Dissonance," *Journal of Personality and Social Psychology,* Vol. 2, No. 6 (1965), 864–868.
50. Donald G. Miles and F. Edward Harris, "An Over-view of Vocational Rehabilitation in the Modern Mental Health Center," Abstract in *Occupational Mental Health Notes* (August, 1966), 0700029660999.
51. James G. Miller, "Information Input Overload," *Self-Organizing Systems* (Washington, 1961), 61.
52. "Nark Presents Awards to Employers of Retarded," Abstract in *Occupational Mental Health Notes* (August, 1966), 0700030735999.
53. J. E. Neighbor, Margaret Beech, Donald T. Brown, David Kevin, and John S. Visher, "An Approach to the Selection of Patients for Group Psychotherapy," *Group Psychotherapy and Group Function,* eds. Max Rosenbaum and Milton Burger (New York: Basic Books, 1963), 413–424.
54. Francis J. O'Neill and David Graubert, "The Sheltered Workshop at Central Islip State Hospital," *Occupational Mental Health Notes* (October, 1966), 0700032763999.
55. Robert Palmer, *et al.,* "Industrial Panel—A Report on Experience in Subcontracting in a Mental Hospital," *Occupational Mental Health Notes* (October, 1966), 0700032767999.
56. Luigi Petrullo and Bernard M. Bass, *Leadership and Interpersonal Behavior* (New York: Holt, Rinehart and Winston, 1961).
57. Bertram H. Raven and Jan Rietsema, "The Effects of Varied Clarity of Group Goal and Group Path upon the Individual and his Relation to his Group," *Group Dynamics,* eds. Dorwin Cartwright and Alvin Zanders (Elmsford, New York: Row, Peterson and Company, 1960), 395–413.
58. R. Reiff and F. Riessman, "The Indigenous Non-Professional," *Community Mental Health Journal,* Monograph No. 1 (1965).
59. ———, "Mental Health Manpower and Institutional Change," *American Psychologist,* Vol. 21, No. 6 (1966), 540–548.
60. David Reisman, *The Lonely Crowd* (New Haven: Yale University Press, 1950).
61. Julius A. Roth, "Review of the Month: Sociology and Rehabilitation," *American Psychologist,* Vol. 27, No. 11 (1966), 333–335.
62. Paul Rothaus, Dale L. Johnson, Philip G. Hanson, Francis A. Lyle, and R. Moyer, "Autonomous and Trainer-led Groups. Houston, Texas, Houston VA Hospital," Paper read at the 72nd Annual Convention of the American Psychological Association, Los Angeles, California (September 4, 1964).

63. Stanley E. Seasore, *Group Cohesiveness in the Industrial Work Group* (Ann Arbor, Michigan: Survey Research Center, University of Michigan, 1954), 11–13.
64. S. Schachter, N. Ellertson, Dorothy McBride, and Doris Gregory, "An Experimental Study of Cohesiveness and Productivity," *Human Relations,* 4 (1951), 229–238.
65. Thomas J. Scheff, "The Role of the Mentally Ill and the Dynamics of Mental Disorder," *Sociometry,* 26 (December, 1963), 436–435.
66. Lawrence Schlesinger, J. M. Jackson, and Jean Buttman, "Leader-Member Interaction in Management Committees," *Journal of Abnormal Social Psychology,* 61 (November, 1960), 360–364.
67. Muzafer Sherif, *The Psychology of Social Norms* (New York: Harper, 1936).
68. Irwin Silverman and Charles Marcantonio, "Demand Characteristics Versus Dissonance Reduction as Determinants of Failure-seeking Behavior," *Journal of Personality and Social Psychology,* Vol. 2, No. 6 (1965), 882–884.
69. Jai B. P. Sinha and Robert J. Wherry, "Determinants of Norm Violating Behavior in a Simulated Industrial Setting," *Occupational Mental Health Notes* (August, 1966), 0700029596999.
70. B. F. Skinner, "Why Teachers Fail," *Saturday Review,* 80 (October 16, 1965).
71. Philip E. Slater, "Contrasting Correlates of Group Size," *Sociometry,* 21 (June, 1958), 129–139.
72. M. B. Smith and N. Hobbs, "The Community and the Community Mental Health Center," *American Psychologist,* Vol. 21, No. 6 (1966), 449–454.
73. Ralph M. Stodgill and Carol L. Shartle, "Patterns of Administrative Performance," *Monograph #81* (Columbus, Ohio: Ohio State University, Bureau of Business Research, 1956).
74. Marvin B. Sussman, ed., *Sociology and Rehabilitation* (Washington: American Sociological Association, 1966). The articles from the Sussman volume listed below deal with the growing problem of dependency in our society and show how dependency of all types is beginning to be thought of as susceptible to rehabilitation:
  74*a*. Samuel W. Bloom, "Rehabilitation as an Interpersonal Process," 114–131.
  74*b*. Eliot Friedson, "Disability as Social Deviance," 71–99.
  74*c*. Jerome K. Myers, "Consequences and Prognoses of Disability," 25–51.
  74*d*. Saad Z. Nagi, "Some Conceptual Issues in Disability and Rehabilitation," 100–113.
  74*e*. Thomas J. Scheff, "Typification in the Diagnostic Practices of Rehabilitation Agencies," 139–147.
  74*f*. Robert A. Scott, "Comments About Interpersonal Processes of Rehabilitation," 132–138.
  74*g*. Robert Strauss, "Social Change and the Rehabilitation Concept," 2–34.
  74*h*. Edward A. Suchman, "A Model for Research and Evaluation on Rehabilitation," 52–70.
  74*i*. Albert F. Wessen, "The Apparatus of Rehabilitation: An Organizational Analysis," 148–178.
75. Joseph J. Tecce, "Relationship of Anxiety (Drive) and Response Competition in Problem Solving," *Occupational Mental Health Notes* (August, 1966), 0700028055999.
76. Robert Theobald, "Should Men Compete with Machines?" *The Nation* (May 9, 1966), 544–550.

77. Edwin J. Thomas, "Effects of Facilitative Role Interdependence on Group Functioning," *Group Dynamics,* eds. Dorwin Cartwright and Alvin Zanders (Elmsford, New York: Row, Peterson and Company, 1960), 449–471.
78. James D. Thompson and William J. McEwen, "Organizational Goals and Environment: Goal-Setting as an Interaction Process," *Group Dynamics,* eds. Dorwin Cartwright and Alvin Zanders (Elmsford, New York: Row, Peterson and Company, 1960), 472–484.
79. Harold M. Visotsky, "New Community Approaches in Rehabilitation," Abstract in *Occupational Mental Health Notes* (August, 1966), 070002-9658999.
80. Paul F. Wernimont, "Intrinsic and Extrinsic Factors in Job Satisfaction," Abstract in *Occupational Mental Health Notes* (August, 1966), 070003-0738999.
81. Western Electric Researches.
82. Jack Wilder, *et al.,* "A Case for a Flexible, Long-Term Sheltered Workshop for Psychiatric Patients," *Occupational Mental Health Notes* (October, 1966), 0700032768999.
83. Donald A. Woolf, "The Management Theory Jungle Revisited," *Occupational Mental Health Notes* (August, 1966), 0700029593999.
84. Yovits, *et al., Self-Organizing Systems* (Washington: Spartan Books, 1962).

THE SYSTEMS ANALYSIS APPROACH TO RELATIONSHIPS BETWEEN AGENCIES FOR THE BLIND AND BLIND PERSONS

Robert A. Scott

This paper is divided into two sections. The first explains some of the thinking that underlies a systems analysis approach and what the potential benefits are which could result from using it for the study of relationships between agencies for the blind and blind persons. The second section evaluates the systems analysis approach contained in the previous paper by Miss Agazarian, and presents some of the findings of a study I recently completed of organizations for the blind in which a systems analysis approach was used.

SYSTEMS ANALYSIS APPROACH

The basic starting point for a systems analysis is the decision as to what the basic components of the system are going to be. They may be people, groups, physical objects, relationships, or even entire societies. We decide what the components will be by referring to the problem we want clarified in the first place.

The systems analysis approach says that components of any system are related to one another in such a way that a change in one part implies some change in all other components; and that the degree of change of each part will vary depending upon how, and how closely the various components are linked.

Second, one of the most important facts about anything that we choose to view in terms of a system—be it a factory, a conference, or a personality—is that it changes. We must therefore have some way of dealing with this fact analytically. We can identify any change that occurs in a system in terms of its effect upon what the system produces or upon the impact of the system on its environment. The technical phrase that is used is "output." Changes in output are attributable to one or both of two factors: changes in the internal relationships within the system; and changes in the amount and kind of information or material that the system is able to extract from its environment and use as input. That means that a factory which begins to produce more cars may be doing so because of a more efficient arrangement and utilization of its internal resources, or because it is commanding more manpower and better resources from its environment, or both. Theoretically it is possible to attribute any change in a system to one or both of these conditions.

Finally, when we start thinking in terms of systems, we cannot limit ourselves just to the unit or group or society or factory that interests us. Unfortunately, this approach is contagious in the sense that it also forces us to look at the surrounding world in terms of systems. This fact suggests an important feature of the systems analysis approach. It is that a component of one system is always seen as a component of other systems as well. Since every system is related in a functional sense to at least one component of another system, we are led to analyze the effects of our present interaction upon other systems in which we are embedded. We cannot be components of the present system without taking time away from our families or work. As a result, being a component of this system is clearly related in important ways to our participation in other systems.

What has all of this got to do with work for the blind? I will try to give you an answer. Those who have spent time in administrative positions have undoubtedly encountered the experience of initiating a program in order to solve one problem, and, in the course of it, finding that another problem more serious than the first has been created. A common cause for this is our inability to keep tabs on everything at once. In formulating policies the exigencies of the situation usually lead us to look at the likely effects that our proposed actions will have on the most immediate problems we face. By the same token our attention is diverted from examining the effects that our actions are likely to have on other seemingly innocuous aspects of the situation. One of the reasons why the systems analysis approach was developed was to overcome this very problem. A systems analysis forces us to identify the likely effects that an action will have on all identifiable components of a system in advance of actually initiating that action. If the approach works, we should be able to anticipate every relevant consequence that will result from any action we propose to take. Moreover, the systems approach allows us to "play around" with alternative planned actions in the sense of trying to measure the differential impact which certain procedures are likely to have on other systems components. Systems analysis is therefore a tool that can be used by the scientist, the administrator, or the technician. It permits him to clarify how all of the factors with which he must deal will interact with one another, what will happen if he changes one component of the system, what effects he can expect from it, and a great deal more.

Clearly, if you can proceed in this fashion, you will be much more effective and successful than if you must continually fall back on educated guesses. Even if your administrative action fails, you will still know where in your program or organization readjustments will probably occur, and this knowledge should enable you to ameliorate at least some of the detrimental effects. For this reason alone it would seem desirable to approach the field of work for the blind, and especially that part of it concerning agency-client relationships, from the systems analysis point of view.

There is a final point to make about this approach. We must be careful to understand that while a systems analysis may be more adequate than most other methods, it is not and cannot be everything; it has definite limitations. A systems analysis, for example, tells us what would happen to components of a system if we were to implement plan A; and how this would be different from the effects that plan B would have. It cannot tell us which course of action we should select, in the sense of which one is morally or otherwise desirable. I raise these points in order to forestall any letdown that may result when it is discovered that systems analysis is not a panacea for this or any field.

Evaluation and Research

With this background material I now turn to a consideration of the previous paper by Miss Agazarian. It is my responsibility to analyze this contribution in order to formulate specific and testable hypotheses about the relationships between agencies for the blind and blind persons. Miss Agazarian attempts to apply the concepts and methods of systems analysis to the agency-client relationship. The first question that must therefore be asked is: "How adequate is the systems analysis that is contained in this paper?" My answer is, "I don't know." Let me explain why.

I do not pretend to be expert enough on the subject of systems analysis to be able to tell you if the particular variant of it which Miss Agazarian has propounded is better or worse than other variants of the approach that might have been used. At the outset, then, I am prepared to acknowledge that my lack of expertise precludes the possibility of a definitive evaluation of her contribution.

While I am not an expert on the subject of systems analysis, I believe that I do qualify as an authority on the subject of relationships between agencies for the blind and blind persons. I have recently completed a study of the entire field of work for the blind in the United States. Part of this study included a careful analysis of all organizations, agencies, and programs for the blind that are currently in operation. The data that I have collected on the organizations provide some scale against which to measure the adequacy of Miss Agazarian's systems analysis approach. A comparison between her framework and my own knowledge of the subject to which she has applied it prompts me to make two general remarks. The first concerns the utility of her approach; the second, its empirical accuracy.

A systems analysis is justified to the extent that it can organize and make better sense out of what is already known; and to the extent that we are led by it to see relationships and to anticipate effects that we would otherwise not have seen. The primary contribution which is made by Miss Agazarian's paper is to describe in terms of systems, selected components of the agency-client relationship. As such, her paper is an attempted transliteration into systems analysis concepts of certain empirical information we have about relationships between clients and agencies. As a transliteration it is incomplete; the areas that are covered are, I believe, covered adequately. I see the paper as a starting point from which we must now proceed. The first step must be to complete the description she has begun; following that, we can then determine, by the two criteria I have cited above, if the systems analysis approach is a fruitful way of looking at work for the blind.

My second comment on her paper will be longer and more involved than the first because I want to challenge an erroneous assumption that has been introduced. Specifically: "It is logical to conclude that the goal of change is a function of both the person's goals and the change agent's goals. The change agent, by virtue of his role in a social change agency, implicitly has change goals that are social. Therefore, in the broadest sense, the goals of the change agent and the person are consistent with the goals of society." The assumption apparently is that there is some consistency between the goals that a blind person wishes to achieve, those which the agency for the blind attempts to set for him, and the ones which society has in mind. I am going to assert that exactly the opposite is the case—what society and agencies for the blind desire for blind people, and what blind people themselves wish, are directly contradictory.

In order to demonstrate this point, I will have to digress into a discussion of the findings of part of my study concerning the relationship between agencies for the blind, the community, and blind persons. I will: (1) present some statistics concerning the characteristics of the blind population of the United States; (2) describe the results of a study I did on agencies for the blind; and (3) make a few concluding remarks about the impact which agencies have on clients. I am doing this not only to refute the assumption in question, but also to bring into the discussion some empirical data upon which a more complete systems analysis can be made.

The number of persons who are blind in the United States is the subject of some dispute. The most reliable estimates of this number were recently made by the National Center for Health Statistics Study of Binocular Visual Acuity. This study showed that for the period 1960–62, there were about 889,000 blind persons in the adult, non-institutionalized population in the age range 18–79 years. If we apply this figure to the comparable United States population census for 1965, we could estimate that there were at that time about 928,000 blind persons in this age range, of which 53 per cent had a corrected visual acuity measured at less than 20/200; the remaining 47 per cent had a corrected visual acuity of 20/200.

A number of facts about this population of blind persons are remarkable. First, a majority of them are elderly persons: 66 per cent are between the ages of 55 and 80 years; another 15 per cent are in the age group of 45–54; 17 per cent of these blind persons are in the age range of 18–44; and only about 2 per cent are children under the age of 18 years. These data show that two-thirds of all blind persons are in age groups where retirement is either pending or a reality; and that only a small minority are in age groups where either employment or education is realistic.

Second, blindness is much more common in women than in men. Seven out of ten cases of blindness in the adult population occur in women, and in all adult age groups there appear to be more blind women than blind men. As one would expect, the sex difference is greatest in the older groups. When we take the factors of age and sex together, we find that 50 per cent of all cases of blindness are found among women 55 years of age and older; another 20 per cent of cases occur among women in the age group 18–54 years. Elderly men account for 18 per cent of all cases, and only 12 per cent of the cases of blindness occur among men 18–54 years of age.

Third, blindness is comparatively rare among children. There are estimated to be only about 27,140 blind youngsters in the United States at the present time. The blindness rate among children is only 0.32 per 1,000 persons. In contrast, the blindness rate for elderly persons is about 33 per 1,000 persons.

Finally, only a small number of blind persons are in fact totally blind; a majority of them have some measurable visual acuity. The data which are available suggest that there is a direct relationship between amount of visual loss and age. The older a blind person is, the more serious his visual loss is likely to be.

Ideally, we would expect services for the blind to reflect the age and sex distribution of the blind population, as well as the respective acuteness of the needs of these groups. A major portion of the financial and manpower resources of work for the blind ought therefore to be invested in programs which are designed to meet the needs of those who cannot be expected to be self-supporting, and more particularly to meet the needs of the elderly. Conversely, a minority of these resources ought to be invested in programs for educating and training children and employable adults.

I made a study of the programs of all direct service agencies listed in the American Foundation for the Blind directory of agencies for the blind in the United States. This list was supplemented by a careful search of the yellow pages of the telephone directories of several major cities. In all, 798 separate agencies, organizations, and service programs for the blind were identified. Of these, 283 are private and 515 governmental. Only 9 per cent of these organizations are concerned primarily with elderly blind persons. By contrast, 67 per cent have programs which are intended primarily for children and employable adults. Another 23 per cent are "mixed" agencies, which offer services to blind persons of all ages. The remaining 1 per cent (11) do not offer direct services to the blind.

An analysis was made of programs in the agencies and organizations which serve elderly blind persons. There are 21 domiciles which house and care for a total of about 1,000 elderly blind persons. The remainder of these organizations are state offices responsible for administering the federal-state welfare assistance programs such as Aid to the Needy Blind. In the mixed agencies which serve blind persons of all ages, programs for the elderly are almost exclusively recreational. These range from organized recreational programs to drop-in clubs where persons may come during the day.

By and large, the only publicly supported services which older blind persons receive are those offered through the welfare department and the Library of Congress. Restorative rehabilitation services are not ordinarily available unless there is a tangible employment objective for either the elderly person or someone on whom he is dependent. In the private sector of work for the blind, elderly blind persons are not automatically ineligible for services. It is simply that the bulk of these programs are clearly intended to serve educable young persons and employable adults. By and large, services for the aged are simply appendages to programs for persons in other age groups. Participation of the elderly in these programs therefore depends upon their having the same general level of health and stamina as those for whom the program is primarily intended. There are some remarkable exceptions to this general pattern. In the state of Massachusetts, for example, comprehensive services are provided to the aged by both public and private agencies. In that state is found one of the few geriatric rehabilitation centers in the country.

There is another fact which is not apparent from these data. Existing programs are not geared to serve all blind persons in a given age group. Numerous services are available for the child who is educable, but very few services exist for the child with multiple handicaps. There are many services for the blind person who is thought to be employable, but few for the one who is thought to be untrainable or for whom employment is an unrealistic goal. Recreation programs for elderly blind persons are located in the agency itself, so that only those older blind persons who are mobile and independent enough to travel can take advantage of them. In effect, programs are geared to serve selected blind persons, and usually those who enjoy the highest probability for success. This point is not insignificant in view of the fact that a very substantial portion of the blind population, in all age groups, have severe and multiple handicaps.

The welfare system for the blind in America is, therefore geared to serve a special and somewhat select portion of the total population of blind persons. Its basic emphasis is upon those who are young, educable, and employable; correspondingly, the system tends to overlook elderly persons who are the bulk of the blind population, and persons of all age groups who are the most seriously disabled by their condition.

Thus far I have compared the distribution of services for the blind in this country with the demographic characteristics of the blind population. Now I want to consider another question. It is the avowed purpose of all programs for the blind to help the individual blind person to function as independently as he can. The question therefore arises: what is the actual impact of agency programs upon the blind persons who do receive services?

In view of the fact that in 1965 there were only about 928,000 blind persons in the entire country, the number of visually impaired individuals living in any particular geographical area is usually quite small. It is estimated that there are only about 40,000–50,000 blind persons in all of New York City, only about 10,000 in Philadelphia, and only about 14,000 in the Boston metropolitan area. Yet, there are nearly 800 separate agencies and organizations for the blind in this country, a majority of which are situated in large urban areas. New York City has 50 separate organizations for the blind, 38 of which offer direct services; Philadelphia has 14 major direct agencies; and there are 13 major agencies in the greater metropolitan area of Boston. Since a majority of these agencies offer services only to children and/or employable adults, there is a very high ratio of agencies to clients. In New York City, for example, there are three major agencies and six smaller ones which offer direct social and educational services to an estimated 1,850 blind children living in the area. Even if we assume that none of these children have multiple handicaps (which we cannot), the agency-client ratio is very large indeed. Twenty-two different organizations and agencies provide direct rehabilitation and vocational services to an estimated 12,000 blind persons who are of working age. This figure is inflated somewhat when we consider that between 50 and 60 per cent of blind persons 18–54 years of age are women, for whom employment is not always a realistic or appropriate objective. There are eleven other organizations which specialize in the production and distribution of braille books and recordings for the blind. In addition, there are a number of statewide and federal services which are available to the blind of New York City.

The fact that there is a disproportionately large number of agencies offering services has many consequences for blind persons, for agencies for the blind, and for the community which supports them. One seemingly inevitable consequence of this situation is that a competition for clients develops among those agencies for the blind situated in the same metropolitan areas. The intensity of this competition varies, of course, with fluctuations in the availability of suitable clients. For example, when the Second World War erupted and jobs for blind persons in commercial industry became widely available, the competition for clients became very intense. By the same token, competition for blind children diminished somewhat when their numbers increased as a result of retrolental fibroplasia. As these children are now moving into adulthood, the intensity of the competition is once again picking up.

The intense and sometimes ruthless competition between social agencies for clients who fit their programs affects the agency's relationship to its clients. When an agency has the opportunity to provide services to a blind person who is suitable for its program, it is reluctant to let him go completely. Finding a suitable replacement for him is always an uncertain matter; and without a substantial number of clients on hand, the agency may find it difficult to justify its expenditures to the public which supports it. Employment is secured for those persons in the agency's sheltered workshops, free recreational services are provided by the agency on an indefinite basis, and residential homes are sometimes maintained as well. Gradually, a greater and greater portion of the client's contact with the larger community becomes mediated, and often determined by the agency until the blind person is literally sequestered from the community. At this point the agency has then completely negated its original objective, which is to help blind persons to become independent, integrated members of the larger community.

These data clearly indicate that the goals which agencies for the blind in fact set for their clients are not necessarily the ones which are most functional for society, or for the blind persons themselves. In fact, the data suggest that the fundamental challenge raised by the welfare problem of blindness in our society is largely unmet; and that in some instances, the responses of society and of the welfare system of services to the blind may have positively injurious effects upon the problem.

The data also argue strongly for a systems analysis approach to this field as being the most effective means by which to correct the inequities I have identified. Miss Agazarian's paper is, I believe, a preliminary step in that general direction.

SESSION REPORT

Peter Kratcoski

During the general discussion period, Miss Yvonne Agazarian suggested to the group that it is more difficult for a visually handicapped or blind person to establish rapport with agency personnel than it is for the sighted person. Ways to overcome this difficulty are not specifically known, and there is a need for research to determine what sort of behavior, communication, and setting can be established to increase the development of rapport between the visually handicapped person and the agency representing him. Proper research might also indicate what sort of behavior would make it easier for blind people to communicate with sighted people in general, and what sort of specific behavior patterns blind people can use to overcome the defensive response of sighted people to avoid them.

The discussion further revealed some discrepancies in statistics and differences of opinion about the number of visually handicapped people and the specific demographic characteristics of this population. These uncertainties indicate a need for further research to provide specific data in these areas.

The majority of programs of existing agencies are designed for the visually handicapped child or the employable adult. Programs for the aged visually handicapped person and the multiple-handicapped person with visual loss as only one of his deficiencies are generally insufficient. Research is needed to determine how many of these people are in need of the services which are offered by the existing agencies and what additional programs are needed. For example, research could discover whether the lack of programs for the aged is attributable to the fact that the aged have adequately adjusted to their loss of sight and therefore have no need for service, or if the present situation is really a misallocation of resources.

Mrs. Sidney Pollack remarked that research in the area of a blind person's "self-conception" might be useful. For many visually handicapped persons who are considered blind in the legal sense there has been no corresponding self-conception of themselves as belonging to this category, and appropriate research might illuminate the process through which a transformation occurs in the person's conception about himself, his deficiencies, and his need for help from an agency.

Agencies develop their goals and policies, according to Robert Lee Robinson, on the bases of what type of clients come to them for help and the demands from publics or groups which give financial support to the agency. Agencies have a tendency, then, to become conservative in their policies and programs and may not adapt themselves rapidly enough to the changing characteristics and needs of the population they serve. Research which focuses on changes in agency policy, on what the process of change entails, and on what influences stimulate change might therefore be especially useful.

Miss Agazarian suggested that perhaps, through the systems analysis approach, research might be conducted which would be geared to help the agency to formulate policies which would be flexible enough to allow for changes in programs automatically occurring as the needs of society and the population being served change. The question, in other words, is: can programs which will automatically adjust to emerging needs be established?

In turn Dr. H. Robert Blank suggested research in the areas which will facilitate and increase the communication between the medical profession and the blind patient as the client of the agency. A large proportion of the visually handicapped population, he asserted, is not receiving services because it has no knowledge of these services, because psychological barriers have been erected against these services, and because the services are inconveniently located for the person involved. Research is needed to determine ways to promote closer cooperation between the medical profession and the agencies, so that blind or visually handicapped people will be introduced to the variety of agency services. Practical research is certainly needed to discover the most suitable geographic or spatial distribution in a city or town according to their accessibility to those who have need of the agencies and agency services.

Dr. Elena Gall expressed the desire for investigations designed to determine how the various concepts and approaches developed and utilized in the various sciences can be stated in terms which in some way have implication for the treatment of the blind. Agency personnel, she said, obviously need terminology in which they can express this knowledge.

Finally, Commissioner Elias S. Cohen thought it important to discover ways to develop greater communication among welfare agencies so that overlapping of programs can be eliminated, with another area for research being the discovery of ways to persuade those in need of services to utilize the services available to them.

PLACEMENT AND OCCUPATION

OCCUPATIONAL PLACEMENT AND CAREER DEVELOPMENT

Albert S. Thompson

Placement in an appropriate occupation is the objective of many of the social betterment programs in existence today. In a way, the basic justification of much of the public education system, the public employment services, the public and private rehabilitation services, and the more recent "anti-poverty" programs is the contribution which the programs make in helping the individual become a more satisfied and effective member of the labor force.

We live in a work oriented society. There are several historical reasons why work is so important in the United States. In addition to the influence of the Puritan principle of work as a duty and as a means of salvation, there were the necessity of denial of present pleasure for future reward and the challenge of conquering a new and hostile environment.

Work has social as well as individual rewards. As Super has written, one's job satisfaction "depends on the extent to which the work, the job, and the way of life that goes with them, enable one to play the kind of role that one wants to play," and "work satisfactions and life satisfactions depend upon his establishment in a type of work, a work situation, and a way of life in which he can play the kind of role which his growth and exploratory experiences have led him to consider congenial and appropriate." [16]

There recently have been predictions that with increasing technological developments the work of the world will be accomplished by a smaller and smaller percentage of the population and with a smaller and smaller percentage of the worker's time. It is then concluded that one's job will take on less significance from a psychological point of view and make much less of a contribution to the total life satisfaction of the individual. I for one am unimpressed by these predictions. In fact, it can easily be argued that the probable changes in the kinds of occupations which will be characteristic of the next generation is in the direction of those occupations which have been held by the most "work oriented" segment of our population. And even if we have a highly structured economic society in which everyone is guaranteed an annual income, and in which the economic motive for work would presumably therefore be reduced, current research would predict that the nature of the job and the extent to which it meets the individual's psychological needs would still be the most important variable in job satisfaction.

Two formulations are relevant at this point. One is the concept utilized by Maslow[11] of a hierarchy of human needs in roughly the following order: (1) physiological needs, (2) security needs, (3) social needs, (4) ego needs, (5) self-fulfillment needs. The hypothesis is that only when the lower needs are met is the individual able to move to the next level. For example, until one's physiological needs are met and until one has a feeling of security, one is less responsive to or influenced by the opportunity for social interaction, social reinforcement, and self-expression.

More recently Herzberg[8] has presented a theory of job satisfaction with evidence to support it. He hypothesizes that there are two kinds of job factors operating, those which he calls "satisfiers" and those which he calls "hygienic factors." Satisfiers are those which have to do with the content or nature of the job tasks and hygienic factors are those which have to do with the context of the job, that is, working conditions, salary, colleagues, equipment, and even supervision. An interesting aspect of his theory is that even ideal conditions of the "context" category do not result in high job satisfaction. That is, even when the general working conditions are quite good, the individual merely has no *dissatisfaction;* conversely, it is only when the job tasks themselves provide an outlet for development of the individual's capacities and interest and when the job provides opportunities for advancement does the individual experience high levels of positive job satisfaction. Likewise, if the content of the job is appropriate, the individual will not experience high levels of dissatisfaction even when the working conditions are relatively poor. It must be pointed out here that other research findings and interpretations are not consistent with respect to this theory.[23]

One of the basic problems of the recent attempts to do something significant about the "hard core" of unemployment has been the development of appropriate work attitudes. In a recent study of those individuals trained under various Manpower Development Training Act programs, it was found that although it was inappropriate to apply the words "alienated" or "unmotivated" to the culturally disadvantaged trainees, it was true that they perceived the system as not really applicable to them. In an abstract sense, they know that success depends on planning and hard work, but they are not certain that they are the masters of their own fate. When asked about the need for personal planning, a majority of trainees chose the response "it is not always a good idea to plan ahead because too many things turn out to be a matter of luck." [21]

CHANGING NATURE OF WORK

It is obvious that we cannot talk about occupational placement in the world of work unless we take into consideration the total occupational structure within which our labor force finds its opportunities (or lack of them). Fortunately, there is a well organized and continually functioning research program carried on by the Bureau of Labor Statistics of the United States Department of Labor. This program has devoted itself to making predictions of the outlook for the thousands of occupations which make up our world of work, based on careful analyses of census data and periodic sample studies. The summary of the outcomes of these studies is contained in the *Occupational Outlook Handbook* which is issued every two years by the Bureau and by the hundreds of separate reports which appear in government publications, particularly in the *Monthly Labor Review*. More recently, the annual *Manpower Report of the President* presents the outstanding facts of particular relevance to our socio-economic development, particularly as it relates to needed legislation at the national level.

There is no need here to present an extended discussion of occupational trends. It will be sufficient to present a few of the most relevant facts from a 1966 projection of manpower requirements over the next decade, as found in the report entitled "1966 Report of the Secretary of Labor on Manpower Research and Training Under the Manpower Development and Training Act of 1962." [21]

1. By 1975 there will be 88.7 million persons in the labor force, about a 25 per cent increase in the total.

2. There will be a continued decline in farm employment, increase in nonfarm goods-producing industries, and an even faster increase in the service-producing sector of our economy.

3. Despite the common predictions of the outcomes of technological developments, the overall demand for less skilled workers will *not*

decrease over the 1965–75 period, although it will decline somewhat as a percentage of the total. The greatest increase will be for professional and technical workers. The white collar group as a whole is expected to expand by nearly two-fifths and to constitute nearly one-half of all the manpower requirements in 1975. Blue collar occupations will grow more slowly but in 1975 will still make up about one-third of the labor force.

4. The changes in occupational requirements have significant implications for certain groups within the labor force. *Nonwhite workers* are disproportionately concentrated in the less skilled occupations which are least likely to grow. If nonwhites do not gain access to white collar and skilled jobs at a faster rate than at present, they will continue to have more serious unemployment problems than white workers.

Young workers are also concentrated in the slower growing, less skilled occupations, and since the supply of young workers will grow quite fast in the next decade (due to the postwar rise in the birth rate), industry will have to take such steps as using younger workers as aides or as assistants and society will have to provide more effective training programs.

Women workers, on the other hand, although they too are increasing faster than the labor force as a whole, are already concentrated in the more rapidly growing white collar occupations. If no changes take place in their proportionate share of jobs in the various occupations, they will have no more serious unemployment problems than they now have. It should be noted, however, that men are increasingly competing for some of the jobs women have traditionally held in such occupations as teaching, social work, library work, and so on.

5. It is obvious that the continued technological developments will create new kinds of jobs as well as influence the total occupational structure. Following are some of the predicted developments: (*a*) Computerization of data processing will continue to be introduced into many industries. (*b*) There will be increasing instrumentation for measurement, sensing, data acquisition, and control. One effect will be to transform the plant operator into a skilled watcher of control panels, with duties demanding patience, alertness to malfunctioning, and a sense of responsibility for costly equipment. (*c*) Advances in communications will create new products for the consumer and improved methods of business operation, through copying machines, tape recorders, teaching machines, and communica-

tions systems. (*d*) Increased mechanization along traditional lines will continue to be an important factor in raising productivity in industries. Textile, meat packing, construction, lumber, printing, and other industries will be increasingly mechanized. (*e*) In general, the overall trend will be one of an increasing proportion of the labor force devoted to the production of services rather than the production of goods. These services will require people at all levels of skill and technical knowledge. In fact, it can be stated that, in the services area, we are still relatively undeveloped and that just as we have seen rapid changes in the goods-producing occupations during the first half of the Twentieth Century, we will see corresponding developments in the service-producing occupations in the second half of the Twentieth Century.

A dramatic illustration of the tremendous possibilities for increased social services was one recent estimate to the effect that half of the current unemployment in the United States could be handled merely by adding a teaching assistant in every classroom in the United States. Likewise, a number of professions are under severe pressure to provide an adequate supply of workers to meet the increasing social needs. In counseling, for example, it is apparent that the current training programs cannot possibly provide enough counselors to meet the positions being created by the various new programs. The Employment Service is now considering a "career ladder" approach to the development of employment counselors, which will include a much larger range of levels of training and skill than are now currently in operation. The same kind of problem exists in practically all of the health and special service professions. Arthur Pearl and Frank Riessman have imaginatively and challengingly pointed out the need for and potential use of the nonprofessional in human services.[13]

CONCEPT OF CAREER DEVELOPMENT

One of the most significant areas of research which has relevance for optimal life satisfaction for the individuals who make up our labor force is that which is devoted to "vocational development." Here the frame of reference is the development of the individual's career as defined by his work life. No longer can we look at the problem of occupational placement as one in which, on the one hand, we have an individual with certain characteristics and, on the other, the world of occupation with certain demands. These two variables are important, but to think of them as static entities which are to be measured and some optimal matching brought about is to provide us with a very limited approach of limited value. A position or a job is the unit within the world of work. It is a particular collection of tasks carried out under certain working conditions at a particular location. A career is a sequence of positions, jobs, or occupations in the life of one person or a group of persons of certain characteristics.

The occupational world has certain basic dimensions. Super's formulation[17] is based upon the three basic dimensions of field, level, and enterprise. Field is based upon the nature of the work that is done, such as selling; level is the scaling of the occupation on some relevant characteristic, such as difficulty, or amount of education required or income level or prestige level; enterprise denotes the source of employment, that is, the kind of employer, whether public or private or profit or nonprofit.

One of the outstanding characteristics of the American labor force, as compared with that of Western Europe, for example, is its rapid mobility. Workers move from one part of the country to another, from one industry to another, from one occupation to another. In fact the predictions are that mobility will increase in the future, and there is already evidence that the "average individual" will hold four or five different kinds of jobs in his career. This mobility presumably results from three factors:

1. The relative free society which we have.

2. The rapid change in the nature of work skills and knowledges resulting from technological developments.

3. The extensive training programs available in educational institutions and provided by the employers themselves. Evidence of the extent of general as well as vocational training available to the American labor force can be found in the studies by Clark and Sloan.[2] From their extensive surveys of training programs in various industries in the United States, they conclude that "we are now witnessing, in the educational activities of American industry, the birth of a great educational force of far-reaching consequences."

The Career Pattern Study[18] being carried out by Super is an example of the kind of research necessary to understand the vocational development of individuals. He intensively studied a group of ninth grade boys in the early 1950's and since then has had periodic follow-ups, sometimes obtaining minimal information and other times retesting, and collecting depth interviews and a wealth of information concerning their vocational lives. An intensive analysis of the patterns of career movements and their outcomes in terms of vocational success and satisfaction is being made. Already significant vocational behaviors such as exploration, establishment, stagnation, and trial have been identified, along with the general stages in an individual's vocational development. So, for example, one can think of having "equity" in one's job, an equity which may be lost if one moves. As we remain in a job, we build up skill, we build up seniority, we may build up status, prestige, and reputation; and whenever a move is made the question can be asked, "What will be lost or gained in terms of the equity built up in my present job?"

Thus, a new frame of reference has been developed for studying the work life of individuals. In contrast to the earlier "occupational model," which was based on the measurement of individual differences and the prediction of potentiality for meeting job demands in a relatively static occupational structure, the "career model" is based on an understanding of the determinants and patterns of movements which characterize an individual's work history.

Recent studies have shown that, for many at present, and for increasing proportions in the future, the individual's career will be multioccupational. That is, the sequence of preparing for, entering upon, and progressing through an occupation will occur several times in his working career. For example, a Department of Labor study[22] was made of the work histories of nearly 2.5 million 18–23-year-olds between February 1963 and February 1965. They found that a considerable amount of shifting from job to job, voluntary and involuntary, takes place in the early years after a young person enters the labor force: these years serve as a time for feeling out the job market, gaining experience, adapting to the discipline of work, and trying to obtain and hold jobs. The ordinary approach, then, of identifying, as early as possible, a particular occupational potentiality, training for this occupation, and then entering and remaining in it until retirement is no longer functional.

NATURE OF THE OCCUPATIONAL WORLD

One of the fundamental problems in relating individuals with their human characteristics to occupations with their duties and demands is that the terms and dimensions used to describe one of these two domains differ from those used in describing the other. So, for example, we speak of an individual as possessing a certain amount of intelligence, as having verbal aptitude, as being interested in interpersonal relations, in being aggressive, in knowing arithmetic. On the other hand, we say that a certain occupation requires that the individual supervise others, run a certain type of machine, inspect certain kinds of objects, prepare layouts, assemble, and repair. What is needed for placement purposes is a description of the world of work in human terms, in terms of what the work requires of the worker rather than what the worker does.

The third edition of the *Dictionary of Occupational Titles* (*D.O.T.*), issued in 1965 by the U.S. Department of Labor, attempts to do just this. It utilizes a new occupational coding system in which the first three digits classify the occupation in terms of its outcomes and the last three digits in terms of its worker functions. The work of the world has been found to involve three large classes of relationships: those having to do with *things;* those having to do with *data;* and those having to do with *people.* Based upon a long series of basic research studies under the direction of Sidney Fine, a hierarchy of worker functions for each of these three major areas of work was developed. Working with data ranges from the simplest kind of function, which is comparing, through increasingly difficult and complex functions such as copying, computing, compiling, analyzing, coordinating, and synthesizing. Likewise, in relation to things, the simplest function is handling, and there is a hierarchy of functions of increasing complexity up to setting up. What the second half of the *D.O.T.* occupational coding system now tells us is the level of difficulty of the occupation on each of these three scales or hierarchies of functions. For example, a gauge inspector in the machine shop industry requires *analyzing* data, no significant relationship with respect to people, and *precision working* with respect to things.

Volume II of *D.O.T.* groups occupations according to these worker functions within 22 large areas of work, areas represented by such categories as art, business relations, engineering, merchandising, and transportation. For each of these worker-trait groups, there is a qualifications profile based on the amount of general education and specific vocational training required, the degree of eleven special aptitudes required, and an indication of the types of interests and temperament traits conducive to success and satisfaction in this occupation. In addition, the occupation is classified according to its physical demands.

These "occupational specifications," although useful, have the obvious limitation that they are quite generalized and are therefore incomplete with respect to the task of placing an individual in a given position. A really successful placement requires an intimate knowledge of the psychological climate as well as of the more objective characteristics of the job.

One important dimension of an occupation is its prestige level. One's job helps determine one's way of life, one's standing in the community, one's social relations. If it is true that one's job satisfaction is a function of the extent to which the job provides a means of expressing one's self-concept, then it is also true that the prestige level of a job helps determine the self-concept of the individuals in that occupation.

A recent large-scale study using public opinion survey techniques presents the relative prestige standing of all the occupations in the Bureau of Census classification system.[14] Just exactly what causes these attitudes is not clear, but prestige level has been shown to be correlated with such factors as level of education required, social level, level of income, and level of independent responsibility required. A striking fact is the stability or rigidity of these attitudes. A number of studies have confirmed the early findings by Deeg and Patterson[3] that prestige level remains relatively constant over long periods of time. Deeg and Patterson found a correlation of 0.98 between the rank order of 25 occupations rated in 1928 with these same occupations rated in 1947, despite the fact that over that 20-year period there had been a major depression, significant changes in the labor force, a world war, and extensive technological developments. These prestige attitudes have negative as well as positive values since a given individual may rule out whole blocks of occupations from consideration as being "beneath him."

PLACEMENT AND SELECTION

It is appropriate at this point to make a distinction between "placement" and "selection." In its simplest form, the distinction is that in selection, the job is the reference point and the task is to choose from a number of possible applicants the one best fitted for that particular job. In placement, on the other hand, the individual is the reference point, and the task is to select from a number of jobs the one which is most appropriate for the individual. Although it is obvious that in both cases the process involves comparing the individual and his characteristics with a job and its demands, the task of placement is in a real sense more complex. Going back to the determinants of success and satisfaction referred to above, the ideal placement is one in which the position makes optimal demands on the individual's strengths, is not influenced by his weaknesses, and provides an outlet for the individual's interest, personality characteristics, and values.

A complicating factor for those involved in the placement of individuals—particularly those with some kind of handicap—is that the employer looks at the situation from a selection point of view rather than a placement point of view. The hiring requirements are therefore influenced by factors which are interfering with or even irrelevant to optimal placement of the individual. Here we see coming to bear, as a barrier to employment, a number of functionally nonrelevant factors, such as various forms of prejudice, inappropriate requirements, peculiar stereotyped attitudes of the hiring officer. It is for these reasons that we have an increasing number of legislated restrictions against various forms of discrimination—particularly racial, and more recently sex and age—and also the public relations campaigns (such as Hire the Handicapped) designed to remind employers that their selection system may be eliminating whole categories of appropriate applicants.

When one takes the selection point of view, a natural tendency is to think in terms of prediction of future job behavior from certain kinds of information available at the time of selection, such as intelligence, special aptitudes, and interests, which are assumed to be relatively stable, and from which predictions can be made. The research paradigm is one of finding out which of the measurable stable characteristics of human beings is correlated with and predictive of later job behavior. The difficulty with this paradigm is that it assumes two relatively static systems: a stable individual, and an unchanging job.

Most of the large-scale studies of long-term prediction of occupational success from tested characteristics have not been particularly successful. The Thorndike-Hagen study,[20] for example, showed that aptitude test scores obtained during Air Force testing were not particularly predictive of success in the individual's occupation 15 years later. The recent summary of the literature on occupational aptitude tests by Ghiselli [7] revealed that although success in training can be predicted fairly well from aptitude tests, the prediction of proficiency on the job itself is much poorer, although frequently better than chance. Ghiselli's conclusion is as follows:

> While there is some evidence that tests, particularly those of intellectual and of spatial and mechanical abilities, can predict general occupational trainability, tests are far less useful in the prediction of general occupational proficiency. Obviously, the selection of the test with the highest validity optimizes the accuracy of the selection of

workers for a particular job. Apparently this is what must be done if one wishes to forecast a worker's success in the performance of that job. But as far as selecting workers for training for that job is concerned, at least moderately good results are likely to be obtained from the use of almost any test of intellectual or of spatial and mechanical abilities. To put it another way, it would appear that the ability and trait requirements are quite specific to the job. On the other hand, the ability and trait requirements for training programs have some measure of generality over a large proportion of jobs.

Special Placement

What is the significance of these findings for occupational placement, particularly of those with special placement needs? In my opinion, it suggests that predictions should be short-term, that long-term goals should be quite general and in terms of a large field and a rough approximation, and that considerable attention should be paid to performance during exploratory situations rather than, or in addition to, the usual kinds of tests. In a recent article in which he identifies four approaches to work evaluation, Walter Neff [12] has very effectively summarized the current situation: (1) the mental testing approach, (2) the job analysis approach, (3) the work sample approach, and (4) the situational assessment approach. Each of these has its strengths and weaknesses and the operational problem is one of identifying which combination of approaches is most appropriate in a given situation.

The "situational approach" is the least well known. It differs from the usual work sample in that its orientation is toward work behavior in general rather than toward concrete work skills. It has been used primarily in rehabilitation situations, such as the Chicago Jewish Vocational Service[6] and in the Jewish Employment and Vocational Service at Philadelphia.[9] In these programs there is an attempt to simulate the total work setting as closely as possible. Wages are paid, real objects are made, the supervision is realistic, and regular working hours are enforced, while still maintaining the vital difference that, in the rehabilitation workshop, assessment is the goal; whereas in ordinary employment production is the goal. As Neff writes, "If we wish to find out whether a given person can work, it seems sensible to put him in a work situation and find out whether he can perform. If we wish to know what it is that prevents him from working efficiently, it seems reasonable to be able to vary his working conditions and discover what it is that produces his difficulty." Neff also states that:

> One of the major stumbling blocks lying in the way of improving our system of vocational evaluation is that we have very meager resources with which to field-test our procedures in actual industrial settings. Once the client leaves the clutches of the evaluation center, we are no longer in a position to observe his future work behavior on an actual job, so that we can ascertain the reason for his success or failure. Our outcome criteria tend, therefore, to be very crude, essentially boiling down to the all or none criterion of employment versus unemployment. We have been able to develop no means of observing our evaluated client in actual employment as intensively as we have observed him during the evaluative phase. It would also be desirable to provide a system of work-trials in unprotected industrial settings, which would provide opportunities for professional observation. At present, however, and for many obvious reasons, once a client is lucky enough to be absorbed by private industry, he disappears from sight. Until the professional evaluator gains some opportunity to observe his clients on an actual job, genuine validation of our evaluation procedures will remain rather inadequate.[12]

One kind of occupational behavior which has only recently been studied from a psychological point of view is the process of job-seeking itself. A recent study by Sheppard and Belitsky[15] of the job-seeking behavior of unemployed workers found that there were three psychological indicators related to success in finding jobs, as follows: (1) achievement motivation (the willingness to persist in efforts to reach a goal), (2) achievement values (the degree of acceptance of social values which emphasize economic success), and (3) job interview anxiety. They found that the unemployed who found their jobs through the public employment service tended to be those with relatively low achievement values and high interview anxiety. Most laid-off workers who scored high in motivation and low in interview anxiety got new jobs through direct application to companies. They also found that the degree of anxiety a job seeker feels in a job interview situation was found to be associated with his success in finding a job as well as his thoroughness in looking for a job.

FUTURE DIRECTIONS

What are the needed future directions for research which would be of greatest value to those involved in the placement of workers in our economy? First, of course, would be the continued testing of the principles or assumptions under which we now operate, as indicated by the statements above. But in addition there are certain research directions which should have high priority.

1. We still need a careful analysis of the basic work operations which make up our occupational system. Our present job descriptions are still too much in terms of the outcomes of work rather than the processes and therefore change rapidly as the products change or as the particular ways of carrying out work operations change. Chalupsky's study[1] which identified four basic factors in clerical work is an example of the need for further identification of the fundamental operations which make up our work. If these were known, then training and work sample evaluation during actual trial could be carried out and become an integral part of guidance, counseling, and placement.

2. We need to know more about the determinants of vocational choice behavior. We know that it is the rare occasion when an individual makes a specific vocational choice in the sense of selecting an occupation and then systematically carrying out a plan of training, entry, and progression in that occupation.

3. We need a more organized interdisciplinary attack on occupational research. An individual's career is influenced by the combined pressures of economic changes, technological advances, social attitudes, and individual needs and motivations. We need a large-scale study of the role and meaning of work in American society and a projection of that role into the future.

4. We need a large-scale attack on the study of occupational prestige. We know that large blocks of occupations are kept out of the psychological life space of the individual because of stereotyped responses to those occupations. We also know that large groups of potential employees—particularly the handicapped, physically as well as socially—are rejected from consideration, again because of stereotyped attitudes toward them. We need to know the genesis of these attitudes, the factors which reinforce them, and effective ways of bringing about public changes in these attitudes. An example is the study by DeLevie[4] in which he found that prejudices toward race and disability were less in the work situation than in the social situation. This finding suggests the hypothesis (which needs further testing) that a breakthrough in attitude change would more likely come through the work situation than through other types of contacts.

5. Finally, we need a systematic study of the placement process itself. Even if placement were restricted to the "matching process," there is need for a careful evaluation and tryout of the new kinds of

information storage and retrieval devices and procedures which are currently being developed. Just as we are now referring to computer-assisted instruction, so we should be making computer-assisted placements.

NOTES

1. A. B. Chalupsky, "Comparative Factor Analyses of Clerical Jobs," *Journal of Applied Psychology,* 46 (1962), 62–66.
2. H. F. Clark and H. S. Sloan, *Classrooms in the Factories* (Rutherford, New Jersey: Fairleigh Dickinson University, 1958), p. 134.
3. M. E. Deeg and D. G. Patterson, "Changes in Social Status of Occupations," *Occupations,* 25 (1947), 205–208.
4. Ari DeLevie, "Attitudes of Laymen and Professionals Toward Physical and Social Disability," (Unpublished Doctoral Dissertation, Teachers' College, Columbia University, 1966).
5. S. Fine and C. A. Heinz, "The Functional Occupational Classification Structure," *Personnel and Guidance Journal,* 37 (1958), 180–192.
6. W. Gellman, H. Gendel, N. M. Glaser, S. B. Friedman, and W. S. Neff, *Adjusting People to Work* (Chicago: Jewish Vocational Service, 1957).
7. E. E. Ghiselli, *The Validity of Occupational Attitude Tests* (New York: John Wiley and Sons, 1966), p. 124.
8. F. Herzberg, B. Mausner and B. Snyderman, *The Motivation to Work* (New York: John Wiley and Sons, 1959).
9. S. Leshner and G. S. Snyderman, "Work Adjustment Training," *Employment Service Review* (January, 1966).
10. *Manpower Report of the President* (Washington: Government Printing Office, 1966), p. xii.
11. A. H. Maslow, "A Theory of Human Motivation," *Psychological Review,* 50 (1943), 370–396.
12. Walter Neff, "Problems of Work Evaluation," *Personnel and Guidance Journal,* 44 (1966), 682–688.
13. A. Pearl and F. Riessman, *New Careers for the Poor* (New York: The Free Press, 1965).
14. A. J. Reiss, Jr., *Occupations and Social Status* (New York: The Free Press, 1961).
15. H. L. Sheppard and H. Belitsky, *The Job Hunt: Job-Seeking Behavior of Unemployed Workers in a Local Economy* (Washington: W. E. Upjohn Institute for Employment Research, 1965).
16. D. E. Super, "A Theory of Vocational Development," *The American Psychologist,* 8 (1953), 185–190.
17. ———, *The Psychology of Careers* (New York: Harper and Brothers, 1957).
18. ———, J. Crites, R. Hummel, H. Moser, P. Overstreet and C. Warnath, *Vocational Development: A Framework for Research* (New York: Columbia University Teachers' College Bureau of Publications, 1957).
19. Albert S. Thompson, "Homo Laborans: An Analysis of the Meaning of Work," *Bulletin of the International Association of Applied Psychology,* 12 (1963), 5–23.
20. R. L. Thorndike and E. Hagen, *Ten Thousand Careers* (New York: John Wiley and Sons, 1959).

21. U.S. Department of Labor, *1966 Report of the Secretary of Labor on Manpower Research and Training under the Manpower Development and Training Act of 1962* (Washington: Government Printing Office, 1966), pp. 71–75, 111–115.
22. U.S. Department of Labor, "Out-of-School Youth—Two Years Later, Special Labor Force Report No. 71," *Monthly Labor Review* (August, 1966).
23. V. H. Vroom, *Work and Motivation* (New York: John Wiley and Sons, 1964), 126–129.

OCCUPATIONS AND PLACEMENT FOR THE BLIND

Norman M. Yoder

THE LONG VIEW

In examining the occupations of the future and the research which may be required to meet the demands of those occupations, we need to evaluate the progress to date and to review those factors which created that progress; for only in so doing can we come to some reasonable conclusions as to the research which may be required to enhance further the employment opportunities for the blind in the next two decades. To this end Dr. Thompson has described in detail, in the previous paper, the changing panorama of employment in the past and the impact of cybernetics and other factors which have, in a sense, recreated and redesigned occupations of the present and which would appear to have a major impact on the design of our occupations for the future.

Accordingly, let us briefly examine the history of employment for the blind and from that background attempt to construct research plans for the future. The annals of the American Association of Workers for the Blind record that, before the turn of the century, professional leadership had three concerns:

1. Adequate educational opportunities for the blind to meet the demands of the time.

2. Adequate employment opportunity for the blind in order that they might assume a responsible position in the economic structure of the day.

3. Adequate social welfare provisions to meet the needs of the blind in the event that opportunities for employment were not available.

Dr. Thompson's paper indicates that these same concerns have been with us whether the particular segment of the population is blind or not. Why else the massive changes under the New Deal, the Fair Deal, the Great Society, and Civil Rights; together with the kaleidoscopic changes in social security, federal aid to education, and public welfare? In each of these, support is offered for the occupationally displaced persons. But within this panorama of change, how much have we done to search out in advance the need for occupational revision? It is true that industry now involves itself in human factors engineering, but the mere process suggests that the opportunities of the future are limited to the superbrain and the highly trained technical person. Are we, therefore, suggesting that our employment needs must require only the best, and that the remainder will find themselves cozily ensconced under the umbrellas of some form of governmental assistance? If this is the direction in which we are pointed, then we have not resolved the prime issues of the 1890's—that is, those regarding education, employment, and social welfare. We have merely confessed that we have failed in finding basic resolutions.

During the final three decades of the 1800's, and the first two decades of the 1900's, employment of the blind was limited to a meager sheltered shop opportunity. Beyond the schools of the day, there was little, if any, opportunity to train. Thus, rug weaving, mat making, chair caning and broom manufacturing established themselves as the traditional trades of the blind.

The labor needs of World War I occasioned some inroads into competitive labor market employment for the blind, again only because of manpower shortages in an industrial complex that was still essentially craft-based and manually operated. But even with these inroads, the employment of the blind in the competitive labor market was short lived; and with the conclusion of the war, there was a mass return to the sheltered workshop or to unemployment. However, simultaneously, educators of the blind exhibited a growing realization that having once demonstrated the capacity of the blind to meet the needs of productive industry without any real training, the time had now arrived for them to provide expanded training opportunities to ensure more adequately the possibilities of placement.

Concurrently, two additional avenues were being explored:

1. The blind did not necessarily need to be trained in schools for the blind, but rather opportunities existed in the public schools in competition with the sighted youngsters provided that certain alterations were made to accommodate the problem of blindness.

2. Blind people might well be trained beyond the high school level and achieve academic status through the acquisition of college degrees.

Both of these concepts contributed materially to the subsequent redesign in the approach to the employment of blind people. Just as there was some evidence of progress, the black days of the early depression years occurred and employment opportunities, not only for the blind, but for all persons, were greatly diminished. Yet under the various emergency programs of the Roosevelt New Deal, blind people once more found themselves discharging tasks which had hitherto been excluded. Just as new social legislation was introduced for the masses, we witnessed within a space of a few years two pieces of federal legislation having major impact on work for the blind: the Randolph-Sheppard Act and the Wagner-O'Day Act. In the former, provision was made for the establishment of vending units on federal property to be operated by the blind. Over the years the Act has been amended, and has provided gross sales of upwards of $70,000,000 and the employment of hundreds of blind persons. To those who engineered the legislation and to those who sponsored it, work for the blind has been deeply indebted.

The Wagner-O'Day Act provided that, all other factors being equal, products manufactured by workshops for the blind were to be purchased by federal agencies. While it took some years to develop, workshops for the blind across the nation are now doing a substantial business with the Federal Government.

These two early pieces of legislation have laid the important blocks in the foundation of employment opportunities for the blind in the past and today and, most assuredly, they will continue to do so in the future.

IMPACT AND IMPETUS

During World War I, adjustment, mobility, and flexibility were segments of vocabulary yet to be introduced into the vocational rehabilitation jargon. However, as the war years closed and American industry shifted its gearing from more and more production of military goods to the requirements of a civilian market starved for consumer goods, major revisions in employment practices were in process. No longer did the employer depend upon government subsidy to carry the load. He was once more a self-dependent competitor and, in order to stay competitive, he had to out-produce, out-advertise and outstrip his fellow manufacturers. This meant that employees now had to be flexible in doing set-up work, handling a variety of jobs, becoming highly productive, and, in the case of the blind, not being so dependent upon fellow workers.

A major shift took place in industry when the agencies for the blind suddenly became aware that in order to remain employed or to become employed, the individual who was blind needed to be thoroughly adjusted to the handicap. That is to say, an attitudinal change in respect to blindness was required. Mobility was essential. Safe travel habits, inside and outside of the plant, were now a requirement. Psychological balance was a prerequisite to continued employment. Finally, the gradual changes in production methods required that training be of primary concern if placements in the future were to be made in the evolving age of automation.

In 1944, 1954, and 1965 amendments to the Vocational Rehabilitation Act were passed; and in each instance, opportunities were enhanced for the the disabled and especially for the blind. To date, we have felt the impact of the stimuli from the 1944 and 1954 amendments. We have not yet felt the full impact of those of 1965.

With the amendments of 1954 and the amendments of 1965, further impetus has been given to the employment of individuals who are blind. These amendments have provided programmatic depth and breadth, the full impact of which has as yet not been fully tested. More importantly, however, these sets of amendments have provided for: (1) assessment and reassessment of the directions in which the employment of the blind is moving; (2) new technological know-how through experimentation; (3) new avenues of research, and (4) fluidity of programs needed to meet the changing demands of our labor market.

However, one major factor in developing future employment opportunities must yet be considered. In most of the public and private agency leadership, there must be a drastic overhaul, and this overhaul must also reach board members, trustees, and others who have been entrenched over the years. Commitment in five areas must be made if we are to survive the challenges of the future, and if we are to provide the basis for research design in occupations that will be meaningful and useful to the blind and visually impaired citizenry of the United States.

1. It is high time that we make a firm commitment to the blind. The attitude of "wardism," "our people," or "the poor blind"

has no place in future occupational development. If we do not have commitments to the total individual who may incidentally be blind, if we do not have confidence in his capacity to produce competitively, if we do not believe in the product we are manufacturing, namely blind labor, then we have no right to be in the competitive labor market. If the professional leadership in work for the blind does not have unflinching and unfaltering belief in the blind, then all of the research, all of the legislation, all of the appropriation will mean very little in resolving future employment problems.

2. If we are attitudinally committed to the capabilities of the blind as a competitive unit of labor, then it follows that the leadership of the public and private agencies must inevitably commit itself to a revision of administrative practices. It would seem to us that we are at the crossroads of choice: (*a*) whether to ply our trade with hat in hand in the posture and attitude of downtrodden social welfare agencies, or whether (*b*) to assume the posture administratively of a soundly operated business and to apply the minimal business practices to the attainment of our objectives.

Why, as public and private agencies in work for the blind, do we become satisfied with less than quality workmanship on our products—namely, blind labor ready for the market? Why do we hesitate to invest time, effort, and money in experimentation, research, and advertising? Why is it that we are afraid to take a long look at future requirements? Is it because to do so demands ingenuity, flexibility, fluidity and commitment? Any business which is successful and tends to remain successful today, must be alert to stay ahead of its market. Can we, in work for the blind, afford to do less?

3. The amendments of 1954 and 1965 added real impetus to research; and yet in work for the blind much of the "research" has traversed the same paths over and over again. This contributes little to the fund of knowledge and far less toward the meeting of demands of the future. Somehow, we have fallen into the trap of thinking that research must be costly. We stay away from it because someone must write the results of research.

A commitment to research does not require that it be done on a grandiose scale; for within the framework of each of our agencies, within the framework of each of our communities, there is much of a basic nature that can be done. We tend to lose ourselves in the ebb and flow of statistics. True, they may be the skeletal framework on which the body hangs, but too frequently we have overlooked the research in the body tissue.

4. Conjointly, we must be committed to experimentation and research at the university level as well as the agency level. However, research without applicability is comparatively useless. We hesitate to innovate, for we feel it may cost us time, money, and perhaps embarrassment. But if, in experimentation, we learn from the failures, then it is money well invested. Conversely, if as a result of experimentation we have improved methods of productivity, if we have improved training facilities, if we have improved placement techniques, then the experimentation has been invaluable.

5. The fifth commitment is one of application. We can commit ourselves to the four situations stated above. But unless we commit ourselves to application, we have done no more than offer lip service, without any real intention to move ahead.

History and the amendments of 1944, of 1954, and of 1965, have made an impact; but it is for us to determine whether or not there shall be a continuing impetus. Let us briefly examine the degree of impetus with which we are thus far involved.

OUR CHANGING TIMES

Some gauge of this impetus may be obtained by examining the caseload characteristics of the rehabilitation agencies over the past two decades. At the outset most of the individuals were given little attention and little effort was made toward adjustment of the total person to a serious disability. Little examination was given to mobility, and certainly not too much interest was accorded advanced training, or necessary retraining, to meet job requirements. Between 1944 and 1954 most of the caseload was moved rapidly from acceptance into employment with perhaps only 1–3 per cent of the individuals placed in advanced training beyond elementary or secondary education. Today, some 15–22 per cent of that same caseload finds itself in advanced training beyond high school.

This shift in caseload does not suggest that we are dealing only with the more adequate person, but it does clearly indicate that we are searching out the most productive talents of each individual and attempting to meet the demands of the labor market with those developed talents. Advanced training is not only the result of market demand, but is, to some extent, also the result of applications of research and experimentation leading to new job opportunities for the blind. The market of tomorrow will demand: (1) a psychologically well adjusted employee, (2) a flexible and trainable employee, (3) an employee who has basic productive skills, (4) an employee who is technically sound and capable of fitting into the ground-floor opportunities.

RESEARCH IN WHAT

Let us for a moment examine each of the principal areas of employment for the blind and suggest where some basic research for the near future may lie.

Industry

With the advent of automation, a variety of jobs which the blind have been doing over the past two decades has disappeared and yet the ever-present manufacturing process continues to be with us. What research have we really carried out as to how to make blind persons more effective in this field of employment? What new measuring devices have we sought to produce? What have we done about schematics, color coding, and assembly? What have we done about job card and job flow of materials? What have we learned about the adaptability and the flexibility of the blind individual in the industrial plant of tomorrow? While the focus of this conference is not on aids and appliances in the field of industrial placement, they are of major concern if we are to remain in industry and improve our position in the future.

Clerical

For the blind person who desires to become employed in the clerical field, we have stuck to (and have been stuck with) the concept of the transcribing typist, limited to taking straight dictation from some machine, hopefully with adequate training. What research have we really done in the following areas:

1. The completion of forms by a blind person.

2. The handling and correction of prepadded and/or precarboned forms.

3. Techniques of erasing and correcting.

4. Filing.

5. Continuation of material in narrative recording.

6. Taking dictation and transcribing dictation from other than voice recorded units.

7. Adequate methods of basic fiscal control in braille, using such equipment as adding machines and calculators.

Small Business

Currently we have redirected our attention to placement in service occupations: hospitals, hotels, laundries, motels, and related fields. Perhaps what I am about to recommend may more properly fall under the caption of small business, and yet it is related to service in its broadest concept. What do we know about opportunities in small apparatus repair? We are training people, but few placements have been made. Why not more? What are the problems? What are we doing about related fields, such as automatic transmission and specialty services? Why was it necessary for the 3M Corporation to develop its current proposals for blind workers, rather than such a proposal coming from work for the blind or from rehabilitation in general? Do we think so lightly of our responsibility that we are dependent upon others to do our advanced thinking and our advanced planning?

Technical Training

Where do we stand in our technical training and our technical placement? There has been a great furor over computer programming as a job opportunity for the blind; and yet modest research and concern has suggested only a few parameters and baselines within which and from which we must operate. At the same time, in our anxiety to take advantage of the field of placement, we are prone to buy inadequate training at the cheapest possible price, only because we have not taken the time to research the basic demands of the industry today and to learn what those demands will be in the future. A prime example of this is a state agency purchasing such training for its blind clients from a school which does not even have access to a computer. Without a computer how can you teach programming?

Professions

Employment possibilities in the professions represent a fruitful area of research for the immediate future and long-range program planning for the blind. A few pertinent questions for consideration are:

1. What do we know about teacher certification for public school teaching, nationally? Why are there so few blind people in this field? What legislative roadblocks exist, and how can they be removed?

2. In the fields of physical and occupational therapy, why should certification or licensing be so stringent that they exclude the blind and visually handicapped? What modifications in equipment, training, and certification ought to be considered to open this field to the blind, particularly when there is a national shortage of practitioners.

3. What have we done to research the basic problems, the basic needs, and the basic methods of training to place more effectively blind people in the professional fields of communication—journalism, radio, and television—an area of economic self-sufficiency?

Apply the same questions, raise the same issues with each of the professional areas of employment, and related research can be developed.

Other Business Activities

Since the inception of vending-stand services under the Randolph-Sheppard Act most of the business opportunities for the blind have been in this area; and yet we know very little about what the blind can do in other business activities. True, there has been some success recorded in insurance sales and management, and modest success in the vending-stand or snack-bar program. How much research has gone into the program? We call conferences to train staff for the Business Enterprises Program, and we discuss methods of dealing with current business problems as they relate to the operation, but we have never really researched the fundamental issues and endeavored to draw some useful guidelines, thereby developing program consistency and stability.

Workshops

The sheltered workshops have been the forerunner of employment opportunities for the blind. Many of them have kept pace with the growing knowledge of production and training. Many of them have failed and are still content to cane chairs, and to attempt competition in the fields of broom making and rug production. These are honorable vocations but they are not solving the modern problem of the production workshop. Decisions must be made, and with respect to the production shop versus therapeutic shop issue, some sound research ought to be undertaken to examine the new minimum wage laws and the Federal Fair Labor Standards Act. Preliminary indications are that both pieces of legislation will have a tremendous impact on the future of the workshop; but unless we begin to put these facts together, unless we research the problems and the implications and take this information to the Congress, we will have lost valuable time, and we will have found that, once more, our programs for the blind are mired in tradition and inertia.

University Research and Agency Needs

Somehow we must relate the university-based research with the agency needs, and we must relate agency research to the expertise of the university staff. If we can sensibly join the research skills of the university staff with the knowledge and research skills of the agency staff, then most assuredly we shall be in a strong position to develop applicable research and experimentation that will solve the problems with which we are now faced.

NOTES

1. Mary K. Bauman and Norman M. Yoder, *Placing the Blind and Visually Handicapped in Clerical, Industrial and Service Fields* (Washington: Vocational Rehabilitation Administration, Department of Health, Education and Welfare, 1966).
2. ———, *Characteristics of Blind and Visually Handicapped People in Professional, Sales and Managerial Work* (Washington: Vocational Rehabilitation Administration, Department of Health, Education and Welfare, 1963).
3. Joseph F. Clunk, "Influence of the Randolph-Sheppard Act on the Em-

ployment of Blind Persons," *Blindness—1966* (Washington: American Association of Workers for the Blind, 1966), 137–146.

4. James F. C. Hyde, Jr., *Law as a Profession for the Blind* (New York: American Foundation for the Blind, 1954).
5. Arthur H. Keeney and Virginia T. Keeney, "Blindness Among Practicing Physicians Who Have Previously Enjoyed Good Vision," *Archives of Ophthalmology* (June, 1950).
6. George A. Magers, "Placement—Key to Employment," *Blindness—1964* (Washington: American Association of Workers for the Blind, 1964), 119–136.
7. Morris Margolin, "Blind Physicians and the Practice of Medicine," *New Outlook for the Blind,* Vol. 53, No. 6 (June, 1959), 199–205.
8. Alex Rosen, "Social Work as a Profession for the Blind," *Proceedings of the Annual Conference, New York State Federation of Workers for the Blind, Inc.* (New York: The Federation, 1965).
9. *Selection and Training of the Blind for Computer Programming* (Washington: Association for Computer Machinery, and American Association of Workers for the Blind, 1966).
10. Anne Whittenbury, "An American Experiment," *New Outlook for the Blind,* Vol. 57, No. 1 (January, 1963), 22–24.
11. Norman M. Yoder, "American Association of Workers for the Blind, 1895–1964," *Blindness—1964* (Washington: American Association of Workers for the Blind, 1964), 151–175.

SESSION REPORT

John Aboud

One of the important problems today in the area of placement and vocation counseling is that of adequately employing the blind client. Industry, according to Dr. Norman M. Yoder, must increase its efforts to provide equipment and training for blind employees and should develop commensurate schematics, such as for color coding. Equally important, emphasis is needed upon training for automated skills, like simple form typing and erasure procedures for secretarial work. Another positive step would be to decrease the size of the braille dictionary. But even these changes would not be enough, and researchers and workers with the blind must learn what other kinds of aids are needed to make blind workers competent in different kinds of jobs. Ninety per cent of small businesses initiated and operated by the blind fail; it is necessary to know why.

According to Dr. Albert S. Thompson, the problems of the blind should be approached through rehabilitation; and careful analysis of work needs is the first step. This analysis would help determine the occupational choice. By viewing the world of work as it changes, and the process by which the handicapped person enters it, rehabilitation centers might be taught how the blind worker can best be trained as he works. Needed to perform this last step is a mass of data describing how people travel through the world of work.

Although considerable research has already been done, investigation must be continued to evaluate that research and to prove its worth. There is a great need to bridge the gap between the findings of basic research and its application in the field.

What kinds of training are most suitable for keeping the blind person flexible and emotionally stable when his job is lost to automation, depression, or other factors? This question raises the second question of how long rehabilitation should last. Why not make it a continuing process, not just a single experience? There is no reason why a case must be closed after one placement. Current research on the best counseling procedures for the blind suggests that continuing rehabilitation or teaching might be fruitful, and further work is being done on the acceptability of this new concept. But in order to check the effectiveness of this and other new concepts, an agency should re-examine the progress of the client every six months to determine what is needed in the way of retraining.

Perhaps there should be different types of agencies: one designed to maintain a positive "public image," for example, and one simply to serve the blind. Still largely unknown are what roles the latter agency must assume, how it should adjust to change, and what other benefits besides workshops it can offer.

Dr. Yoder commented on the structure of these agencies. He believes that they should apply business concepts, and that they should not be social welfare organizations. Their job is rehabilitation; they must perform research and train new workers.

Another approach of possible value is the study of the world of work in terms of operations, rather than individuals. It might also be feasible to do evaluations in the field. By taking groups of actual employers and making them part of a team, the entire spectrum of work could be viewed effectively.

Recently, consideration has been given to the idea of obtaining financial support either from the government or from the Veterans Administration. If one or both of these groups would agree to support employees on the fifth day of the work week, this day could be set aside for training the individuals for future jobs.

Also to be considered are the reactions of the labor force and other community attitudes toward these handicapped workers. After an initial survey to ascertain these attitudes, a demonstration project could be set up in the same city. Then another survey could be taken to evaluate the community attitudes following the demonstration project.

A further area to be explored is that of the blind who have already had successful agency and work experiences. If a study could be designed to show why they are successful—with those who are failures used as a control group—much might be learned.

One final point mentioned during the discussion concerned those people who have gotten jobs without the help of an agency. By examining the characteristics of these people and learning how they got their jobs, and by generalizing their strategies as related to their backgrounds and personalities, a further aid might be evolved to solve the problems in the placement and vocational decisions of the blind.

MULTIPLE-HANDICAPPED BLIND

NEEDED RESEARCH IN THE FIELD OF SERVICES FOR THE MULTIPLE-HANDICAPPED BLIND

*Elena D. Gall**

Nothing in the past two decades of service to the blind has developed so much frenzied activity as have the many efforts in the field of research. Still, a careful study of the findings will reveal that few studies have succeeded in changing practice. Workers with the blind are still seeking fundamental answers to fundamental problems.

Blind persons having additional handicaps represent a group whose limitations and deviations stem mainly from injury to the central nervous system. The National Institute of Neurological Diseases and Blindness of the U.S. Department of Health, Education and Welfare has prepared a series of research profiles[1-10] containing examples of basic research on specific disorders. These research profiles serve to enlighten the practitioner and improve his knowledge in the techniques of diagnosis, treatment, and prevention of the devastating results of disorders of the brain and the central nervous system. Of special interest to workers with the blind are the results of studies concerning the malfunction of the intricate central nervous system which is so tied up with vision, mobility, perception, and coordination.

In one of the studies the various diseases, deformities, and injuries of the eye which can cause visual loss are discussed in relation to directed research for treatment and prevention. The study explains that the eye functions by means of two interrelated processes. The first employs a lens and diaphragm system to focus the light into a clear image at the back of the eye. The second is a chemical conversion of this image into a nervous electric signal

---

* It is with deep regret that we note the recent and tragic death of Dr. Gall and explain that it deprived us of her counsel and her possible revisions as we edited this paper for publication.

which relays the information to the brain. Any disturbance of either of these two processes by disease or other damage to the organs involved results in partial or total loss of sight.[3]

While scientists are attempting to discover, control, and cure defects stemming from impairment of the central nervous system, parents, educators, sociologists, and health and rehabilitation counselors are still groping for methods and materials with which to treat, manage, train, and educate the MHB* of different age groups, of different cultural backgrounds, and of different economic status.

Those employed in work with the disabled, in general, are hampered by the lack of organized, consumable, clear-cut research findings. Some of the obstacles are:

1. The lack of a body of organized data in one or two locations where the teacher, rehabilitation counselor, psychologist, or social worker may turn to discover basic facts concerning blindness and the MHB.

2. The improper and inadequate use of several collections of historical writings, experimental case work reports, and other productions including the so-called quantitative studies which contribute a large body of facts.

3. Data presented are often sparse and, in the field of MHB in particular, they are produced from limited samples. The need for long-range programs established for the field of the visually handicapped is urgent. Particularly, there should be longitudinal studies organized around the service needs of the MHB.

4. The practitioner often finds that authors of research reports are contradictory and prone to conjectural tendencies. Their conclusions, in many cases, are generalizations not based on scientific examination of the data.

5. Definition is one of the major needs in research services for the MHB. Only by common understanding resulting from agreement on terminology can the professions and the public be better equipped to cooperate in research projects for the MHB wherever they may be found.

Another factor which may be responsible for the lag in vision research is the conflict of interest among the professions concerned. Members of the optometry profession, for instance, have found it

* The initials MHB in this paper refer to multiple-handicapped blind persons. The term "blind" includes the partly-seeing persons.

difficult to obtain funds for research; and, as a result, there is a shortage of personnel holding Ph.D. degrees in physiological optics. A national optometric institute has been suggested as a division of the National Institutes of Health, to be responsible for research needs in this field. Such a body should include psychologists, physiologists, biophysicists, pathologists, neuropsychiatrists, as well as optometrists.[11]

It is interesting to note that, in the past, programs of expansion and of refinement of methodology in the fields of research on the handicapped have not emerged from educational and psychological research laboratories in isolation. Observation and recording of behavioral data and charting of psychological processes in the success-and-failure patterns in school task problems have, for the most part, had initial impetus in the classroom. For this reason, in the future, teachers will have the added responsibility of working with specially trained research personnel in order to hasten and encourage research in the improvement of methodology and curricula for the MHB.

Still another source of neglect in research on the MHB is the tendency toward rigidity in existing state laws and agency policies governing the rights and privileges of special handicapped groups. This often tends to deprive the individual who, because he suffers from more than one disability, cannot easily be eligible for any single set of services as prescribed by the law, or as administered by certain private or public agencies.

One of the barriers to research and demonstration is the scant availability of adequate sampling. Despite the fact that the number of MHB cannot be definitely ascertained, it is safe to assume that, with a more enlightened citizenry, better parent education, and improved prenatal and postnatal diagnoses, there will be discovered a larger number of blind children who have additional handicaps. In England, registration of blindness is not compulsory until the age of five; but, for the MHB child, earlier reporting has been urged[12] to establish better parent relationships, to gain the fullest medical and surgical investigations, to try to establish what the dominant handicap is, and to start building up social, medical, and developmental case history.

The problems, consequently, are to discover and identify the MHB at the earliest possible time; to test them as adequately as possible; and to place them in suitable school settings where they can best be trained. Simultaneously, someone must explain them to themselves, to their families (including sibling and other relatives) through skillful counseling, so as to provide them throughout life with rich physical, social, mental, sensory, and communication experiences in a warm, wholesome, and secure environment of training and education until they are capable of independent living. Among the necessary provisions for suitable research in the area of the MHB are the expansion and growth of psychometry and its numerous applications in the fields of education, vocational guidance, industrial personnel, psychiatry, educational adjustment, and evaluation.

Eligible public and private schools, institutions, and agencies should be encouraged to conduct demonstration and research projects in such areas as the development and field testing of special devices for the handicapped, special teaching techniques for children with multiple disabilities, improved methods of training personnel, the causes and solutions to learning problems, and other related areas concerning the educational adjustment of the MHB.[13]

Tests, for the most part, are diagnostic tools for the solution of social, educational, emotional, and vocational problems of the handicapped. They tend to improve the understanding, treatment, and education when interpreted by a team of specialists. The difficulty in administering them and the question of validity should prove to be a challenge rather than a barrier to those working in the field of the MHB.

Some investigations have been suggested in the fields of curriculum and methodology:[14]

1. What specific content and techniques are unique to the education of the MHB or multiple-handicapped seeing children and youth?

2. What are the effects of various classroom and home climates upon the eventual development of the MHB?

3. What are the techniques used for group instruction and those used for individual instruction? What are the advantages of these? In what proportion can they be properly utilized?

Problems in diagnosis and total assessment are of major importance in the education, treatment, and employment of the MHB. Among the unanswered questions are:[14]

1. How may the MHB in the preschool population be identified and diagnosed early?

2. In what ways might early diagnosis of specialized needs of the MHB prevent later educational handicaps?

3. What are the trends in the cause of MHB in infants and preschool children? Are these patterns common to specific racial, socio-economic, or regional groups?

4. Is it possible to assess the perceptual abilities and disabilities of the various sensory modality areas of the brain?

5. Is there a connection between types of MHB and educational needs? What are the effects of such variables as visual acuity, previous visual experience, motivation, maturation, and other relevant conditions?—or of intelligence and parental attitudes?

6. What better testing procedures and instruments are possible for assessing the mental and emotional status and educational potential of the MHB?

7. Given other media for reading and writing, to what extent will a MHB student still find braille a useful tool?

8. How helpful are three-dimensional and enlarged illustrations and diagrams in books for the MHB?

9. Does the use of recorded material, at any grade level, interfere with the rate of reading and comprehension of print or braille?

10. What techniques could be developed for the remedial teaching of cerebral-palsied blind, deaf-blind, or brain-injured, utilizing new technological aids such as computers?

11. What improvements are needed in the quality of existing aids and devices for the MHB, such as pocket braillers, maps, disc recordings, and others?

12. What is the value of electronic aids in a total program of orientation and mobility instruction for the MHB?

In order to bring about practical results, research would be most suitably conducted by a task force of specialists who could pool their resources to develop improved definitions, to study incidence, and to set standards in the discovery, diagnosis, treatment, education, and employment of the MHB. Consultants need to be trained and assigned to local schools in urban and rural centers in order to enable them to facilitate the discovery, training, and integration of MHB children in classes for the normal, or for the blind.

"In the field of education, we identify research with a better understanding of the teaching-learning process, and the conditions under which it is most successfully carried on." [15] There is a dearth of information in connection with classroom teaching, home instruction, and itinerant teaching for the blind as conducted by both public and private agencies. There is a need for investigating the assets of various school and institutional settings by teachers, parents, and school administrators. Some studies are needed to evaluate the present status, and some experimental work should be done with new and dynamic model teaching programs based on learning theories and technological devices which can be utilized by the blind. As an example, ideas need to be explored in regard to the development of a rich variety of auditory and tactual experiences.

Language arts, including the study of foreign languages, represent curriculum areas which can be further explored from the point of view of vocational and social guidance, as well as the provision of a foundation for reading braille and large print.

Multimedia is important in training the MHB. Could a better approach to learning for the MHB be made through several sensory approaches rather than one? What are the advantages of the single channel or medium presentation versus the several approaches? Studies are needed also in setting up systems approaches to instructional problems. What do we teach? How do we teach it? What do we expect the pupil to learn or take on as a result of the lesson? Does the curriculum suit the need of the individual MHB child? These are only a few questions that workers for the MHB are asking themselves as they attempt to use methods and principles in general education and apply them to the education of the MHB.[16]

Of considerable interest are the research bulletins issued by the American Foundation for the Blind.[17] These deal with reports directed mainly to research personnel. They might prove enlightening to educators as well as to psychiatrists, technicians, and sociologists.

However, lack of information regarding the behavior patterns of the MHB is still a drawback in programs of guidance and counseling. This is particularly true in the case of individuals in adolescence. Needed are reports of their capacities, limitations, or the various methods and procedures employed in teaching these youngsters and preparing them for their vocations. They need tryout experiences, school-work programs, and apprenticeships, as well as conventional education, development of hobbies, development of peer identification, and the setting up of some experiences to provide standards for adulthood.

The problems of the MHB adolescent are numerous since such youngsters are faced almost unexpectedly with an additional series of severe adjustment problems, especially those arising from the distressing development period which turns a child into an adult. His appearance, desires, and sexual and emotional attitudes often add to his confusion, feelings of anxiety, and insecurity. He definitely needs counseling. To help him, studies are required which will:

1. Contribute to a growing maturity and self-understanding on the part of the MHB adolescent.

2. Help to sensitize him to cultural and social changes in his present and future environment.

3. Assist the student toward wise educational and vocational choices within the changing occupational structures.

4. Assist the student to learn how to make decisions and to try out the decisions in reality situations even though this involves the realization that he must take risks and learn from failure.

5. Counsel girls realistically about their role in the family and in the labor force.

6. Help the MHB to appreciate and understand themselves as adults and to face psychological realities.

7. Consult with parents and other family members about their role in the adjustment of the MHB person.

8. Serve as liaison between personnel specialists and coordinators of services within the school and within the wider community to facilitate social and economic adjustment.

9. Continue the study of changing characteristics of the student population and interpret the information to the administrative and teaching staffs for use in further curriculum planning and in the development of administrative structures and regulations which will facilitate future programs for the MHB.

It is encouraging to note that research is touching upon the educational needs of the blind and this, in turn, may prove applicable to the MHB. The American Printing House for the Blind recently reported [18] on specific research and development programs which involved perception in braille word recognition, listening in learning by the blind, and problems in nonverbal tactual communication.

In general, current research thinking in the area of the handicapped has not kept pace with that in other scientific fields or with the research developments in industry. Haller[19] has suggested that the following guidelines be observed in order to hasten the process of bringing the results of research to the consumer:

1. Research can be productive only when its objectives are well defined.

2. Some planned duplication is desirable if it is properly controlled.

3. Support should be continued until some tangible and basic knowledge and understanding result.

4. Supervision should stop short of interference.

5. Information we already have must be made easier to find and use.

Services for the MHB would be considerably improved if future researchers would concern themselves with specific needs in broad areas. Particularly needed are research studies of services in the area of the rehabilitation of the MHB. These would include the listing of:

1. Specialized services and facilities and the location where they could be obtained for each type of multiple handicapped person.

2. Available devices in prosthetics, orthotics, and optics.

3. Studies of motivation and dynamics of behavior in the MHB as these affect the rehabilitation process; analysis of employment obstacles of the MHB.

4. Discovery of more ways of shedding light on the manner in which a MHB conceives of himself in his home, on the job, in the community.

Since few institutions are engaged in work with the MHB, and few professionals are specialists in this field, it is somewhat difficult at the present time to conduct effective research. For this reason, dependable findings by existing programs and appropriate supervision of on-going projects are also needed. To add to the effectiveness of research in any specialty there must always take place the evaluation and use of existing scientific information that is germane to the conditions or problems being examined. Haller[19] has stated, "Certainly not only are we failing to use readily available resources, but the mass of information is so great that it can no longer be adequately transmitted by people talking and listening and writing to each other."

Often the worker in a sheltered workshop, institution, or school finds himself alone with the problems of the MHB. He needs to be informed by specially trained consultants or teams of experts familiar with research findings as to what is pertinent and new in the field, as well as where more knowledge is available, and how one utilizes such information in regard to a MHB person.

The critical shortage of specially trained personnel indicates further need to involve the schools—primary, secondary, and college—and their personnel in preventing, correcting, and treating eye defects in an educational setting. While it is apparent that the schools should play a central role in the preventive and remedial efforts in the early school years, it is not clear just how they can improve their efforts to prolong and protect the visual ability of all children while adequately serving those who are diagnosed as blind or MHB. More studies are needed in determining the relationship between low vision or impaired vision and emotional disturbance, delicate health, poor coordination, impaired learning, and educational retardation. Studies of the achievement of the MHB are a rarity in the literature.

Therefore, surveys of common failure, major successes, major satisfactions, or major discouragements among the MHB in school would be helpful in organizing and improving the curriculum and in planning postgraduate and work programs for them. Pupil expectations, pupil anticipation of difficulty, pupil occupational aspirations; what pupils like about special classes, regular classes, itinerant teachers, home teachers, residential schools, length of school day, after-school programs, week-end activities; what teachers view as the most frequently occurring behavior problems of the MHB, are other suggestions worthy of investigation—particularly since what is needed is information regarding the individual's own preferences, motivations, and creative ability.[20]

An interesting approach to research would be a series of studies on the motor characteristics of the MHB. As reported in a recent study,[21] the motor abilities of retarded children are organized in much the same way as in normal children, show similar developmental curves, and are definitely at lower levels than for normal children. It is recommended that with more patience in setting the stage for learning, perhaps retarded children can benefit from the same type of gross physical and manual skill development. Due to the great need all children have for physical activity, the MHB are particularly handicapped when maximum use is not made of their mobility and motor activity. It is equally important to interpret exceptionally well-developed muscular coordination in some MHB—such as manual dexterity—and to channel such ability to the improved adjustment of the child. In a residential setting, for instance, there was the report of a deaf-blind, brain-injured, physically underdeveloped aphasic child who could climb, grasp, and twirl her body in a most exceptional way. Few studies have been made to show any correlation between, for instance, such ability and speed of learning or predictable response to auditory stimulation.

Assuming that research is a search for knowledge, the information which needs to be gathered is that which will lend understanding as well as knowledge. What workers for the visually handicapped need to know is how the nature of the MHB differs from that of other children, why they behave as they do, the ways in which they learn, how they think, how they manage to keep in touch with their environment, how they can develop interpersonal relationships.

The search for such knowledge will lead the investigator, no doubt, in unpredictable directions. Workers with the MHB need to:

1. Accumulate more pertinent information and more adequate methodology to train the MHB to appear, think, learn, feel, and function as near normal as possible.

2. Discover more ways and means by which the public can learn about the abilities, skills, and talents of these individuals so that they may be more readily accepted in their communities and by their friends and families.

3. Enhance professional understanding and improve the knowledge of those in commerce and industry and government toward greater cooperation in programs of training and placement of the MHB in work situations.

4. Devise methods by which one defines blindness in relation to each MHB person, taking into consideration the intellectually gifted, the brain impaired, the deaf, the emotionally disturbed, the orthopedically blind, the neurologically handicapped blind, car-

diopathic blind, mentally retarded blind, and to discover and measure the nature of the disabilities and handicaps as they relate to individual adjustment.

Special methods of parent education, as well as of professional education, are practically unexplored areas in the field of the MHB. They are fertile fields for researchers. How does a teacher explain the child to the parent? How does one involve the parents in the learning process of the brain-injured blind child? It is a difficult enough task, for example, for educators to understand the type of child that Strauss and Lehtinen[22] and Lewis[23] present. However, some teachers have taught such children and have learned to understand them. But how can a parent cope with the nomenclature, the complex nature of the perceptual problems and their understandings? Today, the child with multiple handicaps is often called the child with perceptual difficulties, "the Strauss Child," the minimally brain-injured child, the child with learning difficulties, the neurophrenial child, the hyperkinetic child.

To explain a MHB child to a teacher, parent, or prospective employer may require the combined consultation of an entire clinic staff. Why does he walk this way? How does he see? How much does he hear? What does he retain? Can he eat by himself? Does he choose what he wears? Does he like to sing? How does he feel about the oversolicitude of his parents? What is the extent of his manipulative skills? Can he travel by himself? How does he compare with other MHB's? These are but some of the questions frequently raised by workers with the MHB. If a child is deaf-blind, for example, it will require much knowledge, many discussions, much individual observation, considerable creative thinking, innumerable drill sessions, and much patience and time to enhance the growth and adjustment of a single individual.

Because of the complexity of adjustment, learning, and orientation problems of the MHB, the need for diversity of attack is also paramount in planning research for treatment, and educational and vocational programs for them. Often we are dealing with impairments of speech, ambulation, emotional response, tactile discrimination, and muscular coordination, as well as sensory involvement, in addition to blindness. The educational team, for example, often needs scientific information relating to medicine, psychology, rehabilitation, and technology, and the understanding of such facts, before it can determine the extent and nature of the major handicap and its relationship to the child's capacity for learning, growth, and adjustment.

Should the definition of a MHB be one determined by the educational and training needs? Is a MHB child one who, because of disabilities other than blindness, cannot be served in an educational setting designed for the normal blind child? Does this imply that even if one utilizes existing facilities for the blind, administrators are obliged to provide additional services?

The need for research in perception and learning is of particular importance. The complexity of learning problems in the MHB raises some interesting questions:[14]

1. What is the world like to the MHB?

2. How do the MHB learn? Is learning for them different in kind or degree from that of the average blind or deaf child? Have these ways of learning affected teaching practices?

3. How do the MHB develop concepts about their environment? How realistic are these concepts when compared to the concepts of other children? How useful are these concepts?

4. How much differentiation is made between the educational needs of the congenitally and the adventitiously MHB?

5. Is it possible to increase the overall perceptual development of the MHB through structured and sequential development of all sensory channels?

6. Could the teaching of two-dimensional and three-dimensional forms aid in the perceptual development of the MHB?

7. Does the extended and perhaps excessive listening to talking books and recordings affect the speech development in the deaf-blind?

8. How do the family and community relationships of MHB compare with those of normally seeing children?

9. How early should training begin?

10. How is readiness measured?

DISABILITY SYNDROMES

Probably two-thirds of the MHB population suffers from severe adjustment problems arising from a combination of factors caused by blindness and one or more of the disabilities whose definitions follow. These definitions of disability syndromes, often apparent in the physical, sensory, and intellectual comportment of the MHB, may further highlight the multiplicity of factors which, in various degrees in different persons, cause any or a combination of the following MHB characteristics: bizarre learning behavior, lack of maturity, slowness in comprehension and retention, communication disorders, poor gait and poor posture, defective speech, physical weakness, undesirable mannerisms, emotional disturbances, educational retardation, and social immaturity.

Cerebral Palsy

Cerebral palsy embraces the clinical picture created by injury to the brain, in which one of the components is motor disturbance. Thus, cerebral palsy may be described as a group of conditions, usually originating in childhood, characterized by paralysis, weakness, incoordination, or any other aberration of motor functions caused by pathology of the motor control center of the brain. In addition to such motor dysfunction, cerebral palsy may include learning difficulties, psychological problems, sensory defects, convulsive and behavioral disorders of organic origin.

Brain Injury

The brain-injured child is the child who before, during, or after birth, has received an injury to or suffered an infection of the brain. As a result of such organic impairment, defects of the neuromotor systems may be present or absent; however, such a child may show disturbances in perception, thinking, and emotional behavior, either separately or in combination. These disturbances can be demonstrated by specific tests. The disturbances prevent or impede a normal learning process. Special educational methods have been devised to remedy the specific handicaps.[22]

Mental Retardation

Mental retardation refers to subaverage general intellectual functioning which originates during the developmental period and is associated with impairment in one or more of the following: maturation, learning, and social adjustment.[24]

Aphasia

Aphasia refers to the inability to use and/or understand spoken language as a result of defect or damage in the central nervous system. There are two main types: receptive aphasia (also called sensory or auditory) where the child lacks understanding of spoken language; and expressive aphasia (also called motor or verbal) where the child understands speech but does not talk normally. Central aphasia is a severe disorder where inner language functioning is disturbed. It is an impairment in the ability to communicate with one's self. The term global aphasia is also used by some authorities to describe children who have no inner, receptive, or expressive language function as far as can be determined.[25] In the case of the adult who has loss of speech, we are dealing with modifications of behavior brought about by brain lesions.[26]

Deafness

The deaf are those in whom the sense of hearing is non-functional for the ordinary purpose of life. This general group is made of two distinct classes based entirely on the time of hearing loss. The congenitally deaf are those who were born deaf. The adventitiously deaf are those who were born with normal hearing but in whom the sense of hearing later became nonfunctional through illness or accident. The hard of hearing are those in whom the sense of hearing, although defective, is functional with or without a hearing aid.[27]

CASE STUDIES

The following excerpts from case studies of MHB youngsters illustrate the educational, psychological, and vocational needs of four young people who are categorized as MHB in special school programs.

Case One

> Betty is a 16-year-old in the ninth grade of a special CORE (Slow-Retarded) Program in high school. She has central chorioretinitis toxoplasmosis, nystagmus, and esotropia based on amblyopia. Her primary visual problem has been diagnosed as glaucoma. The prognosis is poor because her central vision will be gone eventually. Her

corrected visual acuity is 10/400 in the right eye and 20/300 in the left. She is allowed only limited gym activities with no vigorous sports. She wears bifocals for close work, telescopic lenses for distance.

Her father is dead and her mother has remarried. Since childhood Betty has been in several foster homes. For the past ten years, she and her 18-year-old sister have been living with a foster parent. Apparently there is sibling rivalry. Betty thinks that her sister is beautiful, smart, attractive; and that she has many friends. Betty is just the opposite. At home, everyone seems to pity her. They repeatedly tell her how hopeless she is, and she, in turn, acts that way.

Betty is a slow learner, but it is debatable if she is to be considered retarded. She is in a special class for borderline retarded children. A factor which makes Betty difficult is that she has been diagnosed as schizophrenic. She rarely trusts anyone working with her. In the past she reported that she had trusted so many people who rejected her later. Now she rarely cooperates with anyone. Her reading and arithmetic last year were on a first-grade level, and she had no desire to learn or even to try.

Betty gives up too quickly when attempting to learn. She resorts to figuring a problem by using her fingers. Feeling embarrassed, she carefully makes sure that the teacher does not see her. But this method almost always rewards her with the correct answer.

In the area of reading, I found that "Dick, Jane, and Spot," was not for a 16-year-old. We often discussed various areas that did not interest her, such as news items and science. One day she told me she had never written a letter and wanted to learn how to do so. I wrote two sample letters with her. To my amazement, I received her first written letter two weeks later.

I constantly try to boost her morale. She has a very poor opinion of herself and refuses to wear glasses because she feels they make her look ugly. She explained that, in the classroom, the wearing of her telescopic glasses helps her to see the board more clearly, but when she looks at her paper (to copy notes) it all becomes a blur. She hates to keep switching glasses and, as a result does not use the telescopic lenses unless she is hearing a lecture or seeing a show.

Betty has proved she can achieve an education that will be suited for her. She is now doing third-grade reading and arithmetic and has gone up two grades in one year. She is doing fourth grade history and science, and is adjusting nicely to the high school. She has also joined the choir.

I am Betty's confidante and am trying to make her realize that she can make something out of her life if she tries. For example, she would never dance at a party. One day, as I casually observed her, she got up and danced, saying, "I'm dancing for someone special." Her handicap is people's inability to accept her as she is.

Betty still needs much help with her reading so that she can read a newspaper by herself. Basic work in mathematics, in order to handle money matters, must be worked on. A basic skill for communication, both that which is written and oral, will be the goal for next year. She still needs constant reassurance that she is wanted and needed.

Case Two

"JB" is an intellectually superior deaf-blind student who presents a challenge to higher education. He is 19 years old, and has been totally blind since birth, with a profound hearing loss since the age of nine. His prognosis is poor. He has excellent general health, does not travel alone, was raised in a rural area, and has attended two residential schools for the blind. He is highly religious and expresses much faith in people.

He has outstanding achievement on the educational level, is an excellent reader, and has adequate social and emotional adjustment. His grades in high school academic subjects averaged more than 90.

His psychological profile is Wechsler-Bellevue 136, Hayes-Binet 138. It is obvious that his multiple handicap has influenced the comprehension sub-test score. He is of superior intelligence, enthusiastic, cooperative, and has considerable potential for higher education.

The manual and mechanical aptitude tests which JB took did not show promise in repetitious type of work in which speed was an important factor. The examiners did not rule out the possibility of employment in a situation that required intelligence, critical judgment, and exactness of detail. By all standards of intellectual capacity, academic preparation, and learning potential, JB should be considered as a most promising candidate for college.

Case Three

Hattie is an example of a child with language disorders and their accompanying educational disabilities. She is ten years old, and was a premature six-month baby. Hattie was in an incubator for a period of two and a half months, with a resultant condition of retrolental fibroplasia. She responds to sounds inconsistently. Hearing loss is bilateral, moderate mixed: right 52 db; left 61 db. Her vision has been corrected to 20/200 in the better eye (left). Future planning in regard to her ability to read ink-print will depend a great deal on her ability to perform. Her eyeballs roll, and she has limited left lateral movements. Tongue movements are slow. Tympanic membranes dull. Normal vestibular responses to rotation.

Her family is cooperative and interested. Psychologically she is cooperative, with rapport easily established. On the Columbia Mental Maturity Scale—a non-verbal test of abstract ability—she attained a mental age of 9 years and 8 months, with an I.Q. of 98. This is functioning on the average level of intelligence. Despite her multiple handicaps, she has shown marked intellectual growth during the past year. It is recommended that she continue her speech therapy program.

Hattie is enrolled in the deaf-blind department of a residential school for the blind, and is showing progress. She has residual hearing that is not yet being used to maximum. She responds well to binaural amplification in the classroom and to individualized instruction. Her speech needs much attention and is interfering with better achievement in arithmetic, science, spelling, and social studies, but her language growth continues to expand on a slow level. There is evidence of confusion and frustration in expressing herself and in receiving oral messages. In reading, her interpretive accomplishment is still on a primary level and her desire to read is extremely limited.

Hattie's teachers are not certain how much of the inability to express herself is due to her hearing loss and how much to known brain damage. Her inability to speak clearly indicates a lack of muscular coordination of the vocal and speech mechanism. Although her I.Q. is that of a normal child, her educational level is from three to four years below average.

Case Four

Peter, aged 15 years, attends a special class for the blind in a public school. He is nervous and insecure. He lacks confidence and continually deprecates himself. He is quite verbal, often volunteering to answer questions without knowing the answers. From his own statement, he spends a great deal of time in study, saying he will study all night if necessary to get his work finished. It is questionable whether he knows how to study, and whether he has the capacity to learn academic subjects. Peter is always polite and does not seem to have any resentment toward his teachers. At present, he is pressuring his home room teacher to promote him to the ninth grade, seemingly without regard to his lack of achievement at the level at which he is now working. He still has difficulty with mobility and orientation in the classroom, moving impulsively with no sense of direction. He is unable to follow simple directions for written work.

His English teacher reports that Peter is able to write coherent sentences but lacks spelling, punctuation, and braille writing skills. His social studies teacher reports that, since achievement in social studies is dependent to a great extent on reading comprehension and some degree of memorization, his performance is very poor. He does not have much ability to reason from facts. He is unable to read maps, seemingly because of poor coordination in hand movements and because of his extreme nervousness.

As far as spelling is concerned, his daily work, which includes word comprehension, is well above passing, as are his weekly tests. However, he failed a recent six-week review test of spelling words. Peter's arithmetic teacher reports that he seems unable to learn computation of numbers. He knows addition combinations but has difficulty in adding a column of figures. Peter is unable to solve subtraction problems unless supervised step by step. He knows nothing about multiplication or division. Occasionally he shows some understanding of the solution of thought or word problems if they are within the field of his experience.

In his science work, Peter responds and participates in the discussion. He does passing work, both oral and written, though sometimes he has difficulty in expressing ideas. He completes his assignments and is never a discipline problem. As far as science is concerned, promotion to a higher class would be considered. His braille teacher reports that he reads passably, but that writing on a braille slate is a real chore. Peter claims the pocket slate is better for him, but his work is still poor on it. He puts forth great effort.

Education

Keeping in mind the learning and adjustment problems of Betty, JB, Hattie, and Peter, the coordinator or educator might raise the following questions in planning the curriculum:

1. What are the essential areas of the curriculum for the MHB? What proportion of time should be spent on each? How important is the teaching of braille writing, large print, reading techniques, hand-writing, science, and health education to the MHB?

2. What procedures are useful in strengthening the psychological adjustment of the MHB? How important is the inclusion of tactual, auditory, sensory training? How can such skills be measured? How can readiness in these be determined?

3. What kinds of educational materials are needed at present and in the foreseeable future? How many students will use these materials? In what form are they needed: tactual, visual, audio?

4. To what extent are students encouraged and prepared to use a variety of materials and aids?

5. Should the development of preschool instruction in orientation and mobility be explored?

6. What constitutes a desirable creative art program?

7. How much special music instruction and braille or large-print music is available?

8. To what extent do MHB children participate in physical education programs in school? By what criteria are they included or excluded?

9. How may the MHB achieve ready access to the quantity, qual-

ity, and variety of educational materials needed in high school programs as well as in adult life?

10. What jobs are open to the MHB?

11. What constitutes a suitable program for the development of personal and social relationships of MHB to the sighted persons around them?

Education for the MHB in general needs to be redefined and analyzed in order to bring sharper focus on the specialized methods, materials, and techniques used in instructing blind children with more then one handicap. The guidance counselor and the placement officer might ask:

1. What are the advantages of placing such children in a school for seeing versus schools for the blind?

2. How early, and to what extent, should orientation and mobility instruction be started with the MHB? What problems may be encountered in the process? How widely do these individuals differ in their mobility needs?

3. What kinds of pre-vocational counseling and preparation are most realistic and helpful for the MHB? When does one start job orientation?

4. How extensive must medical and ophthalmological reports be in order to be of use to workers with the MHB?

5. How does one communicate in the counseling situation?

Those in professional education might wish to ascertain:

1. What factors of personality, philosophy, previous experience, and preparation are likely to produce more effective workers with the MHB?

2. How do competencies and personal characteristics needed by workers with MHB compare with those needed by workers with normally sighted children, or with blind children?

3. What teacher competencies are requisite to enter into specialized teaching, and what might better be developed through inservice seminars or summer studies after teaching experience?

4. Are the roles and functions of teachers in special schools, resource rooms, and itinerant services sufficiently similar that common preparation for all is desirable?

5. What roles and functions are actually carried out by workers in the various types of educational agencies and services?

6. What preparation course work and activities have contributed most and what the least to the later successful functioning of workers in MHB rehabilitation?

7. To what extent should workers be prepared to deal with orientation and mobility of the MHB?

8. What responsibilities do school and agency administrators have for recruiting and preparing special teachers and workers for the MHB?

9. What is the ideal program of field and laboratory experiences and internship?

The administrator of service agencies, schools, and institutions is a key person in the rehabilitation and adjustment of the MHB. As a program planner, he looks into the costs and possible revenue for teaching, training, housing, and feeding of youngsters according to age groups and severity of disability. What are the present and recommended criteria for admission, retention, and referral for educational and vocational services for the MHB? Reports on policy and practices are needed to guide the administrator. He also can utilize information on the changing role of the residential school, the institution, and the special school.

An example of a current trend is the report by Elonen, Polzian, and Zwarensteyn. They reported their experience at the Michigan School for the Blind and confirmed what many educators of the blind suspected—that visually handicapped children are often unjustly committed to institutions for the mentally defective because they apparently do not function in already existing educational settings. For the most part, these represent children who are emotionally handicapped and blind. Once in an institution, such youngsters remain at their low level and even sink lower. However, with enlightened treatment and relaxed, warm understanding and environment, these children are beginning to show evidence of greater potential and of learning.

With the exception of periodic reports of incidence in the deaf-blind population, such data are not reported in the field of the MHB. Directors of programs interested in setting up services for the multiple-handicapped need to know the population that is to be served and whether such persons are enrolled in programs in private or public schools, in residental or day schools, in centers, or in clinics. Of importance, also is information regarding the amount of time that is required in each service program—the average number of days per year, and the number of hours each day.

The age categories into which the MHB fall, as well as the levels of achievement, are necessery items of information for directors and supervisors. Are they in nursery, preschool, elementary school, secondary school? Do they qualify for adult education or college entrance? Would they fall in other service categories, such as hospital schools, home instruction, schools for mentally ill or emotionally disturbed, institutions for the retarded, classes for delinquents, or schools for the deaf? How many are hard-of-hearing blind, orthopedically handicapped blind, cerebral palsied blind, neurologically handicapped blind, or chronically ill blind? How many of the MHB in need of services are economically disadvantaged? How many of them are ambulatory? How many are homeless?

The personnel needed in the care, education, and treatment of MHB is varied in terms of training, background and experience, and function, and in degree of responsibility within a school or sheltered workshop. In order to determine the availability of such personnel, administrators will need to know the appropriate or current salary scale and accepted work load for each job classification.

Today, centers caring for and educating the MHB are lacking in qualified personnel because of noncompetitive salary schedules, lack of certification of requirements, lack of desirable living and working conditions, and lack of organized personnel training programs. On the other hand, little information is available regarding the accepted norms and requirements in these areas.

OTHER NEEDED RESEARCH

How do we finance programs for the MHB? What existing laws provide for such services on the local, state, and federal levels? Can tuition fees become a source of income? Will the community agencies and private foundations be available as supporters of such programs? These questions need to be studied and some guidelines need to be suggested to administrators who are contemplating setting up or extending existing programs for the MHB.

Surveys are needed in order to determine available services in each agency for the MHB and their families. Similarly, studies should be made to determine what further developments should be established in health and recreation services, psychological services, educational and social services, and vocational and placement services. Also needed are surveys of what public and private schools, institutions, and agencies shall become eligible for conducting research and techniques for children with multiple disabilities, the cause and remediation of learning problems, and other related areas concerning the education and adjustment of the MHB.

We need to study the selection, placement, recruitment, and training of manpower on every level of work with the blind and the MHB. We need surveys on the evaluation and improvement of educational, treatment, and training standards. Comprehensive state planning for the MHB is needed to point out methods of implementing existing federal and state legislation. More particularly, for work with the blind a number of regional projects and demonstrations are suggested which would include a meaningful sample of children and adults (including the aged) with more than one disability in addition to blindness. Such projects should be conducted with creativity on an interdisciplinary level by experienced personnel representing sociology, education, psychology, rehabilitation counseling, and medicine. They should include studies which will enlighten the practitioner in matters concerning learning and perception as well as in social adjustment and prevocational placement problems. Investigations into the needs of the MHB should be approached with courage, faith, optimism, and a feeling of challenge.

To economize on time and to utilize human potential to the fullest, it is suggested that those in the teaching profession should take on more responsibility for contributing to the research and dissemination of research findings, possibly through educational organizations and periodicals. Abdication of this responsibility, and relegation of it solely to government and voluntary agencies may remove the research process further from the schools and programs where the MHB should be placed as early as possible.

To achieve these ends, the following lines of research are recommended:

1. The improvement of the self-concept, and an increase in the amount and quality of self-identification, through rich experiences of warm integration and usefulness.

2. Public and professional education in regard to social and economic status, abilities, and skills of the blind in general. What

media can produce information that will lead the public and the professions more accurately to conceive of the totality of the MHB personality?

3. Improved individual instruction to accelerate programs of education, including remedial teaching of basic skills.

4. Raising standards of treatment through humanizing attitudes toward the severely disabled on all intellectual levels.

5. Studies to provide work, residences, human contacts for young adults and older ones who are seeking or are in need of independent living opportunities.

6. Heightened empathy through understanding by parents, siblings, members of the family, and the community at large. How may parents be involved more profitably in the education and care of their MHB?

7. Research for definite age requirements, services, and benefits; and new definitions and classifications as guidelines for administering service programs.

8. Research to provide expansion and improvement of adequate facilities with sufficient equipment to house, educate, and train the MHB regardless of age and degree of disability. Such facilities should include day care centers, research, educational, and custodial care centers.

9. More efficient utilization of the services of aides and volunteers by schools and centers.

10. Studies as to how to strengthen interagency cooperation by coordination of activities and by the analysis of the function of each.

NOTES*

1. Research Profile No. 1: *Summary of Progress at the National Institute of Neurological Diseases and Blindness,* Public Health Service Bulletin No. 1109 (rev.; Washington: Government Printing Office, 1966).
2. Research Profile No. 2: *Cerebrovascular Disorders (Strokes),* Public Health

* *Editor's Note.* Free copies of the extensive bibliography for Dr. Gall's paper will be supplied upon request by: Dr. Maxwell H. Goldberg, The Center for Continuing Liberal Education, 103 Sparks Building, The Pennsylvania State University, University Park, Pennsylvania 16802.

Service Bulletin No. 1154 (Washington: Government Printing Office, 1966).

3. Research Profile No. 3: *Summary of Progress in Eye Disorders,* Public Health Service Bulletin No. 1155 (rev.; Washington: Government Printing Office, 1966).
4. Research Profile No. 4: *Summary of Progress in Hearing, Language, and Speech Disorders,* Public Health Service Bulletin No. 1156 (rev.; Washington: Government Printing Office, 1965).
5. Research Profile No. 5: *Summary of Progress in Mental Retardation,* Public Health Service Bulletin No. 1157 (Washington: Government Printing Office, 1963).
6. Research Profile No. 6: *Summary of Progress in Multiple Sclerosis and Amyotrophic Lateral Sclerosis,* Public Health Service Bulletin No. 1158 (rev.; Washington: Government Printing Office, 1965).
7. Research Profile No. 7: *Summary of Progress in Neuromuscular Disorders,* Public Health Service Bulletin No. 1159 (rev.; Washington: Government Printing Office, 1966).
8. Research Profile No. 8: *Summary of Progress in Parkinson's Disease,* Public Health Service Bulletin No. 1160 (rev.; Washington: Government Printing Office, 1966).
9. Research Profile No. 9: *Summary of Progress in Collaborative Prenatal Research,* Public Health Service Bulletin No. 1161 (Washington: Government Printing Office, 1963).
10. Research Profile No. 10: *Summary of Progress in Epilepsy,* Public Health Service Publication No. 1327 (Washington: Government Printing Office, 1965).
11. Federal Research and Development Programs: U.S. House of Representatives, 88th Congress, First Session. *Hearings Before the Select Committee on Government Research re: House Resolution 504, Part 1* (Washington: Government Printing Office, 1964).
12. M. S. Colborne Brown, "Provision for the Multiply-Handicapped Blind Child in the United Kingdom," *New Beacon* (August–September, 1964). (Mimeographed.)
13. U.S. House of Representatives, *Memo to Members of the Study Panel of the Ad Hoc Subcommittee on Education and Training of the Handicapped* (Brooklyn, New York: Industrial Home for the Blind, 1967).
14. Roberta A. Bowers and Helen Gibbons, *Report of a Conference on Research Needs in the Education of the Partially Seeing and Blind Children* (New York: Center for Urban Education, 1966).
15. John W. Best, *Research in Education* (Englewood Cliffs, New Jersey: Prentice-Hall, 1959).
16. *Symposium on Research and Utilization of Educational Media for Teaching the Hearing Impaired* (Lincoln, Nebraska: Nebraska Center for Continuing Education, 1965).
17. American Foundation for the Blind, *Research Bulletin #2* (New York: The Foundation, 1962).
18. American Printing House for the Blind, *Annual Report—Fiscal 1966* (Louisville, Kentucky: Printing House, 1967).
19. George L. Haller, *Statement Before the Select Committee on Government Research,* November 20, 1963 (Washington: Government Printing Office, 1964).
20. William C. Morse, Richard L. Cutler and Albert H. Fink, *Public School Classes for the Emotionally Handicapped: A Research Analysis* (Washington: The Council for Exceptional Children, 1964).
21. Robert J. Francis and G. Lawrence Rarick, *Motor Characteristics of the*

Mentally Retarded, Cooperative Monograph No. 1, OE-35005, U.S. Department of Health, Education and Welfare (Washington: Government Printing Office, 1947).

22. A. A. Strauss and Laura E. Lehtinen, *Psychopathology and Education of the Brain-Injured Child*, Vol. 1 (New York: Grune and Stratton, 1947).
23. R. S. Lewis with A. A. Strauss and Laura E. Lehtinen, *The Other Child—The Brain-Injured Child* (New York: Grune and Stratton, 1951).
24. Jerome H. Rothstein, ed., *Mental Retardation: Readings and Resources* (New York: Holt, Rinehart and Winston, 1961).
25. Hortense Barry, *The Young Aphasic Child: Evaluation and Training* (Washington: The Alexander Graham Bell Association for the Deaf, 1961).
26. M. Berry and J. Eisenson, *Speech Disorders* (New York: Appleton, Century-Crofts Co., 1956), 387.
27. Merle E. Frampton and Elena D. Gall, eds., *Special Education for the Exceptional*, Vol. 2, p. 148; and Leonard M. Elstad, *The Deaf* (Boston: Porter Sargent, 1955).

REACTION TO LOSS OF BODY PARTS, OR FUNCTIONS-RESEARCH PRIORITIES IN REHABILITATION

H. Robert Blank

Unfortunately, the preceding paper by Dr. Gall, although excellent, is not organized around any gradient of priorities that would take into account at least the following areas: existing knowledge and the failures in its transmission for optimal services, teaching, and research; the serious paucity of professional personnel in general and the even more serious paucity of personnel interested in work with the MHB; the current deployment of research and training subsidies in the field versus more efficient use of funds and professional personnel; and the psychosocial and political determinants of who gets what services, and of what research is favored by grant allocation.

I shall therefore confine myself to discussion of certain priorities that are fundamental to the solution of many of the problems presented and implied in Dr. Gall's contribution.

In my clinical experience with the psychological problems of blind and other handicapped persons and in work with hospitals, social agencies, schools, and rehabilitation centers, I have noted that many blocks and failures in education and rehabilitation are primarily attributable to factors other than the handicaps per se, notably:

1. Failure adequately to prepare patient and family for the eventual handicap when such preparation was possible.

2. Failure to deal promptly, and in a sustained fashion, with the predictable major emotional disturbances in patient and family in those cases in which there is no opportunity to prepare them for the handicap; for example, in congenital blindness or in blindness due to accident.

The net result of the operation of these adverse factors is that, in the typical case of a child, when the worker in rehabilitation first sees the client he is confronted with an impossible etiologic diagnostic problem: that of differentiating the combination of severe learning disability, mental retardation, and personality disorder attributable to blindness plus brain damage from that attributable to inadequate mothering followed by several years of deprivation of adequate and consistent social and educational stimulation. From six months to a year of a therapeutic trial, with a child in a good home, in a good residential school, and with a therapeutic program geared to his needs, can clarify the prognosis as to educability and reversibility of damage.[6] Often the damage is irreversible. Adequate therapeutic trials of this kind are unavailable for most severely disabled multiple-handicapped children; and adequate long-term multidisciplinary treatment facilities are almost nonexistent. Most of these children become state hospital or state "school" custodial cases.

To restate the thesis: Prevention is the most important focus. Psychologically sound work with patient and family during the medical and surgical treatment phase is essential to the later definitive education or rehabilitation of the handicapped person, child or adult. Because this critical aspect of *prevention* of educational and rehabilitational failure is so widely ignored, I shall now give it more detailed consideration as it pertains to the handicapped child.

REACTIONS OF CHILDREN TO LOSS OF BODY PARTS OR FUNCTIONS—TREATMENT, TEACHING, AND RESEARCH CONSIDERATIONS

The reactions of children (and their parents) to loss of body parts or body functions is virtually an unexplored field in terms of *systematic* teaching and research. As an example of an appropriate treatment teaching and research model for medical centers, I have suggested that the research team (representing the disciplines of psychoanalysis and psychiatry, clinical psychology, social case work, sociology and rehabilitation counseling) study the following four categories of children:

1. Those with congenital blindness, deafness, malformation, and other disorders. A congenital handicap, often multiple, represents initially a severely traumatizing loss for the parents, especially for the mother; and careful interpretive and supportive help for the parents is essential as soon as the diagnosis is made. If such help is not provided, the child will not receive optimal mothering, and its

optimal development and the results of education and specific treatment will be compromised.

2. Children suffering accidental loss of body parts or functions. Obviously, in these cases, as in the case of congenital defect, there is no opportunity to provide child and parents with preparation for the loss. Psychologic study, treatment, and research with these children and their parents should begin in the hospital emergency room, continue throughout the hospital stay and during the outpatient rehabilitation period.

3. Children requiring surgery that results in loss of a body part or function, including cases in which the only external sign of a loss is a prominent scar, and those who have to be immobilized for prolonged periods.

4. Children suffering from diseases that predictably are fatal or lead to blindness, deafness, or paralysis.

In the last two categories, there is obviously opportunity to prepare child and parents for the loss, as well as to help them cope with the loss *post facto*. For example, in the case of infants and children with limited verbal capacity, we should strive to preclude separation from the mother during hospitalization. If rooming-in is unavailable, the periods of separation from the mother should be minimal throughout the entire hospitalization.

Clinical Considerations

Psychologic preparation of child and parents for the loss is the primary responsibility of the physician in charge of the case. The psychiatrist can provide insight and guidance for the physician on the timing and technique for such preparation. He can provide the necessary psychotherapy that is frequently indicated even with the best preparation. Many later complications and failures in education and rehabilitation are attributable to grossly inadequate psychologic preparation for loss which left the patient anxiously confused and hostile to all physicians and anything associated with hospitals, agencies, and other institutions. In contrast the following cases are instructive.

CASE HISTORIES

Case One. An ophthalmologist consulted me about a ten-year-old boy, blinded accidentally in one eye two weeks previously. The ophthalmologist now felt it was urgent for the blind eye to be enucleated, but he was "panicked" at the idea of telling the boy to whom he had become deeply attached. The boy and his parents were intelligent, stable personalities and most cooperative with treatment thus far. It was recommended that, after prior "clearance" with the parents, the ophthalmologist interpret the situation to the boy in the presence of his parents. Accordingly, the child was told that there was no chance of restoring vision to the eye; that it had to be removed because it endangered the normal eye, that it was necessary cosmetically; and that he would be fitted with a prosthetic eye that would match his normal eye. The ophthalmologist had been prepared for a more serious reaction than the boy's relatively mild anxious depressive response. Surgery was performed the next day. Net result: an actively cooperative patient and family.

In similar medical situations, because of neurotic predisposition and other factors, the surgery might be resisted, or it might be followed by prolonged severe depressive reaction in spite of skillful honest interpretation prior to surgery. But the physician in charge is in a far better position to deal with the total problem, including successful referral for psychotherapy, if *he* emerges from the traumatic situation as someone who can be trusted, and who will continue to help the patient live and develop productively with the handicap.

I prefer not to use the terms *handicap* and *disability* synonymously. The handicap is the objective limitation that has to be accepted as a fact if rehabilitation is to succeed. The disability of a handicapped child or adult, although frequently attributed to the handicap, is often chiefly the result of serious personality problems that are not obvious, or far less obvious than the handicap. Such disability can be markedly reduced preventively by adequate interpretation, beginning with the initial contacts of the physician with the child and his parents.

Case Two. A colleague consulted me about the case of a 13-year-old boy with ulcerative colitis, treated for six years by an internist. After the latest and almost fatal recurrence and subsidence of colitis, the findings seemed to indicate resection of the bowel, and the physician was preparing the boy physically but not psychologically, for the surgery. The psychiatrist was called in "to get the child's agitated mother off the internist's neck."

I suggested that it was essential for the internist to give the boy and the parents a simple and direct anatomic and physiologic interpretation of the illness. And, if surgery was decided upon, both parents and the patient should know what was going to be done and the net result. It was clear that the mother would need prolonged psychotherapy, but it appeared that the internist would be able to handle the emotional repercussions in the boy.

The suggestions were followed. The boy, an undersized constricted personality, had established a passively dependent and compliant relationship with his doctor and the hospital staff. Outside he was depressed and asocial, subtly provoking his mother's demands on the internist. Medical frankness with the patient and his family, and psychotherapy for the mother, resulted in marked improvement in the emotional climate of the home and in the boy's total functioning. He became more active, alert and sociable, and his physical condition improved surprisingly. Even though he was prepared for surgery, it proved to be unnecessary. This continued to be the status one year after our initial consultation.

It is no more than suggested that the sustained physical improvement was related to the improved psychologic handling of child and family. What is emphasized is that, with or without surgery, honest interpretation is far more likely to produce a responsibly cooperating patient and family than evasiveness and false reassurance.

Often in consultations and in seminars on the subject of preparing child and family for the loss of body part or function, the question is asked, "What do you tell them?" especially in cases where blindness is anticipated or an amputation has to be performed. If the physician clearly understands that a grief reaction, a manifest depression, is the normal reaction to loss of a body part or function (as it is to loss of a loved one), and that he can materially help the patient through the reaction, he will have less difficulty in finding the appropriate words. If, in a given case, the physician has reason to suspect that child or parent is predisposed to pathologic reactions to loss, it is all the more important not to evade the issue, but first to consult with a psychiatrist.

It cannot be overemphasized that the child's worst fear is the fear of abandonment, not the fear of death, which, to the extent that it can be conceptualized, tends to be reacted to in terms of abandonment. What is more difficult for parent and physician to understand is that, in spite of their physical presence, disturbed communication between parent and child, between physician and child, constitutes a form of abandonment to which the child is very vulnerable.

APPLICATION TO ADULT HANDICAPPED

What has been said about prevention of psychologically determined disability in the medical-surgical treatment of the handicapped child applies also to the handicapped adult. Space does not permit more than a brief case history to highlight the application.

A 58-year-old diabetic man, blind for four years with a preceding six-year history of retinitis, was brought by his wife and son for consultation because of a chronic severe depression and angry resentful intolerence of any attempts at rehabilitation. He had been a successful businessman, more than adequate as husband and father, until visual impairment made it impossible for him to work. His internist and ophthalmologist had never honestly interpreted to the patient or his family the nature of the illness and possible permanent visual impairment. Rather, they handled the situation with pollyannaish optimism until the man was almost totally blind; whereupon both patient and family were rather abruptly told that it was unlikely his vision would improve. The man was then referred to a rehabilitation agency. This produced a severe state of shock and depression, with the patient angrily refusing rehabilitative help and refusing to see his doctors. Aided and abetted by his family he embarked on years of medical shopping over the U.S. for the magical cure for blindness, the patient rationalizing that he was not blind because of his variable (but completely useless) light perception. When he was finally convinced the quest was hopeless, he was taken to a rehabilitation agency where his hostile, depressed, and demoralized state made psychiatric consultation imperative. Prognosis for social and vocational rehabilitation was poor.

THE GENERIC APPROACH

In my outline of the multidisciplinary diagnostic-treatment-teaching-research team[3,7,8,9] approach, in my stress on the application and expansion of existing knowledge, and in my case examples, it should be clear that the psychological principles and their psychotherapeutic use to prevent and treat serious psychogenic disability applies to any handicap. This in no way denies that every handicap provides specific problems or that every handicapped person has his unique assets and limitations. But delineation of what is specific to a given handicap is hardly possible without knowing the generic predictables that can be anticipated in dealing with any person who has suffered a serious loss, and with his family. Thus we still hear about traits and personality disorders attributed to blindness that have no such specificity.

For example, in previous discussions of sudden blindness,[5,8] I indicated a characteristic sequence of severe psychological reactions: an acute depersonalization followed by a more prolonged depression. If my experience had been limited to blinded persons, I might have been convinced that the sequence was specific for sudden blindness. However, I had observed the depersonalization-depression sequence after traumatic leg amputation, and in two patients following bowel resection and colostomy for which they had not been prepared. Hence my conclusion that the sequence tends to be evoked by the *sudden loss of any major body part or function.* That the depression following such loss represents a state of mourning for the lost part is directly indicated by the frequent use among handicapped persons of the expressions, "my dead arm," "my dead ears," and "my dead eyes."

My emphasis here, and in most of my papers on the subject, on the need for generic professional training receives strong support from Scott.[18] His intensive study of agencies serving the blind reveals that many individuals in control of agencies have "highly specialized expertise" but lack generic professional training. Their limitations are hallmarked by rigidity and resistance to change, and they are incapable of functioning outside of their ingrained boundaries.

The teaching of generic knowledge applicable to handicapped persons in general should begin during the education of physicians, teachers, nurses, case workers, and other workers involved in rehabilitation. In postgraduate work and training, the learning under expert supervision of the specifics about particular handicaps can then proceed on a more solid base.

It is my conviction that this goal is a *sine qua non* for the recruiting and training of competent professionals for work with the multiple-handicapped. It is essential for optimal intercommunication and collaboration among workers in different fields of rehabilitation who now tend to be isolated and insulated in their respective fields.

NOTES

1. L. Bellak, ed., *Psychology of Physical Illness* (New York: Grune and Stratton, 1952).
2. E. P. Bernabeu, "The Effects of Severe Crippling on the Development of a Group of Children," *Psychiatry*, 21 (1958), 169–194.
3. H. Robert Blank, "The Integration of Psychiatric Services in a Casework Agency for the Blind," *New Outlook for the Blind*, 46 (1952), 229–231.
4. ———, "Psychoanalytic Considerations for Professional Workers in the Prevention of Blindness," *The Sight Saving Review*, Vol. 25, No. 2 (1955); also published in *Social Casework*, Vol. 36, No. 7 (July, 1955).
5. ———, "Psychoanalysis and Blindness," *The Psychoanalytic Quarterly*, 26 (1957), 1024.
6. ———, "Psychiatric Problems Associated with Congenital Blindness Due to Retrolental Fibroplasia," *New Outlook for the Blind*, 53 (1959), 237–244. This paper presents an instructive case in some detail, discusses multiple etiology and the problem of reversibility of functional damage, and deals with some of the intrinsic reasons for the paucity of professional workers with the MHB.
7. ———, "The Multidisciplinary Treatment and Research Team," *New Outlook for the Blind*, 54 (1960), 115–118.
8. ———, "The Challenge of Rehabilitation," *Israel Medical Journal*, 20 (1961), 127–142.

9. Thomas J. Carroll, *Blindness: What It Is, What It Does, and How to Live With It* (Boston: Little, Brown, 1961), 382.
10. P. Chodaff, S. B. Friedman, and D. A. Hamburg, "Stress Defence and Coping Behavior," *American Journal of Psychology*, 120 (1964), 743–749.
11. Sigmund Freud, "Mourning and Melancholia," in the Standard Edition of *The Complete Psychological Works of Freud,* ed. J. Strachey (London: Hogarth, 1957).
12. S. B. Friedman, P. Chodaff, J. U. Mason, and D. A. Hamburg, "Behavioral Observation in Parents Anticipating the Death of a Child," *Pediatrics,* 32 (1963), 610–625.
13. J. F. Garrett and Edna S. Levine, eds., *Psychological Practices with the Physically Disabled* (New York: Columbia University Press, 1962).
14. T. F. Graham, "Mind Over Malignancy," *The Physician's Panorama* (January, 1966), 13–16.
15. M. R. Karon, "Truth Sustains Leukemic Children," *Medical World News* (September 3, 1965).
16. L. C. Kolb, "Disturbances of the Body Image," *American Handbook of Psychiatry,* ed. S. Arieti (New York: Basic Books, 1959).
17. E. Lindemann, "Symptomatology and Management of Acute Grief," *American Journal of Psychology,* 101 (1944), 141–148.
18. Robert A. Scott, "The Selection of Clients by Social Welfare Agencies: The Case of the Blind," *Social Problems,* 14 (1967), 248–257.
19. V. Tisza, "Management of the Parents of the Chronically Ill Child," *American Journal of Orthopsychology,* 32 (1962), 53.

EMPHASIS: THE DEAF-BLIND

Edward J. Waterhouse

In popular usage, the deaf-blind are persons who are wholly without sight or hearing. Such individuals, however, represent a very small minority of the group with whom we have to be concerned.

In her paper Dr. Gall includes "definition" among the obstacles standing "in the way of further utilization of research results." The very paucity of services for those loosely called "deaf-blind" does simplify the matter of definition for this group. However, even in this small field in which organized research is scarcely a decade old, there have already been two distinct and probably incompatible approaches towards defining what deaf-blindness should mean to persons and agencies providing services to its victims. The two approaches are perhaps explained by the different outlook of those whose experience is with adults and those who are concerned with children.

Chronologically, the definition for deaf-blind children came first. On January 26, 1954, the National Study Committee on Education of Deaf-Blind Children (which included representatives of all known groups in the United States with programs for deaf-blind children) meeting at the Iowa School for the Deaf in Council Bluffs, Iowa, placed on record its recognition that "there is a wide range of disabilities involved in this double handicap," and proceeded to define a deaf-blind child as "one whose combination of handicaps prevents him from profiting satisfactorily from educational programs provided for the blind child or the deaf child."

This functional definition has served, and is serving, to reduce the number of children in danger of rejection from programs for the deaf or blind. It is receiving wide support both in the United States and Canada and in a growing number of overseas countries. It recognizes that a combination of visual and auditory handicaps, either of which might be quite slight and which singly would not be serious, can in combination have grave effects.

A second approach is recorded in Volume I of the series of admirable manuals on the Rehabilitation of Deaf-Blind persons published in 1958 by the Industrial Home for the Blind at Brooklyn, New York. In his introduction to Volume I, Alexander F. Handel, Research Sociology Consultant for the study project, confines himself to definitions of deafness and blindness. He writes, "For purposes of this study, the term deaf has been defined to mean: Inability to understand connected discourse through the ear." The definition of blindness is the generally accepted "legal" definition: "Central visual acuity of 20/200 or less in the better eye, with correcting glasses; or central visual acuity of more than 20/200 if there is a field defect in which the peripheral field has been contracted to such an extent that the widest diameter of visual fields subtends an angular distance no greater than 20 degrees."

It should be noted that this statement actually avoids defining deaf-blindness. The implication, however, that persons whose handicaps fall within both the above categories are the people to be considered as deaf-blind is clear. However, even in the study project a great deal of latitude has been permitted and it does seem safe to say that, in practice, criteria adopted for deaf-blind adults are far more akin to those in use for deaf-blind children than is suggested by considering the degree of each handicap separately and limiting the clients to those whose handicaps are as severe as the above statement suggests.

No less an authority than Dr. Peter J. Salmon, the Executive Director of the Industrial Home for the Blind, in his foreword to the first volume of this study states, "There have been so many discussions as to what deafness and blindness is and so many approaches to the problems arising out of the combination of these two handicaps, that it might be well to say here, even though it may seem frightening, that I have learned that deaf-blindness is not just two disabilities—deafness added to blindness; but is instead a third and totally separate disability."

Within the field of deaf-blindness, there have been attempts to set up subdivisions with their own definitions. In *New Frontiers for Research on Deaf-Blindness,* published also by the Industrial Home for the Blind in 1966, attention is given to differentiating between the deaf-blind and the blind-deaf: "Members of the seminar perceived important differences between clients whose deafness preceded their blindness (the deaf-blind) and clients whose blindness preceded their deafness (the blind-deaf)."

While Dr. Gall has exercised admirable restraint in presenting her ideas and suggestions almost exclusively in terms of the MHB (and I will follow her lead in using this abbreviation for the multiple-handicapped blind), she is clearly aware of the fact that handicapped persons are indeed persons. The student of a special group must acquaint himself with what is new in research findings concerning human beings as a whole. Research into the development of deaf-blind children must use what is known about child development—a vast field indeed. When Dr. Gall asks, "What is the world like to the MHB?", she raises the question, "What is the world like to the average child?" How much do we know of that?

Success as a worker with the deaf-blind depends largely on the understanding a worker possesses of problems common to all persons. Specialized knowledge of the handicapped can be only an extension of his knowledge of such wide subjects as physiology, psychology, and sociology. Educational and rehabilitation principles and techniques which are effective with the handicapped are almost without exception adaptations of those used in more general programs. The vast amount of knowledge that should be gained and made available to the appropriate workers, as indicated by Dr. Gall, cannot be a substitute for a more general education, but is a necessary addition to it.

As I look over the topics Dr. Gall included in her paper and think of them in terms of the variables that have diversified the thirty or more children found in any one year in the Department for Deaf-Blind Children at the Perkins School for the Blind, I find myself hoping for the aid of a computer to analyze and correlate even such few facts as are already now available. For in this group, the range of degree of deafness exceeds what would usually be found in a school for the deaf; and the range of blindness exceeds that normally encountered in a school for the blind. The age of onset of each handicap affects the impact of the other. Since also the impact of a deaf-blind child on a family is likely to be far greater than that of a child with a single handicap, family problems can be expected to be both intensified and of greater variety. In no group is it truer that every single child has unique problems and unique needs.

To my knowledge, the only formal program in the world that seeks to train teachers for the deaf-blind at present is at Boston College and Perkins School for the Blind. Planning funds, however, have been granted to George Peabody College for Teachers in Nashville, Tennessee, and to San Francisco State College for Teacher-Training Programs which, hopefully, will get under way in a few months. Some in-service training is given teachers in a few schools that enroll deaf-blind children both in the United States and in Europe. In-service training for rehabilitation workers and volunteers is given at the Industrial

Home for the Blind in Brooklyn, New York. The time for expanding these services seems to be ripe. Far more interest in deaf-blind children is being evidenced at home and abroad than ever before.

In my opinion, one of the most important passages in Dr. Gall's paper is the reference to the work of Elonen, Polzien, and Zwarensteyn. This report indicates that, given a suitable program, children with severe multiple handicaps can make significant progress. This points up the need for determining what program is most suitable for a handicapped child, including, of course, a deaf-blind child. It is perhaps going to be more difficult, as it is certainly just as important, for these needs to be identified for the deaf-blind as for any other group.

One of the special features of the group of children who are deaf-blind is in the smallness of its numbers. This is, indeed, fortunate when looked at from the point of view of those who are not deaf-blind; but it creates serious problems for those who are unfortunate enough to be included in the small group. Were there as many deaf-blind children as mentally retarded children for example, society would have taken steps long before now to devote more attention to them. Dr. Gall points out that "One of the barriers to research and demonstration is the scant availability of adequate sampling." At Perkins, where we have made considerable efforts to evaluate as many deaf-blind children as possible, we are faced with problems arising from the smallness of the group. There have never been, at one time, as many as forty deaf-blind children in the school. The next largest group in the world is in Alabama and the numbers there, I believe, have never reached thirty. In England, where all deaf-blind children are brought together at Condover Hall School for Blind Children with Additional Handicaps, the number is less than twenty.

The Register of Deaf-Blind Children kept by the American Foundation for the Blind has listed as many as 400 names. Many of these are believed to be ineducable. It has been difficult to arrange for evaluation in many cases because of the small number of persons who are trained to carry out this function adequately.

As a result of the rubella epidemic of several years ago, the number of deaf-blind children in the United States has increased. Nobody knows how many defective children resulted from maternal rubella at this time, though estimates have gone as high as 30,000. Of these, again, no one knows how many have a combination of deafness and blindness. However, agencies like Perkins which are known to be concerned with the deaf-blind, are finding that inquiries and appeals for help are coming in the mail in increasing quantities.

Two research workers on the Perkins Staff, Miss Nan Robbins and Mrs. Gertrude Stenquist, have made a somewhat intensive study of the rubella deaf-blind children who have come under their notice in recent years. Their report will be available shortly.

As a result of the smallness in the numbers of deaf-blind children and adults, it is inevitable also that the numbers of those who are working with them should be small. The Industrial Home for the Blind has had a program which has offered services to the deaf-blind for nearly fifty years and has been carrying out a project since 1962 with the support of the Vocational Rehabilitation Administration. During this time great efforts have been made to arouse interest in this group. Nevertheless, when a seminar on "New Frontiers for Research on Deaf-Blindness" was held in Brooklyn in April 1966 during the celebration of the Centennial of the birth of Anne Sullivan, the number of those attending who could be said to have had experience with this group was extremely small. A similar seminar on the education of the deaf-blind child, held at Perkins during the same celebration week, also brought a disappointing response from educators and administrators. Perhaps, again, the increase in the number of deaf-blind children as a result of the rubella epidemics may bring about a marked change in this situation.

I would like to refer to the paragraph in which Dr. Gall observes, "Multimedia is important in training the MHB. Could a better approach to learning for the MHB be made through several sensory approaches rather than one?" This seems to me to be particularly applicable to the deaf-blind. As Dr. Gall indicates elsewhere, a blind child with an additional handicap is also likely to have a third. Certainly this is true of the majority of deaf-blind children who have come to our attention. As already indicated, there are many children coming under the definition which I have adopted for this paper who have considerable vision. Also many of them have residual hearing. The adaptation of audio-visual techniques to these children is indeed an approach which might produce significant results. The emphasis placed on the use of vibration for the deaf-blind, not only in reading speech and in the development of speech by the child, but in the development of rhythm, might hold some promise for handicapped children of other categories.

I am also pleased to find that Dr. Gall does give particular attention to studies on the motor characteristics of the multiple-handicapped blind. Among the deaf-blind children that have come to our attention are many who have motor inadequacies, and it would be helpful to know whether, as she suggests, there is any correlation between motor dexterity and "speed of learning or predictable response to auditory stimulation."

Dr. Gall has not forgotten the parent. She asks the question, "How does a teacher explain the child to the parent?" This, to me, is one of the most important questions we can ask. How can we train our teachers to interpret what they know about the children in a way which is intelligible not only to parents but to fellow workers and perhaps to the children themselves. A complement of this, of course, would be to know how can parents be trained to report accurately on their children to educators. Surely among the most inaccurate records on file anywhere are parents' reports on handicapped children in connection with their admission to schools.

Dr. Gall finishes her paper with a challenge to teachers to participate more fully in research and in the dissemination of their observations of children to others. She points out, in particular, the necessity for "research leading to the improvement of the self-concept and the extent and quality of self-identification through rich experiences of warm integration and usefulness." Indeed, I would like to see her ten recommendations at the end of the paper made available to all teachers and workers with the multiple-handicapped. It summarizes the general fields of concern which we should have, not only for the MHB child, but for the services we offer them and the organizations under which these services function, and it concludes with the all important recommendation that we "study how to strengthen interagency cooperation by coordination of activities and by the analysis of the function of each."

SUGGESTED RESEARCH IN THE FIELD OF SERVICES FOR THE ORTHOPEDICALLY HANDICAPPED BLIND

Lee H. Lacey

My specific assignment is to address myself to the identification of "future research areas in problems associated with blindness and to develop them to the point of proposing relevant hypotheses and methodologies" for the orthopedic blind individual, but I may stray into the area of other multiple-handicapped blind categories with my references and suggestions.

These are the primary goals selected for discussion in this paper:

1. The collection at one location of sufficient case record material for concentrated analysis, to determine the variety of needs of such a group of individuals as are included in the category of MHB (multiple-handicapped blind).

2. The assembly of representative, successful, experienced specialists in the various phases of diagnostic, treatment, educational, and rehabilitation services for the blind and multiple-handicapped individuals; and to have them compile a guideline document for the successful delivery of services to the MHB individual and his immediate family.

3. The initiation of specialized services located geographically around the country in centers of concentrated population.

4. The utilization of selected specialized agencies, which now primarily serve the physically disabled, the psychiatrically disabled, or the blind, to serve MHB, adding capability in their missing areas of services; or the close integration and coordination of two special-

ized agencies staffed substantially to provide the services needed by the MHB clients.

Separate considerations should be given to research in the areas where multiple handicapping conditions occur at birth or in early childhood and where similar multiple handicapping conditions occur in adolescence or later in the person's life.

COLLECTION OF DATA

My study of the problems presented has led me to identify sparsity as a major problem. I mean the sparsity of orthopedic or multiple-handicapped blind with whom to work to learn their needs. There is a sparsity of professional specialists who have knowledge or experience in working with such a group. And for the blind with other significant handicaps, there is a sparsity of institutions that are willing and able to serve such individuals. It is fortunate for individuals and families that there are not many blind persons with orthopedic disability. However, this very situation complicates and compounds the problem of learning what their needs are and how to serve them effectively so as to minimize their disability.

While there is limited information about the needs of, and services for, the orthopedically disabled blind, there is some; and it would seem to be productive to study as much of this information as possible. The sources of the information are probably concentrated in selected public and private agencies serving children and adult blind. In conducting such a study, it would be essential to consider all agencies and programs where the individuals selected for study were served.

To implement such study, a research task force composed of experienced specialists in fields related to serving blind clients or clients with multiple disabilities should be established. One phase would be to collect case records and analyze the services and results of services to MHB. These materials should concentrate on cases served since World War II and should include services provided to such clients as children, and to clients becoming blind by all causes as adults. The analysis should focus on identifying the required constellation of services; their timing and coordination that resulted in successful maximum independence; and personal, social and vocational adjustment of the individuals studied.

Another phase might have the same task force identify educational and rehabilitation agencies currently serving MHB of all ages, and identify their current philosophy, methods, and results. This operation should employ the same methodology as used in the previous phase where similar services, conditions, and objectives are concerned. This is essential in order to carry out the next step.

The third phase would entail compiling the record of all the findings classified as to apparent successful or unproductive theories and procedures and developing a set of guidelines that appear to yield most successful results in terms of the patient's independence and personal, social, and vocational adjustment.

The fourth and final phase should entail a reasonable period of implementation of the guidelines in educational and rehabilitation agencies, covering all ages, to confirm the productive approaches, to develop modifications, and to eliminate approaches found to be unproductive.

The findings that result should then be utilized in the most significant way by private and public educational and rehabilitation agencies serving MHB persons. Those agencies responsible for raising or setting standards of services to be provided to MHB would be concerned with their continued implementation and improvement.

VALUE OF PROFESSIONAL WORKSHOPS

At the present time, it would appear that if significant knowledge of the techniques and procedures for effectively serving the MHB exists, it must be in the minds of practitioners. Because of the sparsity of known MHB and their geographic dispersion, it is difficult to identify their needs or to know how to serve them most effectively. The professional person working with this problem has access to the knowledge of but a few consultants, and the limited published material is likely to be too specialized, even if the professional locates it.

One familiar way to collect such information is through an institute or workshop. Select experienced professional specialists. Include a structured pre-conference activity for the participants in preparation for the program. Encourage the workshop participants to document basic techniques and procedures used for delivering needed services to MHB. Organize the collected material into a resource manual that could be useful to all personnel engaged in serving the MHB. With the many methods of recording and reproducing materials currently available, the experience of many specialists might be captured in one week.

During such a workshop advantage should be taken of the availability of the specialists to secure information regarding laws and regulations of federal and state agencies affecting services to the MHB. While it is not likely that this group could give "chapter and verse" from either the law or regulations, they could very well point out the difficulties that have been barriers to providing adequate and timely service. A compilation of these difficulties could be followed up by a special study in this particular area.

So far, the focus of my remarks has been on capturing as much present information as possible. This is to be done by a study and an analysis of current recorded information, plus an institute or workshop to document the successful techniques and procedures currently used by the most knowledgeable, experienced practitioners.

GEOGRAPHICALLY CONCENTRATED PROGRAMS

All age groups should be served in specialized programs with special emphasis on ages up to 25 years. It is understood that to accomplish this would necessitate multiple direct-service agency participation. In addition, a diversity of primary emphases would be required among the group of participating agencies—general and special hospitals, and public and private educational and rehabilitation agencies serving children and adults. Case finding and referral agency resources should be an integral part of such a coordinated service. Special attention should be devoted to providing for progressive movement between agencies to maintain, as nearly as possible, an unbroken continuum of services to the individuals and their families, as long as services are needed.

Significant data should be collected in the areas of client progress and adjustment, so that it might be possible to coordinate the initial findings to give better direction to succeeding periods of study, both with the same participants, and with ones who would be added each year. With a large enough sample in all age categories, and with a standardized format for collection of data, pertinent findings should begin to appear by the third year. These findings would be most useful in the work of the previously discussed task force effort.

In developing areas of service to be provided in each of these geographically concentrated programs, it is suggested that they fall generally into the following areas: medical evaluation and treatment; psychological and psychiatric study of the child and family, with diagnostic emphasis on family members and diagnosis and treatment as indicated for the child; and a complete social study of the child and his family, including both maternal and paternal grandparents. Such a study should include the accumulation of all available definitive medical data, which might prove useful in subsequent phases of the study. The final general areas to be explored would be educational and vocational.

The basic approach to the child would have to be adjusted according to chronological age and functional level of the child at a given time. The younger the child, the more emphasis on diagnosis and prevention in the medical area would seem appropriate. This emphasis should decline with the increase in the age of the child, but the trend could be reversed if the individual was involved or subsequently became involved with a progressive or new medical problem. More extensive work with parents and family members would be indicated in the earlier ages, with appropriate continuation throughout the child's developmental period. Vocational emphasis would not seem appropriate until a chronological age of twelve years or later, depending on the physical, functional, and intellectual potential of the child.

A secondary, but important, advantage of centralizing services to the MHB in larger metropolitan areas is that the breadwinner of the family should be able to maintain steady employment and opportunities for advancement without having to locate himself away from the needed service. The services for the child and the family could be maintained on a more continuous basis, at least through the crucial developmental periods of the child. The agency serving the child and the family will be well advised to establish a good relationship with the public and private employment services in order to meet this need smoothly when it occurs. This assumes that the child-family relationship is a positive contributing one that should be closely maintained at least to the teenage years.

In planning for, and providing services to the MHB, recognition of the logical priority of services to be rendered to the disabled individual must be carefully scheduled. This will be complicated by the feelings of the staff members, as well as by the specific problems presented by the MHB person. If it is difficult for the professional staff to know in what order, and with which services to serve such an individual, imagine how much more difficult it is for the person and the family involved. If treatment is attempted to resolve too many problems at the same time, the patient is likely to be too frustrated to progress. In most instances, the resolution of the medical problems of diagnosis, treatment and prevention, followed by special services or training related to blindness should be the general pattern to follow. One other word of caution: be sure the program meets the needs of the MHB individual and not the needs of the family or the staff.

Up to this point in my discussion, reference has been directed primarily to the congenitally multiple-handicapped blind, or to children who become so disabled at an early age. It has been my observation that, when the multiple disability occurs after the individual has passed into adulthood, there is a different set of circumstances to resolve for the individual and for the professional team working with him. A major difference is the self-image the client has prior to disability and following disability. There is also the difference in the image the client's immediate family has of him, both before and after the disability, and the image that the client and the family have of a person disabled in a manner similar to that now characterizing the client. If the family's image of a blind person is based on their contact with an individual who had been a self-sufficient business or professional person, their image of the client as a blind person will be positive. However, if their contact has been limited to an individual who has been homebound, or who has been seen soliciting funds on the streets of their home community, their image of the client will be negative.

SPECIALIZED AGENCIES

The incidence of blindness in adults occurs in conjunction with many different pathologic conditions which frequently bring about co-existing losses in neuromuscular function or necessitate amputation of extremities. Another source of blindness and multiple disability is, of course, accidents.[1]

In two different studies[2,3] of groups of blind individuals—one a selective sample and one a random sample—approximately 30 per cent of the individuals lost or began loss of sight after 19 years of age. The incidence by age further indicates that the period between 20 years and 44 years of age accounts for approximately 25 per cent of all blindness occurring after the age of 19 years. These are the years when higher education, marriage, birth of children, and vocational achievement normally occur. This is the period of maximum achievement of social and economic independence. Add to this the number of other people affected—family members, for example—and their loss could be even greater than that for the larger group of MHB who have lost their vision before reaching 19 years of age.

In meeting the needs of adults who become disabled the first step appears to be the earliest possible contact with the patient and family to give them assurance that something can be done to maintain their self-image at an acceptable level. The next important thing is to assist the MHB to regain as near normal function as the condition will permit. For the blind person, this may mean moving about in his home, in his community, and on the job, in an acceptable manner. For the person with medical and physical disabilities, it means the regaining of any loss of function or control so he can present himself to his family and community in as near normal a manner as possible.

Under the present circumstances, the problem of locating the adult MHB individual need not be so difficult. The availability of rehabilitation services, pensions from public sources (including social security disability coverage for the wage earner and his family) and extra income tax credit, give the client and family incentive to make their plight known to one or several agencies in their community. However, finding these individuals on a timely basis may be another matter.

Aside from the prevention of disability, including blindness, the greatest need with the adult group is for the skilled professional specialists to give assistance to the client and his family in making the necessary emotional, intellectual, and physical adjustments resulting from disability. The significant loss of sight is designated by the most recent Veterans Rehabilitation Administration amendments as constituting a "catastrophic disability." There is little question that most sighted adults would consider the loss of sight the greatest possible loss that could be experienced. For this reason and others, including the client's feelings of the change in self-image and his changed status within the family and community, the period of adjustment extends over too long a period of time. Add to this the loss of part or all of an extremity, or the loss of the normal use of body parts, and even greater negative reaction to loss will be observed.

Research in the methods most successful, efficient, and of shortest duration to effect adjustment and remobilization of the MHB individuals should be pursued. An additional area would be to study the dynamics, both of the staff implementing the procedures and of the disabled individual, to identify those personality dynamics that appear to be most conducive for effective assistance in the adjustment period.

In her paper, Dr. Gall accurately identifies existing problems of referral and service when an individual with an orthopedic disability is also blind. Such an individual may not be accepted for service by either the nonblind orthopedic oriented agency or the agency for the blind. This is a game those of us in agencies many times get caught up in because of our concern to identify, for the record, what the primary diagnosis or disability is. We seldom stop to think that it makes little difference in a given situation, that an individual with diabetes becomes blind as a result of that condition and also may require an amputation. In such an instance, what is the primary diagnosis?

It should be stated that vocational rehabilitation services at the federal and state level do not ordinarily make this problem difficult. The criteria for both the general rehabilitation services and the program for the blind, if they are separate, usually overlap sufficiently for either agency to provide orthopedic or other special medical services. I think this problem becomes more noticeable as the agency, at the patient service level, becomes more specialized. The orthopedic agency and specialist become overly concerned when their patient is blind. I suspect that the specializing agency and professional in the field of work for the blind become overly concerned with the presence of an amputation, particularly during the period of fitting and training of the blind client in the use of a prosthesis.

Another way of stating this problem is that the greater the specialization of an agency or its staff, the more difficult it is going to be for the MHB individual or his family to be served adequately. A major factor in this is that specializing needs of the professional, or the agency, are not readily met by such a multiple demand. Therefore, it would be essential to study the characteristics of the more successful agencies and staff members who have achieved good results in serving such clients.

In our era of specialization of services, professional personnel, and agency programming, the MHB is a "misfit" who will frequently be overtreated in one phase of his multiple needs with little coordination of his total needs or who will be rejected by the various agencies and fields of specializations. The real solution may lie in the establishment of services and facilities for the MHB on a national or regional basis. The model would be that of a Mayo Clinic, a Warm Springs or a Menninger Clinic, providing comprehensive diagnosis and/or treatment to the MHB and to the immediate members of the household. There should be emphasis that such facilities must be appropriate for the MHB and that skilled services to the non-MHB members of the household, including the children, be provided.

NOTES

1. Mary K. Bauman, *Adjustment to Blindness, A Study as Reported by the Committee to Study Adjustment to Blindness* (Harrisburg: State Council for

the Blind, Department of Welfare, Commonwealth of Pennsylvania, 1954), 157, Table 21.
2. Ibid., 162, Table 28.
3. ———, *Characteristics of Blind and Visually Handicapped People in Professional, Sales and Managerial Work* (Harrisburg: Pennsylvania Office for the Blind, 1963), 105, Table 6.

HUMAN VALUES AND THE RESEARCH FRONTIER

VALUES, MODELS AND, RESEARCH,

Maxwell H. Goldberg

Through much of the planning for this Consultation, a session was allocated to explore what we of the conventionally designated "Humanities"—the literary, historical, and philosophical humanities—might contribute to this worthy effort. In this intended session we were to consider how the Humanities might be brought more effectively to bear on continual enrichment toward fullness of living on the part of the blind. But more urgent matters kept coming to the fore and so this concern was moved to the periphery.

Yet the hope continues to be strong that, before long, some occasion will be provided—perhaps through our Center here—at which we practitioners of the Humanities will have the opportunity to do our share. So I would like now to enter a word on behalf of just such an inquiry, whether we call it a "consultation," or a "seminar," or a "colloquium."

This inquiry would not be dedicated exclusively to the practitioners of the Humanities in dialogue with professional workers with the blind. To do that would be specialistic and, as such, would violate both the spirit that has shaped our present Consultation and the spirit of the Humanities viewed as liberal studies. For the spirit of the Humanities, which Mary Bauman has so sensitively, eloquently, and realistically voiced, is a holistic spirit. The goal of the Humanities is to see the individual whole and to enable him to live his life with a sense of wholeness.

This Humanities-focused inquiry, then, would provide an opportunity where, in concert with their academic colleagues from other disciplines and with leaders whose work deals with problems related to blindness, the practitioners of the Humanities could explore ways for their discipline to contribute toward that fullness of life which should be our shared ideal.

IMPLICATIONS OF TECHNOLOGICAL CHANGE

First, I want to correct any misconceptions my response to Dean Mallinson's query at the opening session may have encouraged. Dean Mallinson wanted to know why we had no provision for a consideration of the relationships between (1) developments in technological "hardware" and research in the "hard sciences" and (2) research into problems associated with blindness. I bluntly replied that representatives of those "interfaces" had been ruled out as a matter of deliberate policy by the Planning Committee—on the grounds, as Dr. MacFarland added, that already there had been a number of conferences dealing with the hard sciences and the hardware.

Actually, I was very much in sympathy with the apparent intention of Dean Mallinson's query—namely, to stress the importance of an inter-relational, transactional kind of probing and inquiry which would force us in the Humanities and the "soft sciences" to draw out the *human* implications, for research in problems associated with blindness, of the relevant technological and hard science developments. An index to this awareness of the urgency of this concern may be found in the often-cited statement that the sheer rate of *speed-up* of technological change is to be regarded as exponential, producing not just quantitative but qualitative modifications, like biological mutations or quantum jumps in nuclear physics. This index is to be found also in corresponding statements about the rate of speed-up in industrial and social change.

This emphasis is due to a strong impression gained both from nearly four years of effort, with other groups, to face up to the implications of such intensive technological change, and from observations here. This impression is that many of us still have not begun to confront the present and impending implications of these still dramatically accelerating technological changes and their concomitants or sequels in other areas of change, especially industrial, social, and educational. For example, there has been little to assure us that —not in a visionary way, but realistically—we have begun to recognize the implications of the developments in bionics, in social, biological, and psychological engineering.

Again, we have hardly begun to draw out the research implications, for problems associated with blindness, of Russell Williams' reference to the modern technology of learning and the applications of latest technological developments to the teaching-learning process. The same holds for our immediate responses to the references of William Usdane, Albert Thompson, and others to the implications, for research in problems related to blindness, of the revolutions in data processing and information collection, storage, retrieval, and dissemination—both as effected by the computer and by the laser, already threatening, in some areas, to push the precocious computer to one side.

In view of such impressions, one might say that all we have done here, in probing the implications that the electronic revolutions have for new directions for research as to problems associated with blindness, is to run the gamut from A to B. In saying this, more is in view than the exploitation of the products of this revolution in research processes themselves, and in strengthening the practical, day-to-day functioning of the blind. There are also probes which, in terms of human values and human dignity—personal dignity, would explore the implications of the electronic and other advanced technological revolutions for individuals who happen to be blind.

So far as this sort of normative or axiological probing is concerned, Arnold Barach gave us our point of departure when he declared that as a result of the new electronic technologies, values would inevitably have to be changed. Thus, C. Tibbetts suggests as a major area for study, "the examination of the impact of the evolving economies and the transition from handwork to automation and cybernation in the place of the elderly in society today"; and, according to Elias Cohen, he suggests that "these factors may be even more important than the demographic factors of birth rates, migrations, distributions, and comparisons of population components."

At this Consultation we do not seem to have squarely faced the normative or values issue. The same thing has happened with other groups when presented with this challenge.

One instance during a group session involved an engineering graduate, now president of a small but prosperous company manufacturing industrial machinery. This industrialist resorted to nearly every dodge he could think of to avoid direct, realistic confrontation of the implications, for himself and his firm, of the cybernetic revolution as applied to industry. When it was pointed out that his competitors among the great companies were already far advanced in the installation of numeric-control systems, he said: "We'll put an end to that by law." When it was pointed out that such laws could neither control the advance nor combat the systems of numeric-control already set up in competitive industries abroad, he said: "Okay, then, the big sharks will smell the blood and will gobble us little guys up." He was reminded that this was evasion rather than real confrontation of the issue at hand.

We have not followed such a pattern of regressive evasion. But we, too, have yet to address ourselves realistically to the host of new or radically altered questions posed by advanced technological change, with its breathtaking rate of acceleration, and with its pervasive impact upon the individual and society.

This prompts a disturbing thought: it may be later than we think.[1] Three years ago, we were speaking to middle management groups about what advanced automation and numeric-control were already doing, or what they were going to do, by way of job dislocations and displacements in business and industry. The attitude of these middle management people was one of self-satisfaction and sympathy for those experiencing such dislocation or displacement. Then, suddenly, middle management itself felt the changes brought about by advanced cybernation. The reactions were often surprise, consternation, fear for the outcome, often of anger at not having been warned (so they claimed!).

Nor has this sort of resistance to making the personal application been limited to middle management. The same sort of thing may be seen among other lay and professional leadership groups. There may be seen, also, the same failure to make intelligent and informed provisions for creative accommodation to the ultra-rapid changes.

Hopefully, we here will constitute an exception to the customary modes of response to the impact of technological change; and hopefully we will exemplify the suggested constructive reactions. Those concerned with problems associated with blindness ought to take a cue from what is going on in the automotive industry. Current operations and plans for the immediate future assume the continuation of gasoline-powered cars as the "staple." Yet there are researchers assigned to the task of considering, on a middle-range or long-range basis, various alternatives, among them the electric-powered car. Such explorations are in the province of Research and Development (R&D); and the suggestion is sound that has been made here to the effect that there ought to be a similar R&D group addressing itself solely to opening up and exploring nonroutine possibilities—however "far out" some of them at the moment may appear—with regard to the applications and implications of vaulting technological change to research in problems associated with blindness.[2]

Side by side with this R&D group, we need a group to look after another concern—this one likewise aggravated by the phenomenal speed-up in the rate of technological change and pressures for industrial, social, educational and, notably, psycho-ethical change—particularly through counseling and education.

We often anxiously express our sense of this terrific pressure for drastic psycho-ethical change by referring to "value concepts," "value structures," "value systems," and to "human values"—frequently specified as "social values," "cultural values," "values for living," and "moral or ethical values." The pressures for change in them seem to threaten their vigor, their strength, and their viability. Hence they seem to threaten us who have cherished these values as providing our central sanctioning, evaluative, and motive power toward the goal of the good man, the good life, the good society. Our anxiety often seems to go deeper when we are told that, in view of the drastic changes in our total environment and our circumstances, we must be prepared to scrap our traditionally cherished or respected values in favor of new "values"—claimed to be, if not better, at least as good as those which have nourished and sustained us.[3]

In this respect, too, there seems to have been a strong tendency at this Consultation to evade direct confrontation with the whole matter of values. It has been wryly amusing and not a little worrying to see how, often, we flirted with the topic of "values," only to flit away from it before we could get closely involved. We used that tried-and-true semantic dodge: "Let's not get bogged down in definitions." It is a dodge, because frequently, when we say this, the difficulty we are trying to avoid is not one of definition *per se*. Rather, the verbal difficulty is often merely the more or less superficial symptom of far more deeply originating difficulties—emotional, psychic, social, and ethical. They are difficulties at the core of our very idea of what constitutes the good life—what are the relationships between the creature-comfort values and the beauty-nourishing values; or between the creature-comfort values and the character-forming and character-enhancing values—the values that enhance the individual's sense of human dignity and personal worth—of integrity and wholeness—the values that may call for inconvenience, discomfort, pain, suffering, self-denial, self-sacrifice.

Hence it is that, as Elias Cohen has pointed out, "in a society which apparently places a high value on work, some investigators have given high priority to inquiry on the issue of the value system," especially in connection with the problems of the aging and the aged, whose "role and adjustment to society is so much a function of culture values and the status accorded the aged by society at large."

WORK ETHIC: LEISURE ETHIC

By way of illustration let us consider the tensional twist that is getting more painful for more and more people in our "advanced" societies. As many here have indicated, there are two major intersecting components that produce this torque. First, there is the thrust of the new and, to a great extent, technologically induced leisure-oriented ethic and style of life, which is fast building up its momentum, especially because of the surge of advanced automation and numeric control and of advanced electronic innovation and information handling. Second, there is the massive inertia of the traditional work-ethic and its life styles for centuries sanctioned by religion; for generations, in more recent times, secularly sanctioned by our modern business-industry civilization.

Here, on the one hand, we have an ethic which—to refer to Aaron Levenstein's *Why People Work*—as far back as Hebraic times has sanctified work as a mode of worshipping God; an ethic which—as Thomas Carlyle was so fond of stressing—has had behind it the Christian *laborare est orare* ("to work is to pray"); an ethic which has had behind it the Calvinistic-Puritan exaltation of work as meeting a prime requirement imposed by God on man ("by the sweat of thy brow!"); and an ethic which—as Ben Seligman has so vividly brought out—has behind it the sanctioning force both of the business-industrial cult of success through competition in the "free market," and the political cult of success through competition in the open arena.

Here, on the other hand, we have an ethic which, to be sure, goes back to the Aristotelian, aristocratic ethic of leisure; yet which, in modern terms, has been adapted to stress the right of the individual, of whatever class or station in life, to those modes of self-realization or self-fulfillment largely or exclusively outside the domain of the market economy and the power structure. This ethic turns away from stress on success as measured in terms of dollars gained through the production and distribution of goods and the rendering of services; or success as measured in terms of power to manipulate or control material resources, people, agencies and organizations.

It is an ethic that asserts the right of the individual to that sort of self-esteem and the esteem shown him by others which is gained through the constructive use to which he puts his open hours and days in terms of creative self-development. These open hours and days are outside the orbit of the labor market and the market economy.

They are evaluated in terms of states or qualities of experiencing, in terms of actions and accomplishments—including services to others —which may have little or no income value in the market. Ideally, this ethic yields what Goethe called "the significant individual," living the significant life.

However misguided, however sentimental and romantic, however irritating or annoying they may at times become, the genuine "hippies" and the "flower children" are a pathetic yet eloquent witness to the primal psychic needs and aspirations of which the leisure ethic is a perenially recurring formulation.

Already it is being pointed out that whole categories of our population must be encouraged to find their self-identification, their sense of personal dignity—through the second of these modes of personal satisfaction—the mode that takes us into the heartland of leisure— both voluntary and involuntary. Among these categories are: many of our recent school and college graduates who find it increasingly difficult to gain an opening into the market economy world of work; members of ethnic and other minority "out-groups" such as Negroes, Puerto Ricans, and Orientals; many of those who may still regard themselves as in the prime of middle age, yet who are being "plateaued" in favor of younger individuals or who are being coerced into early withdrawal from the market economy through early retirement; and last, but most significant for the particular concerns of this Consultation—the *handicapped*.

Hence, a crucial question asked by many: What if this new leisure-oriented ethic is reinforced by something like a guaranteed minimum annual income (or "negative income") as a matter of Constitutional right—on democratic, or altruistic humanitarian grounds, or on grounds of the enlightened self-interest of a market economy depending upon ever-increasing *consumption* of goods and services by the total population? What if it gains sufficient momentum to prove a necessary, or at least a truly viable, alternative to that sort of self-identification and self-realization conventionally sought through the struggle for success in the competitive world of the market economy (including the professional "helping" services for such an economy)? What would happen to our fundamental thinking and planning about the blind; our fundamental rationale for research in connection with problems associated with blindness?

Such a fundamental re-orientation might set up two master models of the self-realizing unsighted person—in place of the one model that now seems to exercise a monopoly on our thinking and our researching. The one model would continue to be that of the victor in the conventional competitive world of the market economy with its professional adjuncts, and of the socio-political arena. The other model would be quite different: that of the inwardly nurtured and developed yet socially related and contributing individual whose worth lies in what he is, whether "profitable" in and for the market economy or not; of the quality of his personality and character, of the refinement and strength of his esthetic and intellectual development; of his capacity to enjoy the cultural life, and to enjoy and be a source of enjoyment for others.

A good example is the blind-deaf poet recently interviewed on NBC's *Today* program. What impressed me most about him was the creative force he displayed in his poetry; and the astonishingly moving, rhythmical eloquence with which he gave oral readings of his poetry. In such an individual we have perhaps a model for an increasingly viable alternative to the conventional model, which overwhelmingly stresses success through competition in the market economy, and which, at this Consultation, has been the master model dominating our thinking, imagining, and projecting into the future.

What might be the implications of the acceptance of this alternative model as possible—as centrally relevant to our studies having to do with new practices and directions in research with regard to problems of blindness? It suggests the useful role we practitioners of the Humanities might play in educating both youth and adults for such a leisure-oriented life of self-realization and self-fulfillment. A main problem would be to win our colleagues in the Humanities over to research and educational efforts of this kind. For, right now, many of the practitioners of the Humanities are themselves largely dominated by the market economy and power-structure values. At the moment, there are far more immediately lucrative and professionally rewarding projects luring them.

Among other things, to achieve this re-orientation we would have to strengthen the whole educational endeavor we now more and more frequently designate "Continuing Liberal Education." This is education viewed as a lifelong, cumulative, developmental process.

Hence, some of those charged with responsibility for advancing the frontier of research in problems related to blindness should constitute themselves a kind of R & D group to feel out the implications of the increasing assertiveness of a leisure-oriented ethic—hence of a leisure-oriented life-style, hence of a leisure-oriented lifelong education in and for mature self-realization. This group should give its boldest and most imaginative thought to probing the possibilities of such a life-style as a viable alternative to the conventional work-ethic.

One of the most challenging among the questions for such an "axiological R & D group"—technically engaged in normative inquiry—would be that of how to adopt, as a major concern and enterprise, the extraordinarily difficult job of changing fundamental attitudes that have powerful momentum or massive inertia. As Mr. Robinson has put it: in our culture, a mature person is expected to pay his way; and he rightly asks: how deeply rooted in "universal nature" is this? How much is it an acquired factor of our culture, hence amenable to change?

A few illustrations taken from our present Consultation will serve to show just how difficult and radical (in the sense of "going to the roots") a task this is.

Our attention has been called, for example, to the disappearance from the scene with the advent of automation of a variety of jobs which the blind have been doing for the past two decades. But what are the inferences we have been asked to draw from this? Not that we ought to explore the possibilities and the desirability of other motivations, other goals, and other means for giving to the blind a sense of self-sufficiency, self-fulfillment, and self-respect—in addition to the goals of successful competition in the market economy. Rather, what we have been urged to address ourselves to is "the application of research and experimentation leading to new opportunities for the blind in our automated world of today." We have been urged to continue to think in terms of the business ethic, with its "fundamental axiom" of knowing "what your customer wants and will need and then to design your product to meet these wants and needs as they occur." We have been urged to continue to keep ourselves "attitudinally committed to the capabilities of the blind as a competitive unit of labor."

Now, in citing the preceding, the intent is not to imply that the path to self-satisfaction for the blind through competition in the market economy should be blocked. Yet some group among those concerned with research in problems associated with blindness should give major attention to the alternative routes—particularly that of the leisure-oriented ethic as sketched above, with its implications for life-style, self-concept, social status, and recognition.

In our Consultation papers we do have situations which, if their implications were opened up, might lead to inquiries of the type called for as viable alternative models of ethic and life-style. In one of the papers, we have, for example, the following: "If we do not have commitments to the total individual who may incidentally be blind, if we do not have confidence in his capacity to produce competitively, namely blind labor, then we have no right to be in the competitive labor market."

This can evoke a double reaction. Let us by all means do all that we can to make those among the blind who are fitted for it as competent as possible to produce competitively, and to push for success in the competitive labor market. But let us not adopt this as our sole pattern to be held up to the blind as *the* way to the satisfying life. Let us open up routes other than that leading right through the market economy—especially the alternative route of the leisure-oriented ethic (so long as we provide an adequately challenging, adequately dignified and dignifying concept of the motivations, means, and ends for such a leisure-oriented ethic quite different from the notion of leisure as time to be killed).

When, moreover, it is recommended that our proposed axiological R & D group, give its thoughts to this leisure pattern of self-fulfillment for the blind, it is not meant that this is to be solely or dominantly with the older person in mind. In two respects, at least, these thoughts include more than the already aging or aged blind. To prepare the individual for meaningful leisure in old age, we would need to start with the earliest phases of his education as a youngster. We would need to continue such foresighted, anticipatory education through young adulthood and the middle years. Then we could really provide the sort of meaningful continuing education for self-realization in the advanced years. Included are the many young people and people of the middle years, who, for various reasons, are not fit candidates for being tooled into competitive units within our labor economy or market economy. A wise leisure-oriented ethic would be much more useful, productive, and profitable (in coinage of *human values*) for many of the blind unsuited either by lack of capacity or perhaps by sheer temperamental bent, to becoming successful competitors in the labor market.

What is needed here, above all, is a fundamental change of attitude in our society—an attitude which does not arbitrarily and dogmatically demean all who are not units of the labor economy. It is a change of attitude which resists the temptation automatically to condemn, through stereotypic labeling, anyone who gives himself seriously to self-fulfillment and social contribution through responsible self-development with a genuinely humanistic life-style sanctioned and motivated by a worthy leisure ethic. It is a change of attitude which curbs the stereotypic impulse to label, out of hand, as "dilettantes" "drones," "parasites," "goldbrickers" or "goof-offs" any and all who are not centrally involved in the "rat race" of the labor economy, the market economy; and which is slow to come to the judgment that such a leisure-shaped individual is unworthy of social maintenance, social respect, and other social rewards.

But it is going to take a lot of doing to bring about, if deemed desirable, a fundamental shift of attitude which would regard a leisure-oriented ethic as a viable alternative to a labor-economy, work-oriented ethic for the blind. In such a conference as this, set up under the co-sponsorship of the HEW Vocational Rehabilitation Administration, it is not at all surprising that we should give major emphasis to work-oriented, market economy-oriented problems associated with blindness. It is not surprising to have references to the "race toward successful employment and living in society," or to the "lower self-concept" characteristic of "ethnic and racial minorities who have not been given the opportunity to participate in the harness race towards the goal of occupational and social mobility."

There are less obvious references, however, which demonstrate how deeply ingrained within us is the very idiom and imagery of the market economy and the conventional work ethic, extended to include even the most intimate aspects of our personal lives. Our personal living itself, we have been told, is a business—a "process of bargaining." Again, our pattern of reactions in the presence of death and its aftermath is referred to not as the "celebration" of mourning, but as "the work of mourning." "The work of mourning is an extended job of parting with the persistent image of the loved one." So mourning, too, becomes something we work at; and it is observed, about death itself, that our "knowledge about how to *handle* the end of life is limited." (Italics mine.)

One of the recommendations Douglas MacFarland has made in his analyst's paper helps to emphasize how important to the further-range concerns of this Consultation is this matter of value-laden attitudes and their modification. In one place, Dr. MacFarland has called for "an attitudinal study of a random sample of sighted persons to determine the attributes they feel a blind person ought to have in order to be fully accepted in society." During much, or most, of our inquiry and discussion, we seem to have held the assumption that one of these attributes should be successful competition in the labor market and the market economy. Actually, this assumption may now only in part be tenable; and, before long, as it stands, it may be quite untenable. For already too much favorable publicity has been given to the alternative modular attribute—namely, that of self-responsible and socially related, socially contributing self-realization within the leisure life-style.

My guess is that the attitudinal study called for by Dr. MacFarland would reveal that a process of change is going on as to the attributes favored by society, and hence as to those attributes the blind should have in order to be "fully accepted by society." The change is one which is to the advantage of that attribute or group of attributes which enables an individual to achieve "success" under the sanction and with the inspiration of a leisure-oriented ethic and a leisure-shaped life-style. This tendency of change, being much to the advantage of the blind, should be encouraged by all those who work with problems associated with blindness.

Agenda for future research in problems associated with blindness should, then, include the following:

1. How may we speed up the change of attitude which will make a worthy leisure model of the good man and the good life much more widely known, understood, and accepted by society?

2. How may we get our colleagues working with the blind and the problems related to blindness to accept this leisure model as a viable alternative to the conventional work-ethic, money-measured, power-measured success model?

3. How may we help the blind themselves to accept this alternative leisure model and to strive toward self-realization through it?

Much of this sort of research would call for team organization between those working with problems associated with blindness and those who, like us of the Center for Continuing Liberal Education, are doing R & D work in developing new programs of informal liberal studies for adults. Key questions might be:

1. How can we educate the sighted adults—the family, the neighborhood, the community, the nation—to appreciation of a worthy leisure-model as a legitimate, even laudable alternative to the work-for-pay model of the good man, the good life, the good society?

2. How can we re-educate the teachers, the opinion shapers, the decision makers to the same sort of appreciation, and to the application of this in their personal, professional, and civic endeavors?

3. How can we do the same with those who work with the blind?

4. How can we do the same with the blind themselves?

Not that the parallel job that has to be done with youth is to be belittled. On the contrary, as has already been indicated, to achieve a total societal reorientation of attitude with regard to the work-ethic model and a worthy leisure model, we have to start with the youngster in kindergarten; and, beginning there, make far-reaching changes, all along the line, in the educative process—so that there is a cumulative readying of the individual for a worthy adult life of self-realizing, socially-related, and socially-responsible leisure. And these changes, too, call for a vast deal of research at the frontiers. But here the adult phases of continuous education for leisure are being stressed, for at least two main reasons:

1. Because of our work and responsibilities here at the Center for Continuing Liberal Education, we are more intimately acquainted with both the problems and the potentialities of such education in the adult phases of our maturation.

2. Because the logic of some of the demographic figures cited in our Consultation papers is so cogent. Consider Commissioner Cohen's statement: "The political power of the elderly will continue to shift in their favor in the environment of the future. Whereas the aged represent about 15 per cent of those eligible to vote today, in the future they will begin to approximate 25 per cent."

There also is the stress made in several of our Consultation papers that the largest percentage of our blind are in the late-adult age brackets and that, precisely because they are not good investments for successful competition in the labor market and the market economy, the least investment is being made toward their true well-being. What this amounts to is that they are sadly neglected. It is this neglect and consequent atrophy, rather than the mental decline or decay caused by factors of outright physical, physiological degeneration, that makes the lives of so many of the aged or aging so futile and empty.

Such an assurance as a "pension for the blind" is an important contribution to the self-image and the image held of him by society. This may become a real status symbol. This may provide a firm base for the raising of the self-image and for motivational thrusts toward personal self-development—in terms other than of the market economy, of professional striving, of the political arena. The absorption of this pension system for the blind into a comprehensive national system, such as that of the "demogrant" referred to by Mr. Robinson, might make an even greater contribution to the elevation of the self-image of the blind and the image held of him by society. Yet we would then merely become free for the more difficult, the less palpable axiological problems involved. As Commissioner Cohen has stated, we would be dealing with the value systems of the future—the culture value systems—with the qualities of life as formulated in telic goals.

According to Mr. Cohen, "some of us policymakers and program implementers have been sloppy about formulating end goals." Hence, our proposed axiological R & D group would have, as one of its prime functions, to replace such sloppiness with persistent, sustained, disciplined, yet imaginative projective thinking and telic model-making and testing.

This R & D group, as Mr. Cohen suggests, would need to involve "the populations" themselves in this axiological effort. We would need to learn, from the aging and the aged themselves, an appreciation of how it feels to be getting older—and unsighted.

We need, also, to take full advantage of the opportunities provided by literature and the fine arts for empathic understanding. Here, indeed, is where the professional practitioners of the Humanities, the Arts included, may render signal service. True, as Dr. Kent has observed, we have to accept certain experiential limitations on insight. Yet, fortunately, we have available to us the full range of vicarious experience and insight provided by the cumulative and ever unfolding record of man's myriad feelings and attitudes, embodied in literature and the arts.

Take, for example, John Milton's *Samson Agonistes*. This tragic masterpiece furnishes moving documentation of Mary K. Bauman's description, based on Louis Rives' account, of how it feels to be blind; it also provides a memorable exemplification of Herbert Rusalem's observation, "The patient must die as a sighted person in order to be reborn as a blind person."

For that matter, the mature study of imaginative literature provides a wealth of dramatic or otherwise vivifying realizations of the dynamics of those emotion-linked values, which are dealt with in so rigorous and scientific a fashion and yet, in so imaginative, sensitive, and humanistic a fashion in the monograph, *Adjustment to Misfortune*. Such literary and dramatic realizations, particularly when augmented by historical and philosophical studies on an interdisciplinary and integrative basis, can contribute substantially toward the fashioning and recreative experiences of researchers, as well as of workers with the blind.

Something else should fall within the purview of our proposed axiological R & D group, which should deal, as Dean Roose has recommended, with "the quality of life" in the future. This is the concept of man's basic nature that is being assumed in our inquiries concerning future research and in the research itself. It has been stressed that we ought to do research on how to improve the quality—that is, the accuracy—of the ophthalmological data upon which so much of our subsequent research rests. At the other end of the spectrum, we need to exercise like rigor as to the imponderables that go into the context and texture of the research. One of the most crucial among these is the idea of man that is assumed. As implicit presupposition, axiom, premise, the basic idea of man that we entertain invisibly saturates our proposed research methodologies, hypotheses, and projects. Hence the importance of continual re-examination of our thinking so that we may identify this pervasive idea of man, and make due allowance for it.

At this Consultation we have had two master images or models of man either recommended to us or implicitly functional. One of these is cynical, tough-minded, hard-boiled, "realistic." It depicts man as being, basically, an egoistic predator. It is an image of man compounded of elements from the jungle, the arena, the marketplace, and the forum. According to this picture, man is always trying, through force and/or cunning, to pull deals that will yield him the biggest payoff—in money, and power.

Of equally distinguished traditional lineage and stature, and often entertained, too, by men of intelligence and authority, has been a quite different fundamental reading of the nature of man. This is the reading found, for example, in Kropotkin's influential treatise on mutual aid. It is the reading suggested, too, in the opening paper that set the societal and cultural stage for this Consultation: Arnold Barach's report on his findings among youth questioned, for Kiplinger's *Changing Times,* as to why they have joined such enterprises as the Youth Corps.

Among these findings, Mr. Barach stressed that those questioned have often listed two basic motivations, self-education and service to society. (This second point is all the more noteworthy since many of the young men and women questioned have come, not from Michael Harrington's *Other America,* but from John Kenneth Galbraith's *Affluent Society.*) On the one hand, those questioned have declared that they have wanted to find out who they themselves are (to establish their own self-identity); and they have wanted the experience of doing a job responsibly. Of such opportunity, they have maintained, they have been largely deprived by this Affluent Society which, ironically, has given them so much.

On the other hand, when they have returned from a tour of duty with the Youth Corps, these young men and women have insisted that they want to render humanitarian service; they want to help fellow human beings. They have rejected "making a buck" as their dominant drive.

Which of these two readings of the basic nature of man—the egoistic or the altruistic—is the one to be accepted as valid? This is not the place to make and defend such a determination; nor to defend a compromise. Nor should we now try to gain definitive acceptance for a compromise view of another sort. That is the view that even those impulses and acts which appear to be most sympathetic, most compassionate are intrinsically egoistic. Let us not try to gain acceptance of this paradoxic view. We need not here consider an acceptance of the Epicurean rationale, which states that one's efforts to relieve another of pain are due to his selfish desire to be relieved of the discomfort he himself experiences as he identifies himself, vicariously, with the person who is actually suffering; nor the Benthamite variation of the Epicurean formula; that of enlightened self-interest and the greatest good for the greatest number.

The point is that, so far, not one of these models of the basic nature of man has been definitively validated by modern positivistic research, by empirically disciplined systematic inquiry, as *the* model to rule our minds—our hypotheses, our researches. Hence, as we discuss research at the frontiers concerning problems associated with blindness, we must not accept any one of these models offhandedly and as self-evident. We need a continuous scrutiny maintained by our axiological R & D group with regard to the picture of man's fundamental nature assumed in our thinking about research and in our research itself.

Scholarly devotion to intellectual truth and justness calls for this ongoing critical scrutiny. So does devotion to the practical ends for which this Consultation has been convened. For the pre-suppositional reading of man's nature that is implicit in one's whole approach to research as to problems associated with blindness may have far-reaching practical implications both for those who work at these problems and for the good of the blind themselves.

Putting the question of cultural ideals and aspirations to one side, the blind, practically, have much to lose from dominance of the egoistic model of man's nature; and, conversely, they have much to gain from the dominance of the compassionate model. In a word, the dominance of the compassionate model is to their own enlightened self-interest. Ralph M. Stodgill and Carol L. Shartle, cited by Yvonne Agazarian, seem to be signaling in this direction when they point to the possible "ultimate dominance of the new view that rehabilitation is no longer tied to manpower needs and today requires a humanitarian ethos based in *productive living* rather than *productive output*."

A compassionate, but not a sentimental model! For, as has been pointed out at our planning sessions, those who, however well-intentioned, sentimentalize their relations with the blind do much harm. They may thus habituate the blind person to being overprotected against reality; they may blanket his own impulses toward self-reliance.

The wise compassionateness here advocated takes into account certain admonitions that have been voiced; for example, the laudable desire, in the blind themselves, not to be obliged to woo the world into loving them: "Don't try to get everyone to love you. So long as they let you have the freedom you want—that's enough." Yet this compassionateness hastens to add: "And so long as you handle that freedom within the constraints of capacity and circumstance." Further, this compassionateness is quite different from the depersonalized "compassionateness" of the big organization or agency—what Dr. Roy Buck likes to call "cool and calculated corporate compassionateness." [4]

The desired compassionateness is personalized. It is sensitive to that *"x"* factor Elena Gall has described as functional only through personalized relations between, say, the counselor and the counseled. It sympathizes, moreover, with the desire that the blind have, as has been so simply yet eloquently put at one of our sessions: "I want to be me." It is the desire that wants at least occasional freedom from the burden so often placed upon the blind: to remember, always, that each is responsible for the image the public has of the blind. It is the desire that wants to be free from "the responsibility of educating the whole wide world" to a favorable impression of the blind.

Not that a dog-eat-dog atmosphere is any better than mawkish sentimentality. Such an atmosphere may well depress the morale of the blind person. It will practically and seriously disadvantage him. It might well be said with John Donne: *if you diminish one, you diminish all.* If you denigrate the general image of man, by assuming him to be basically "short, nasty and brutish," you diminish all men thereby, and this means too, a diminishment for the blind. Again, what has been applied elsewhere applies here. It has been observed at this conference that, when you label a "hesitant youngster" a "stutterer," you make him a stutterer. Similarly, if you label a man a "predator," you make him become that. So both the image of man as basically "short, nasty, and brutish" and experiences at the hands of those dominated by this image may well fill the blind person with an added burden of anxieties and fears, frustrations, resentments, angers. They may tend, strongly, to make him, too, that which he fears and hates, a psychic predator, "red in tooth and claw."

What is to the advantage of the blind—in terms both of his material and his psychic "economy"—is what James Copp has referred to as a "faith in the goodness of the world," an atmosphere of sensed human solidarity and tempered compassionateness—prudent, sagacious. It would be the task of our axiological R & D group to concern itself with these implicative aspects of the implicit model of man held by those working with the blind or on research problems associated with blindness. With admitted hyperbole, one might say: *as the model goes, so goes the research.*

SYSTEMS THINKING: RESERVATIONS

Speaking of models, let us add one more item to these notes toward an agenda for our axiological R & D group. This has to do with the systems-thinking that has played such a prominent part in our papers and our sessions. Indeed, one may seem to be a "square" if he does not go along with this vogue for systems-thinking. Yet it should be one of the functions of our axiological R & D group to risk the embarrassment of being labeled "square," and to subject this systems "style" to the same sort of critical scrutiny it is to apply to readings of the fundamental nature of man. It is one thing to borrow from cybernetics its concepts, its formulations, its idiom, and its imagery. It is another thing to let this cybernetic "universe of discourse" take over and dominate your own symbolic universe and the very picture of reality which constitutes your map of man and society, or your map of man *in* society.

So tangled a map do your systems networks become that, eventually, you lose all sense of the actual, living human being, the actual living groups of human beings behind the map; and both your cognitive and your cogitative world are more and more abstracted from actuality. Mere models became apotheosized—or deified—as reality itself. Further, what started out as cybernetic metaphor, simile, or analogy goes literal. What was set up as fiction—more or less fruitful —comes to be treated as fact. The institution, organization, agency, bureau, neighborhood, family—each is simplistically reduced to just a cybernetic system and no more. Finally, the living individual is leached away. What a diminishment of man—to the cost of all men and, particularly, of such men as the blind.

Where we have systems-thinking and the homeostatic concept, we are likely to get a strong impulse toward putting the system under the sort of control which will be optimum for such homeostasis. And when we get a strong impulse to control, we get a strong tendency toward a mechanistic reading of man's nature, a strong tendency to reduce man to the status of a machine—to be ecologically and psychologically manipulated for the optimum workings of the homeostatic impulsion.

This tendency should be of grave concern to us. Whatever encourages the conception of man as a machine—and no more—a mechanism merely, a mechanical system to be manipulated is a potential threat particularly to the blind. It has serious negative import for those who work with the blind, or who are involved in research with problems associated with blindness.

So there are plenty of items for the agenda of our axiological R & D group: there is plenty of work for it to do. How much is suggested in Tamara Dembo's observation that, inevitably, the adjustment to blindness involves value adjustments—both for the blind and for those around him, and both externally and at the core of the self. And these value adjustments are intimately implicated in changes of attitude. The question has been put: how deeply rooted in "universal nature" is our work-success ethic, how much is it a factor of our culture and hence variable, hence amenable to change? It is a crucial question, for, as has been pointed out, the answer bears directly on the self-image the blind entertains—both actual and telic—and the normative image society entertains of him. In partial response, Dr. Blank has both encouraged and discouraged us. On the one hand, he has told us that, at any given moment, we cannot control our affective behavior. On the other hand, he has told us that we can successfully attenuate such behavior, if deemed undesirable—through application of reasoning, as in checking the virulence of the egoistic, sadistic, xenophobic impulse to persecute minorities. We have hard work ahead of us just to follow out the implications of these questions and observations concerning changing attitude in relation to changing values.

NOTES

1. In their prize-winning *Ferment in Medicine* (Philadelphia: Saunders, 1966), Richard M. Magraw and Daniel B. Magraw make observations pertinent to this point. Treating the topic of "Automating Medicine," they admit that it "is difficult to predict how rapidly changes will come in medical practice as a result of the innovations" in electronic measurement, automation, and computerization or cybernation. "At the moment," they note, "it appears that any sweeping change in the procedures of medical diagnosis and treatment as a consequence of automation is at least ten

or fifteen years away." They immediately add, however: " . . . *but similar estimates in regard to automation in other fields have usually been far too conservative.*" (Italics mine.) They then offer this explanation: "Propelled by demands of the space race and of business efficiency and economy, automation has progressed so rapidly since World War II that even the most optimistic guesses of the time required to reach certain goals have been grossly in error." (Quoted in *Saturday Review*, October 7, 1967, p. 66.) *Ferment in Medicine* won the 1966 Norman A. Welch Memorial Award for the year's "most scholarly and meritorious contribution to the literature of medical economies."

2. Cf. Herbert Kupferberg, "Bionics: A New Science Helps the Blind to 'See,' " *Parade* (October 8, 1967), 14–16. On page 16 there is a picture of Consultation participant Russell Williams, explaining the "laser cane" to Representative Dorn of South Carolina. The caption states that the cane "emits three light beams to detect impediments, indicates them by vibrations in the handle."
3. Cf. "The Achievement of Values in Architecture," address by Dr. Joseph W. Sittler, Professor of Systematic Theology, The Divinity School of the University of Chicago, to appear in the Proceedings of the 1967 International Congress on Religion, Architecture and the Visual Arts.
4. In his book, *The Automated State: Computer Systems as a New Force in Society* (Philadelphia: Chilton, 1967), Robert O. MacBride presents the Defense Department as providing an admirable model of the effective computer system. As such, he regards it as "the intellectual sword of the republic, and the true cradle of the future." In giving a profile of this "splendid example," Mr. MacBride notes that the Defense Department is both "authoritarian" and "compassionate": "For example, it will see to it that the humblest private is flown halfway around the world to be at the bedside of a dying relative. It does not even limit its compassion to its own; its millions having succored flooded Dutchmen, rescued Arab pilgrims stranded on the road to Mecca, dropped hay to snowbound Canadian elk, dispatched ships to the aid of Greek earthquake victims." So enthusiastic is Mr. MacBride about this exemplary model that he exclaims: "Who, indeed, can point to a better working model of the Good Society?"

For Background and Context

William R. Brickman and Stanley Lehrer, eds., *Automation, Education, and Human Values* (New York: School and Society Books, 1966) consists largely of papers developed through the CCLE-IBM Humanities Project on Technological Change, Center for Continuing Liberal Education, The Pennsylvania State University, introduction and conclusion by project director, Maxwell H. Goldberg, who supervised "Bibliography and Appendix containing Points of View—Prophetic or Provocative?"

Maxwell H. Goldberg, "Unity of Knowledge," *The University Today: Its Role and Place in Society* (Geneva, Switzerland, 1960).

——— "The Humanities, Critical Issues, and the Quest for Wholeness," *Critical Issues and Decisions* (Washington: USDA Graduate School, 1962).

——— "The Humanities and the Discovery of New Knowledge," *Current Issues in Higher Education,* ed. G. Kerry Smith (Washington: Association for Higher Education, 1963).

——— "The Humanities as Heuristics," *CEA Critic* (June, 1963).

——— "General Education and the Explosion of Knowledge," *General Education: Current Ideas and Concerns,* ed. James Rice (Washington: Association for Higher Education, 1964).

——— *Meaning and Metaphor,* Notes and Essays on Education for Adults No. 45 (Brookline, Massachusetts: Center for the Study of Liberal Education for Adults, 1965).

——— "Continuous Education as a Way of Life," *Adult Education* (Autumn, 1965).

——— "The Impact of Technological Change on the Humanities," *The Educational Record* (Fall, 1965), 388–399.

——— "Education for Human Competence in a Scientific Age," *Impact of Science on Society* (Oak Ridge Institute of Nuclear Studies, November, 1965), 138–148.

——— "The Displacement of Human Labor," *The Evolving Society* (New York: The I.C.R. Press, 1966). [I.C.R. = Institute for Cybercultural Research].

——— *Technological Change and Human Dignity: A Study in Human Values* (Center for Continuing Liberal Education, University Park, Pennsylvania, 1966) (Editorial Associate, Patricia Kochanek).

——— "Expectations and Responsibilities of Higher Education for the Mature American," *Wayne State University Graduate Comment,* Vol. 9, No. 3, 191–197. Article is a revision of a paper which first appeared in *Current Issues in Higher Education* (Washington, 1966).

——— "Human Values, Telic Models, and the Self-Renewing Society," *Proceedings, CCLE Seminar on Urban Policy, New Castle,* ed. Dr. Roy C. Buck (Center for Continuing Liberal Education, University Park, Pennsylvania, Spring, 1966).

——— "The Agony, The Ecstasy . . . and The Big If," *Penn State Alumni News* (January, 1967), 8–12. (Article concerns technological change, human values, and the survival of man).

——— "Human Values for Human Beings: The Role of Telic Models for the Self-Renewing Community," *Adult Leadership,* 15 (February, 1967), 270.

——— "Religious Education as a Humanity," *School and Society,* Vol. 95, No. 2288 (February 18, 1967), 123–124.

——— "The Humanities and the Alienated Adolescent," *School and Society,* Vol. 95, No. 2292 (April, 1967), 257–261.

——— "Cybernation: The Dilemma of Control," *Spectrum* (Magazine of the Colleges of Engineering, and Mineral Industries and Sciences, The Pennsylvania State University) Vol. 7, No. 1 (October, 1967).

——— "Higher Education: Equalization of Opportunity," *The American University and the World of Scholars,* eds. Ardath W. Burks, David Cayer, and T. Hall Wilson (New Jersey: The Rutgers University Press, 1967), 97–108.

——— "Technological Mythmaking and Humanities Teaching," *School and Society,* Vol. 96, No. 2300 (February 17, 1968).

——— "Automation, Manpower, and Education," *Adult Leadership,* Vol. 16, No. 9 (March, 1968), 341–342, 346.

——— "Liberal Education, Academic Governance, and the Bed of Procrustes," *School and Society,* Vol. 96, No. 2303, Feb. 17, 1968, pp. 98–99.

Forthcoming

——— "Structures and Problems of Human Values: 2000 A.D." Concluding paper, *Symposium on Technology and Education in the 21st Century,* ed. Donald Strel (Center for Technological Education, The San Francisco State College, Daly City).

——— "Socrates, the Computer, and Ivied Walls," *School and Society,* Fall, 1968.

——— "Technology and Urban Issues"—Report, National Consultation on Technology and Human Values, National Council of Churches of Christ in America, prepared May, 1967. An adapted version of this report appears in: *Human Values and Advancing Technology,* compiled by Cameron P. Hall (New York: Friendship Press, 1967).

——— "Heart Transplants for the Humanities," *Liberal Education,* Fall, 1968.

——— "1967 Books on Higher Education: A Selective and Projective View," *Current Issues in Higher Education: 1968* (Washington: American Association for Higher Education, Fall, 1968).

Recent and Relevant: A Bibliography

For the comprehensive bibliography on Technological Change and Human Values see: Brickman, William and Stanley Lehrer, eds. *Automation, Education, and Human Values* (New York: School and Society Books, 1966).

The following are some additional items recently published:

Issue devoted to "The Electronic Revolution," *American Scholar,* Vol. 35, No. 2 (Spring, 1966).

Bazelon, David T. *Power in America* (New York: New American Library, 1967).

Bronowski, J. *The Identity of Man* (Garden City, New York: American Museum of Science Books, 1965).

Brown, George W., James G. Miller, and Thomas A. Keenan. *Edunet: Report of the Summer Study on Education Networks* (New York: The Interuniversity Communications Council, 1967).

Issue devoted to "Toward the Year 2000: Work in Progress," *Daedalus* (Summer, 1967).

Efron, Arthur. "Technology and the Future of Art," *Massachusetts Review,* Vol. 7, No. 4 (Autumn, 1966), 677–710.

Ewald, William R., Jr., ed. *Environment for Man: The Next Fifty Years* (Bloomington, Indiana: Indiana University Press Midland Book, 1967).

Galbraith, John Kenneth. *The New Industrial State* (Boston: Houghton Mifflin, 1967).

Hilton, Alice Mary, ed. *The Evolving Society, Proceedings of the First Conference on the Cybercultural Revolution* (New York: The I. C. R. Press, 1966).

Hall, Cameron P., ed. *Human Values and Advancing Technology* (New York: Friendship Press, 1967).

Kahn, Herman and Anthony J. Wiener, *The Year 2000. A Framework for Speculation on the Next Thirty-Three Years* (New York: Macmillan, 1967).

MacBride, Robert O. *The Automated State: Computer Systems as a New Force in Society* (Philadelphia: Chilton, 1967). This volume contains the "Memorandum" and the complete list of the members of the Ad Hoc Committee on The Triple Revolution; the Report of the National Commission on Technology, Automation, and Economic Progress; the National Data Center Proposals; and the Statement of Senator Edward Kennedy on

"A Bill to Authorize a [National] Computerized Information Center."

Matson, Floyd M. *The Broken Image: Man, Science and Society* (Garden City, New York: Doubleday Anchor Books, 1966).

Platt, John R. *The Step to Man* (New York: John Wiley and Sons, 1966).

Obenhaus, Victor. *Ethics for an Industrial Age: A Christian Inquiry* (New York: John Wiley and Sons, 1967).

Rosenberg, Jerry M. *Automation, Manpower, and Education* (New York: Random House, 1966).

Issue devoted to "The New Computerized Age," *Saturday Review* (July 23, 1966).

Seligman, Ben B. *Most Notorious Victory: Man in an Age of Automation* (New York: Free Press, 1966).

Theobold, Robert, ed. *Dialogue on Education* (Indianapolis: The Bobbs-Merrill Co., 1967).

Westin, Alan F. *Privacy and Freedom* (Boston: Atheneum, 1967), financed by the Carnegie Corporation of New York and sponsored by the Special Committee on Science and Law of the New York City Bar Association.

THE TOTAL PERSON, THE TOTAL CULTURE, AND HUMAN VALUES

Mary K. Bauman

I would take issue with something that was said in one of the meetings. Someone was regretting that, after 20 or 30 years in work with the blind, he heard us seeking information about the opportunities to do something about the same things we were trying to get information about and do something about when he began in the field. We are, he said, still talking about education for the blind, welfare for the blind, and job placement for the blind. I say I think we should. I think we should be talking about these problems a hundred years from now. Not because we have made no progress—because I think we have made great progress in these 30 years and will in the next—but because we should never stop. And so, for our research and work frontiers there will be no end for us as long as there is blindness. Although we will never arrive, the important thing is never to stop going.

And there are a couple of pleas I would especially like to make. One of them is for us to proceed in our thinking of research and of people to consideration of the opportunity for blind people to have total careers. A career is a part of the whole person, not just his job. There is a very big difference between a career and a job, and so many of the blind people with whom I have talked have not had a career. Even when they had a profession they did not have a career because they were not doing what they most wanted to do—perhaps, even what they had spent some years learning to do. They had been forced into the available job. Until we, in work with the blind, have dealt with this and all the ramifications in regard to the public view, we will not have reached, by any means, the end of our work.

To do that I think we need leadership of ever-growing breadth, and it has been my pleasure in the years I have been in this field to see such leadership getting constantly better and better. Of course, I do not demean those who are gone, and who have made their great contribution. I just say that people with more knowledge, more interest, and more education constantly keep coming into the field. The only thing I regret is that their hands are so often tied by the routines which waste their time. I hear of the wonderful computers where one feeds everything in and pushes a button and what he needs comes out. I only wish we would get enough computers to do the routine work of our administrators. I wish every federal and state agency administrator could push buttons that would alleviate his daily struggle with routine and the occasional struggle with the legislature, which I see wasting the emotional and physical energies of so many of the good people in the field.

We do need to use all available knowledge to solve our problems and we need more knowledge, but there are always going to be gaps. Into these gaps go values, because the only way one can tolerate ambiguity is to have some sense of worth which helps him through that knowledge gap.

But what values? Well, I have just alluded to the idea of the "total person." I think it matters very much to consider human values. And I would like to use the multiple-handicapped individuals as one of those dream examples. We have always had multiple-handicapped people in our culture, which traditionally has centered on the closely knit family unit. In such a culture an individual with handicaps had a place. There was, for example, the old person who could not do this or that, but she belonged in the family, and had a place and a value, and was absorbed by the family and the community, as she, in turn, was absorbed in whatever she could do for them.

One of our growing difficulties in working with multiple-handicapped people is that our families are less and less close. We are now a culture in which people move a lot; they live in apartments; they do not have space; they do not have time; and everyone is rushing somewhere. Someone has to be left by the wayside.

And yet there are, I think, encouraging signs in our society. The growth of the service industries and increased opportunities to place people in service occupations seem to me to show that we are using the services that used to be maintained within the family unit in a larger cultural unit. I think we are only beginning to learn how to use it—in some cases serving ourselves with machines and in other cases serving ourselves with people in service industries. Perhaps we could find a way for even our multiple-handicapped people to find the equivalent place in the larger culture where they have a value, and where they are human beings who can love and respond and care. I think that if we are imaginative enough, we can find that, within the total culture, they are still valued and still loved and still needed and will have their place.

SESSION REPORT

Conrad Raabe and John R. Swinton

Dr. Magner began the closing session by asking for comments concerning any areas which the participants felt deserved more emphasis, or which were not brought out formally.

George Park briefly commented that he would like to see a conference devoted to the attitudes of the seeing *toward* the blind and the effect of these attitudes on the blind.

By way of addition to the above comment, Dr. Tamara Dembo observed that the problem of the relationship between the client and the agency worker ought to be explored. As her final point she brought up the problem to which almost every participant had alluded at one time or another: the problem of how to relate research, both current and past, to the operation in the agencies. The consensus was that this is a very grave problem in the field of working with the blind. For example, as Dr. William Usdane mentioned, there is a five to ten-year gap between basic research discoveries and their application in the field. In terms of applied research, the problem does not seem to be much better. As an example, he cited a study by Edward Glazer entitled *Application of Research Results* which attempted to relate applied research to agency operations.

This problem of research application is directly related to that of "research awareness." If the agency workers are not aware of the research being done, how are they to apply it? Several solutions were suggested:

1. A bibliography of research being done or accomplished in the area.

2. A central storage area for research information.

3. A committee (already in existence) of university, in-service-training personnel and administrators to aid in research data collection and interpretation. (For information contact Mr. Henry

Williams, Department of Health, Education and Welfare, Regional Office, Region 11, 42 Broadway, New York 10004).

4. The creation of a system that would make data, research, and general information quickly available through a storage-retrieval system.

5. The cataloging and use of operating agency records as sources of information.

6. Increased precision of language and terminology to decrease ambiguity in the transmission of information.

Other problems in the research area dealt with the inspiration of research topics and areas. In a more general sense Dr. Geraldine Scholl and Dr. H. Robert Blank suggested that a continuity between the medical and rehabilitation dimensions of the handicapped be kept. In the same vein Dr. Francis M. Andrews felt that medical schools ought to devote a few lectures to the "normal handicapped" as well as making use of nearby schools for the handicapped for first-hand observation.

Dr. Richard M. Lundy commented that research stemmed from the availability of funds and the availability of tools, and from "fads." Specifically, he felt that conferences such as this one could start fads and encourage the flow of money in certain directions. He urged a problem-solving approach to research.

Dr. Albert Thompson urged that researchers examine the relevance of 20th century problems to rehabilitation of the handicapped. In addition to the revolution in data collection, storage, and retrieval, he suggested examining the environment control techniques which have been developed, the change in the nature of the role of "work" in society, and an examination of the factors concerning attitude change using group techniques for example.

Lee H. Lacey advocated holding a conference dedicated to public education by bringing together the editors of national newspapers and magazines with rehabilitation workers. In addition he expressed a desire to see a program of continuing education conferences to bring workers in the field up-to-date on new techniques and ideas, and to make this mandatory as part of a licensing procedure.

In general and in summary the most often recurring points of discussion dealt with the application of research findings to the operating agency's procedure and with the problem of defining research areas. Crucial to both these interrelated problems is ready communication both within the field and with the public at large.

To close the general discussion, Dr. Elena Gall contributed the following extemporaneous remarks:

> To make a person aware, to create appreciation in him, and possibly to awaken in him the incentive to discover how he can use what he observes around him to serve people who may need help —such goals as these are brought about, of course, by a person's environment, and especially the sort of environment which, for generations, has set the tone of this university.
>
> Now, during this Consultation I have made a discovery which I can express after the fashion of Mary Bauman: You can classify information, knowledge, and attitudes in terms of history, culture, and the social patterns. In her opening address, Mary Bauman also emphasized the need for understanding blindness as a very personal thing and not as something that is superimposed on, taken out of, or associated with an individual. This message, I think, has provided the motivation behind much of the thinking that has gone on here.
>
> Still, I have been somewhat frustrated by the "numbers game" which has been played at every session I have attended. I know that those of you who attended the same sessions have heard me inveigh against a concentration solely upon the numbers of blind people we have or can expect to have. Perhaps I have not been able to make my position clear, for I must admit that we *do* have problems of numbers in the education and care of the blind, but we *also* have to contend with the extremely diversified problems that each individual presents; so we must deal with both of these kinds of problems in a variety of fashions. Certainly we should not, then, be motivated by any one single concept, either of numbers or of the individual's difficulties.
>
> The need for coordinated effort has been mentioned over and over again. The willing help of the members of the allied professions can contribute much to the understanding of the educators. This point has been stressed by all of us, so I can safely say that any party who brings about coordinated effort and collaborative research will earn the gratitude of each of us.
>
> We have talked about the needs for specialized materials, and methods, and trained personnel; and we have talked about the fact that public education can be formalized to include the meaning of blindness in the same way that it includes the meanings in science and in language arts, as well as those meanings that are basic to the understanding of our social pattern.
>
> One of the most interesting points of discussion has centered on "bad" terminology—if I may use that phrase—or terminology that should no longer be used, or terminology for which people apologize constantly. I do not think we are in any position to reject those words or structures that have been used in the past. We are in such dire need of new patterns that, it seems to me, we ought to collect all that we have, good and bad, and examine it in terms of what new areas of study can be elicited and how these areas can be implemented.

I think "manipulating the environment," for instance, is a fine phrase to use when you talk to teachers of the brain-injured or the brain-impaired; for unless you sensitize the environment somehow to reach them, there is nothing but chaos. My opinions were strengthened by Dr. Cofer when he claimed that the new theory of motivation is probably even more important than the older theory, and that we can probably stimulate people from without much more than we can from within. It seems to me important to bear in mind that, in some professions, manipulating the environment is a constructive skill, while in others it can certainly be extremely hazardous.

Another word is "priority." In child development it is probably possible to discover priority needs in a child and, in designing an instrument or a structure, one knows what he must learn before he proceeds to a more complete understanding. The uneven pattern which our handicapped people follow toward normality is, in fact, a basic challenge to understanding and patience—with regard to the fact that maybe this child will react immediately in the way that you would have expected him to react in five years, or that you expect him to have attained the ability to react in a certain way today but he is still clearly unable to react in that manner.

If it is ever possible to have another conference like this, I would like something to be included in terms of "prevention." We have not discussed all the ways science has discovered to prevent neurological, sensory, and physical disabling, and how teachers and other workers in family groups can immediately get to work on the symptomatology or the preparation of the public for such preventive measures.

CONTRIBUTORS

Aboud, John (Session Recorder)—Graduate Student, Department of Psychology, College of the Liberal Arts, The Pennsylvania State University.

Agazarian, Yvonne M. ("The Agency: Agent of Change")—Consultant, specializing in group psychotherapy, to the Hallmercer Community Health Center, Pennsylvania Hospital, Philadelphia.

Ashcroft, S. C. ("Social Participation, Citizenship, and the Visually Handicapped")—Chairman, Department of Special Education, George Peabody College for Teachers, Nashville, Tennessee.

Barach, Arnold B. ("Technological and Social Changes Ahead")—Senior Editor of the Kiplinger Magazine, *Changing Times,* and the author of the book *1975: And the Changes to Come.*

Bauman, Mary K. ("Welcoming Remarks on Behalf of the Committee for Research in Problems Related to Blindness"; "Dimensions of Blindness"; and "The Total Person, the Total Culture, and Human Values")—Director of the Personnel Research Center, Philadelphia, and co-author (with Norman M. Yoder) of the recent book *Adjustment to Blindness Re-viewed.*

Blank, H. Robert ("Reaction to Loss of Body Parts or Functions—Research Priorities in Rehabilitation")—Associate Clinical Professor of Psychiatry, Albert Einstein Medical College, New York City, and Associate Editor of *Psychoanalytic Quarterly.*

Cofer, Charles N. ("Motivation and Motivational Theory")—Head, Department of Psychology, University of Maryland, and the co-author (with M. H. Appley) of the volume *Motivation: Theory and Research.*

Cohen, Elias S. ("Research Needs and Developments in Gerontology")—Commissioner, Office for the Aging, Department of Public Welfare, Commonwealth of Pennsylvania, Harrisburg.

Copp, James H. ("An Interpretative Review of Research Dealing with Social Participation and Citizenship")—Chief, Human Resources Branch, United States Department of Agriculture, Washington, D.C., and the editor of the book *Our Changing Rural Society*.

Davis, Carl J. ("Adjustment of the Blind Adolescent")—Head, Department of Psychology and Guidance, Perkins School for the Blind, Watertown, Massachusetts.

Dembo, Tamara (Co-author of "Adjustment to Misfortune—A Problem of Social-Psychological Rehabilitation")—Professor of Psychology, Clark University, Worcester, Massachusetts.

Ford, Donald H. (Co-author of "A Conceptual Framework and Research Approaches for Evaluating Counselling")—Dean, College of Human Development, The Pennsylvania State University and co-editor (with Hugh B. Urban) of the book *Systems of Psychotherapy: A Comparative Study*.

Gall, Elena D. ("Needed Research in the Field of Services for the Multiple-Handicapped Blind") was, at the time of her recent death, Education Consultant to the New York Institute for the Education of the Blind; a member of Mayor John V. Lindsay's Committee on Mental Retardation for the City of New York; and Associate Professor of Education, Hunter College, New York City.

Goldberg, Maxwell H. ("Values, Models, and Research" and "Introduction")—Professor of Humanities; Associate Director for the Humanities at the Center for Continuing Liberal Education; Chairman of the Council on the Humanities, College of the Liberal Arts, The Pennsylvania State University; and General Chairman, "Blindness Research Consultation" project.

Granberg, Donald (Session Recorder)—Graduate Student, Department of Sociology and Anthropology, College of the Liberal Arts, The Pennsylvania State University.

Hager, Cyril F. ("Welcoming Remarks on Behalf of the Center for Continuing Liberal Education")—Associate Dean, College of the Liberal Arts and Director, Center for Continuing Liberal Education, The Pennsylvania State University.

Kratcoski, Peter (Session Recorder)—Instructor, Department of Sociology and Anthropology, College of the Liberal Arts, The Pennsylvania State University.

Lacey, Lee H. ("Suggested Research in the Field of Services for the Orthopedically Handicapped Blind")—Executive Director of the Harmarville Rehabilitation Center, Pittsburgh, Pennsylvania.

Leviton, Gloria Ladieu (Co-author of "Adjustment to Misfortune—A Problem of Social-Psychological Rehabilitation") was, at the time of this study, a psychological researcher and a psychologist practicing in LaGrange, Illinois.

Little, Adrienne V. (Session Recorder)—Graduate Student, Department of Sociology and Anthropology, College of the Liberal Arts, The Pennsylvania State University.

MacFarland, Douglas C. ("Counseling the Blind")—Chief, Division of Services to the Blind, Vocational Rehabilitation Administration, Department of Health, Education and Welfare, Washington, D.C.

Nolan, Carson Y. ("Research in Education of the Visually Handicapped")—Director, Department of Educational Research, American Printing House for the Blind, Louisville, Kentucky.

Raabe, Conrad (Session Recorder)—Graduate Student, Department of Political Science, College of the Liberal Arts, The Pennsylvania State University.

Robinson, Robert L. ("Blindness and Stress: Catastrophic and Continuing")—Research Associate, Department of Research, The American Foundation for the Blind, New York City.

Rusalem, Herbert ("The Role of Motivation in the Rehabilitation of Blind Persons")—Research Consultant to the Industrial Home for the Blind, Syracuse University; to the Columbia University College of Physicians and Surgeons; and to National Industries for the Blind. He is also Visiting Associate Professor, Columbia University Teachers' College and full-time Associate Professor of Education, Hunter College, New York City.

Sarup, Gian (Session Recorder)—Graduate Student, Department of Sociology and Anthropology, College of the Liberal Arts, The Pennsylvania State University.

Saterbak, Melvin E. ("Developments and Research Needs in Work with the Aged Blind")—Director, Vocational Rehabilitation Administration Research and Demonstration Project, The Minneapolis Society for the Blind, Minneapolis, Minnesota.

Scholl, Geraldine T. ("A Selectively Drawn Picture of Research in Education and Special Education")—Associate Professor of Education, School of Education, University of Michigan, Ann Arbor.

Scott, Robert A. ("The Systems Analysis Approach to Relationships Between Agencies for the Blind and Blind Persons")—Assistant Professor of Sociology, Princeton University, Princeton, New Jersey.

Sherif, Carolyn W. ("Needed Research on Adolescents: Seeing and Blind")—Associate Professor of Psychology, College of the Liberal Arts, The Pennsylvania State University and collaborator (with her husband Muzafer) on several books including *Groups in Harmony and Tension.*

Sussman, Marvin B. ("Family Structure, Parent-Child Relationship, and Disability")—Chairman, Department of Sociology and Anthropology, Western Reserve University, Cleveland; Consultant to the Vocational Rehabilitation Administration and Welfare Administration, Department of Health, Education and Welfare, Washington, D.C.; and Editor of the *Journal of Marriage and the Family.*

Swinton, John R. (Session Recorder)—Editorial Assistant, Center for Continuing Liberal Education, College of the Liberal Arts, The Pennsylvania State University.

Switzer, Mary E. ("Foreword")—Administrator, Social and Rehabilitation Services, Department of Health, Education and Welfare, Washington, D.C.

Thompson, Albert S. ("Occupational Placement and Career Development")—Professor of Psychology and Education, Columbia University Teachers' College, New York City.

Thompson, R. Paul ("Parent-Child Relationships and Visual Loss") —Executive Director, American Association of Instructors of the Blind, Inc., Washington, D.C.

Urban, Hugh B. (Co-author of "A Conceptual Framework and Research Approaches for Evaluating Counseling")—Psychologist and Coordinator of the Psychotherapy Program, The Pennsylvania State University Division of Counseling, and co-editor (with Donald H. Ford) of the book *Systems of Psychotherapy: A Comparative Study*.

Waterhouse, Edward J. ("Emphasis: The Deaf-Blind")—Director, Perkins School for the Blind, Watertown, Massachusetts.

Wright, Beatrice A. (Co-author of "Adjustment to Misfortune—A Problem of Social-Psychological Rehabilitation") was, at the time of this study, Research Fellow in Psychology, University of Kansas, Lawrence, Kansas.

Yoder, Norman M. ("Occupations and Placement for the Blind")—Commissioner for the Blind, Department of Public Welfare, Commonwealth of Pennsylvania, Harrisburg, and co-author (with Mary K. Bauman) of the recent book *Adjustment to Blindness Re-viewed*.

Session Leaders

Bernreuter, Robert G.—Vice President for Student Affairs and Professor of Psychology Emeritus, The Pennsylvania State University.

Gorlow, Leon—Associate Professor of Psychology, College of the Liberal Arts, The Pennsylvania State University.

Harris, Dale B.—Head, Department of Psychology, College of the Liberal Arts, The Pennsylvania State University.

Hylbert, Kenneth W.—Associate Professor of Education, College of Education, The Pennsylvania State University.

John, M. E.—Head, Department of Agricultural Economics and Rural Sociology, College of Agriculture, The Pennsylvania State University.

Kent, Donald P.—Head, Department of Sociology and Anthropology, College of the Liberal Arts, The Pennsylvania State University.

Lundy, Richard M.—Professor of Psychology, College of the Liberal Arts, The Pennsylvania State University.

Magner, Thomas F.—Associate Dean for Research and Graduate

Study, College of the Liberal Arts, The Pennsylvania State University.

Monat, William R.—Professor and Associate Director, Institute of Public Administration, College of the Liberal Arts, The Pennsylvania State University.

Morgan, Winona L.—Professor and Director of the Nursery School, College of Human Development, The Pennsylvania State University.

Roose, Kenneth D.—Dean, College of the Liberal Arts, The Pennsylvania State University.

Usdane, William—Chief, Division of Research and Demonstration, Vocational Rehabilitation Administration, Department of Health, Education and Welfare, Washington, D.C.

Consultation Planning Committee

Bauman, Mary K., Committee for Research In Problems Related to Blindness, and Director of the Personnel Research Center.

Buck, Roy C., Associate Director for the Social Sciences, Center for Continuing Liberal Education, and Professor of Sociology, The Pennsylvania State University.

Cohen, Sidney, Executive Secretary, American Association of Workers for the Blind.

Goldberg, Maxwell H., Associate Director for the Humanities, Center for Continuing Liberal Education, and Professor of Humanities, The Pennsylvania State University.

Hager, Cyril F., Associate Dean, College of the Liberal Arts, and Director of the Center for Continuing Liberal Education, The Pennsylvania State University.

MacFarland, Douglas C., Chief, Division of Services to the Blind, Vocational Rehabilitation Administration, United States Department of Health, Education and Welfare.

Rives, Louis H., Jr., President, American Association of Workers for the Blind.

Yoder, Norman M., Commissioner for the Blind, Department of Public Welfare, Commonwealth of Pennsylvania.

INDEX